Artificial Intelligence for Oral Health Care

Falk Schwendicke
Prabhat Kumar Chaudhari
Kunaal Dhingra • Sergio E. Uribe
Manal Hamdan
Editors

Artificial Intelligence for Oral Health Care

Applications and Future Prospects

Springer

Editors
Falk Schwendicke
Conservative Dentistry
and Periodontology
LMU Klinikum, LMU Munich
Munich, Germany

Kunaal Dhingra
Division of Periodontics, Centre
for Dental Education and Research
(CDER)
All India Institute of Medical Sciences
New Delhi, Delhi, India

Manal Hamdan
Department of Surgical and Diagnostic
Sciences
Marquette University School
of Dentistry
Milwaukee, WI, USA

Prabhat Kumar Chaudhari
Division of Orthodontics
and Dentofacial Deformities, Centre for
Dental Education Research (CDER)
All India Institute of Medical
Sciences, New Delhi
New Delhi, Delhi, India

Sergio E. Uribe
Department of Conservative
Dentistry and Oral Health
Riga Stradins University,
Latvia / Conservative Dentistry and
Periodontology, LMU Klinikum,
LMU Munich
Munich, Germany

ISBN 978-3-031-84046-3 ISBN 978-3-031-84047-0 (eBook)
https://doi.org/10.1007/978-3-031-84047-0

This Springer imprint is published by the registered company Springer Nature Switzerland AG
The registered company address is: Gewerbestrasse 11, 6330 Cham, Switzerland

Contents

1 Artificial Intelligence in Oral Health

Harisankar Binod, T. Shithij, Antonin Tichy, and Subhankar Mishra

1.1 Introduction

Artificial intelligence (AI), especially machine learning (ML) and its subfield, deep learning (DL), have revolutionized several industries. DL has recently delivered cutting-edge performance in speech processing, text analytics, and computer vision. The widespread use of AI algorithms across many fields has made these technologies indispensable to daily life. Healthcare, a sector historically immune to significant technological upheavals, is now starting to be impacted by AI systems as well [1]. However, their application is associated with several problems and challenges, including safety, privacy, and ethical considerations. Another major problem faced in AI applications in healthcare is the limited availability of representative, diverse, and high-quality data, which is crucial for training accurate and reliable ML models. The lack of enthusiasm to implement data exchange standards in wider healthcare industry is also hindering the efficacy of ML systems [1].

Recent studies on this topic include a scoping review conducted by Arsiwala-Scheppach et al. [2], published in 2023, which attempted to characterize the overall body of evidence concerning dental ML tasks. The review also assessed types of tasks, their distribution in different dental fields, the risk of bias and reporting quality, as well as the applied metrics. A similar work was done by Leite et al. [3], but it also investigated the applications of radiomics in the field of oral healthcare. The paper emphasizes the promising results achieved through the integration of radiomics and ML, showcasing their ability to improve accuracy, early detection, and personalized treatment strategies.

The objective of this chapter is to conduct a comprehensive review of the applications of AI in oral health. Prior to that, Sect. 1.2 provides the reader with basic information about ML and DL, presenting common machine learning

Harisankar Binod and T. Shithij contributed equally with all other contributors.

H. Binod · T. Shithij · S. Mishra (✉)
National Institute of Science Education and Research, Jatani, Bhubaneswar, Odisha, India
e-mail: harisankar.b@niser.ac.in; shithij.t@niser.ac.in; smishra@niser.ac.in

A. Tichy
Charles University, Prague, Czech Republic

First Faculty of Medicine, Charles University, Prague, Czech Republic and LMU University Hospital, Munich, Germany

General University Hospital in Prague, Prague, Czech Republic

Ludwig-Maximilians-Universität München, Munich, Germany

Tokyo Medical and Dental University, Tokyo, Japan
e-mail: Antonin.Tichy@med.uni-muenchen.de

F. Schwendicke et al. (eds.), *Artificial Intelligence for Oral Health Care*,
https://doi.org/10.1007/978-3-031-84047-0_1

tasks, DL model architectures and metrics, as well as considerations on privacy and adversarial attacks.

1.2 Basics of Machine Learning for Medical Applications

Massive amounts of data are produced in healthcare, and ML can assist in their processing, which is challenging using "traditional methods." The benefits of ML and DL have been particularly marked in medical image analysis, delivering human-level performance across various fields, e.g., in clinical pathology, radiology, ophthalmology, and dermatology. Recent breakthroughs in ML techniques have yielded remarkable outcomes in tasks like organ recognition [4], interstitial lung disease classification [5], lung nodule detection [6], medical image reconstruction [7], and brain tumor segmentation [8]. These advancements significantly impacted prognosis, diagnosis, therapy, and clinical workflow.

1.2.1 Machine Learning Tasks in Medical Image Analysis

Image analysis is one of the primary applications of ML in the medical field. It aims to support clinicians and radiologists in determining the diagnosis. Various imaging methods can be analyzed by ML, e.g., magnetic resonance imaging (MRI), radiography, computed tomography (CT), ultrasound, and positron emission tomography (PET). The tasks performed include image enhancement, detection, classification, segmentation, retrieval, reconstruction, and treatment analysis, as discussed below and summarized in Table 1.1.

Table 1.1 Methods in medical image analysis

Task	Description
Enhancement	Techniques to improve the quality of medical images for better diagnosis
Detection	Detection and identification of specific abnormalities in medical images
Classification	Categorization of medical images based on specific criteria or classes
Segmentation	Partitioning of medical images into meaningful regions or subjects
Reconstruction	Creation of interpretable images from raw medical data
Report drafting	Report generation from imaging modalities

Enhancement is a critical preprocessing stage of improving the quality of medical images which may be compromised by artifacts and noise, which in turn hamper image analysis. Various DL models are used for denoising medical images, such as *Convolutional Denoising Encoders* and *Generative Adversarial Networks* (GAN) [9]. These methods can also reduce the cost of MRI imaging, as they can obtain super-resolution (SR) from low-resolution MRI images, which do not require such strong background magnetic field and associated pulse sequences [10].

Detection is the process of identifying specific disease patterns or abnormalities, which conventionally involves expert radiologists and physicians. With a large number of reports to check daily, this requires much time and effort and is also susceptible to human error. On the other hand, DL-based methods have shown high potential in such task, and other ML methods such as *k-nearest neighbor* (k-NN) and *decision trees* (DT) were also successful in some cases, for example, the detection of dermatological diseases [11].

Unlike (object) detection, which includes the localization of a pathology in the analyzed image, classification models only determine if the pathology is present or not. The performance of classifiers based on DL, such as *convolutional neural networks* (CNN), has been shown to be superior to other non-learning-based methods. CNNs have been used extensively in recognizing body organs, abnormalities in medical imaging, and modality classification [1]. DL models can also be used in a popular technique called *transfer learning* [12]—a model pre-trained on a big set of different data is applied and fine-tuned on a relatively modest set of target data, i.e., medical images. Methods like *synergic deep learning* have also proven efficient in medical image classification [13]. A review article by Cai et al. [14] explored the use of transfer learning in image classification for detecting fundus related diseases.

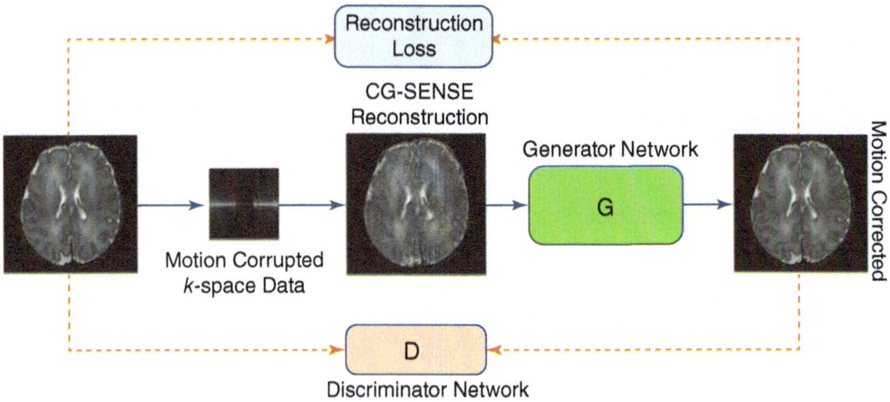

Fig. 1.1 Reconstruction of motion-corrupted images using GAN [19]

Segmentation is the process of dividing a picture into distinct nonoverlapping portions based on predefined criteria such as color, texture, and contrast. In the study of medical image analysis, segmentation is crucial. Sarraf et al. [15] have segmented brain MRIs to facilitate early detection of Alzheimer's disease. Various DL models, such as CNNs and *recurrent neural network* (RNNs), are used for segmentation [16], and several DL architectures are being developed for multimodal and volumetric image segmentation [17]. Segmentation will be further discussed in Sect. 1.2.1.1.

Medical image reconstruction helps generate clear and interpretable images from raw data. By speeding up the traditionally slow process of determining the original system inputs from the output results, DL models aid in the early detection while also saving time and reducing storage requirements. As an example, GANs were employed for the reconstruction of motion-corrupted brain MRI [18], a simplified scheme of the process is presented in Fig. 1.1.

Lastly, DL can be used for drafting the reports of image analysis. Writing the reports is very time-consuming and tedious, and it may be difficult for inexperienced radiologists and pathologists or even for experienced experts under time pressure. Various researchers have attempted to resolve this issue with the help of *natural language processing* (NLP) models, which can be used to annotate clinical radiology or pathology reports. Besides, DL architectures like *long short-term memory* (LSTM) network, CNNs, and RNNs are developed for automatic report generation. Figure 1.2 shows a report generated for chest X-rays [21].

1.2.1.1 Comparison of Object Detection and Segmentation

Object detection is a computer vision technique that deals with locating object instances in images or videos [19]. *You only look once* (YOLO) and *deep residual networks* are widely used DL architectures for object detection, while popular training datasets include COCO, ImageNet, etc.

Segmentation categorizes the image at pixel level. *Semantic segmentation* classifies the pixels based on their semantic meaning, treating all objects within a category as one entity, as opposed to *instance segmentation*, which differentiates between individual instances of the same category, enabling more accurate identification of objects.

Many real-world applications utilize semantic segmentation, such as self-driving cars, pedestrian detection, and diagnostic purposes. Other DL systems can use this pixel-level semantic data to grasp spatial positions and make judgments [22]. A popular segmentation model called *U-Net* was created for biomedical image segmentation and used, for example, in a study of oral lesions [23], where segmentation was performed along with object detection using YOLO. Figure 1.3 illustrates the differences between object detection and semantic segmentation.

The applications of instance segmentation include robotics, autonomous self-driving surveillance, medical diagnosis, etc. [17]. A common instance segmentation framework is mask R-CNN

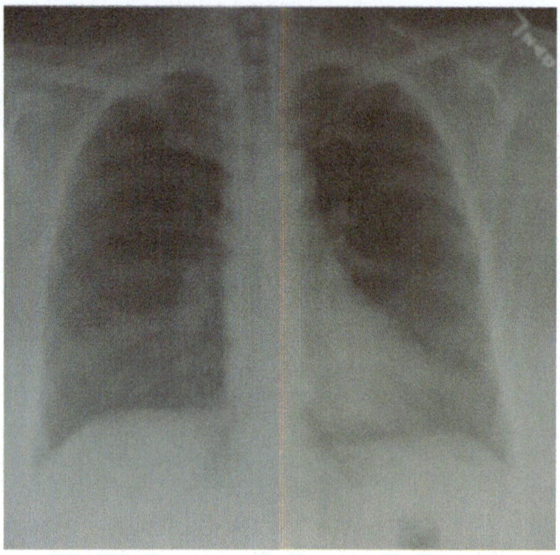

Fig. 1.2 Frontal chest X-rays of a patient, alongside the findings and annotated tags [20]

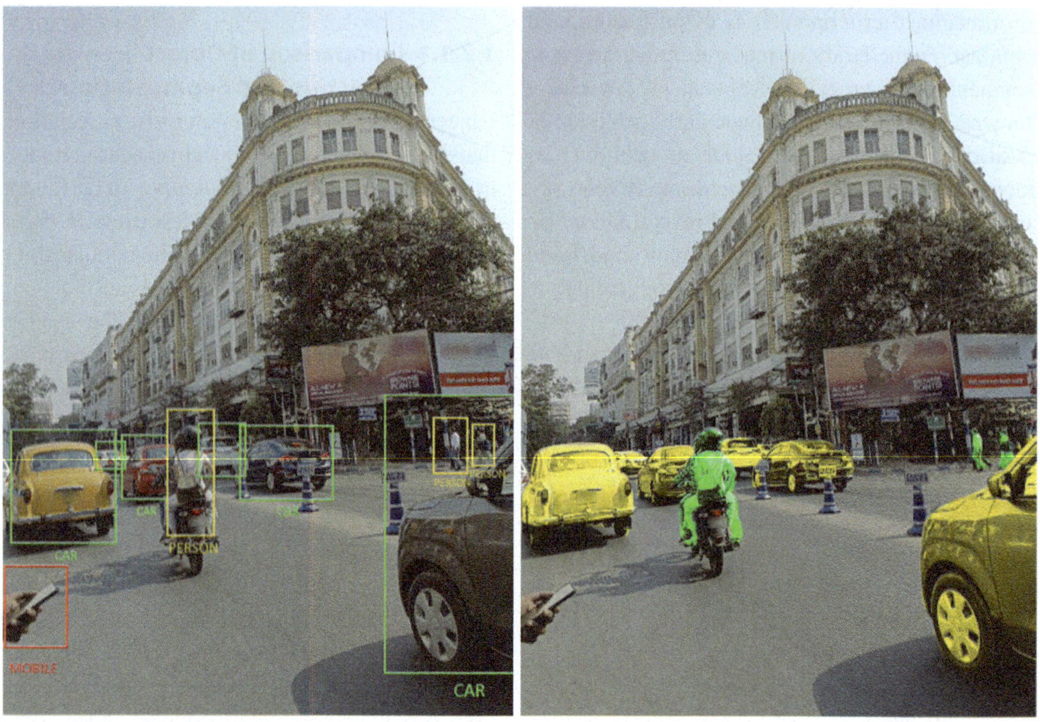

Fig. 1.3 On the left, object detection localizes the different objects in the scene using a bounding box. On the right, semantic segmentation labels every pixel of the identified objects but has no notion of separate instances of the same entity

[24]. For each object instance, it predicts a bounding box, a class name, and a pixel-level mask. The Detectron2 model developed by Facebook was used to construct Mask R-CNN with three distinct *ResNet Feature Pyramid Network* (FPN) backbones.

1.2.2 Deep Learning Architectures

In this subsection, DL architectures including DenseNet, ResNet, U-Net, mask R-CNN, and YOLO (Fig. 1.4) will be presented in detail, as

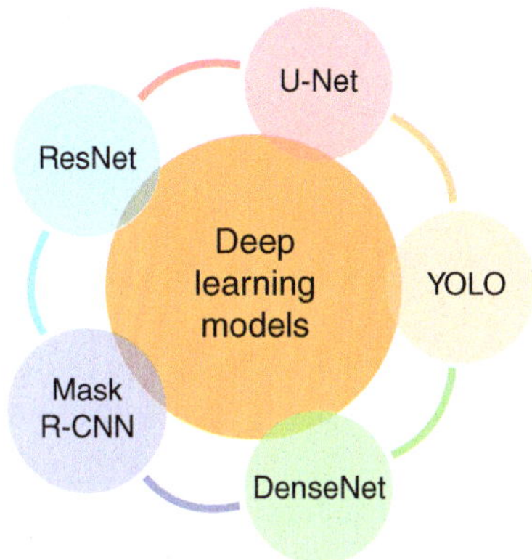

Fig. 1.4 DL architectures frequently used in oral health

they have been demonstrated to be very successful in various oral health applications.

DenseNet, an abbreviation of *dense convolutional network*, is a deep learning architecture that has gained significant attention and popularity in computer vision. DenseNet differs from traditional CNNs by introducing direct connections between every layer, creating a densely connected network. These connections enable each layer to receive direct input from all preceding layers, resulting in feature reuse and enhancing gradient flow. This architecture promotes more robust feature propagation, encourages feature extraction at multiple scales, and improves overall network efficiency. DenseNet has demonstrated impressive performance on various visual recognition tasks, often achieving state-of-the-art results with fewer parameters than other models. Its dense connectivity and efficient parameter usage make it an appealing choice in all computer vision tasks. Figure 1.5 presents a diagram representing the DenseNet architecture.

ResNet, short for *residual neural networks*, was proposed by He et al. [26] and has since become a cornerstone in many state-of-the-art image classification and object recognition tasks. Traditional deep neural networks suffer from the degradation problem, where the model's accuracy decreases as the depth increases. ResNet addresses this issue by introducing skip connections that allow information to flow directly from one layer to another, bypassing a few intermediate layers. ResNet allows the training of very deep neural networks with hundreds or even thousands of layers (Fig. 1.6).

U-Net is a widely used CNN architecture designed specifically for image segmentation tasks. U-Net's name is derived from its U-shaped architecture, which consists of an encoder path and a corresponding decoder path. The encoder path performs downsampling operations to extract high-level features and capture contextual information from the input image. The decoder path then uses upsampling and skip connections to recover spatial information and generate segmentation masks with fine-grained details. The skip connections enable the network to fuse low-level and high-level features, facilitating precise localization of objects. Figure 1.7 depicts the U-Net architecture.

Mask R-CNN, i.e., *mask region-based convolutional neural network*, is a state-of-the-art DL model that combines object detection and instance segmentation abilities. The model consists of two main components: a region proposal network (RPN) that generates potential object regions and a network head that simultaneously predicts bounding box coordinates, class labels, and object masks. By incorporating a fully convolutional network into the architecture (Fig. 1.8), mask R-CNN enables accurate instance segmentation while maintaining real-time inference speeds.

YOLO, *you only look once* in full, is an object detection architecture that has gained popularity for its real-time performance and high accuracy. It was introduced by Redmon et al. [28] in 2015. The key idea behind YOLO is to approach object detection as a single regression problem. The image is divided into a grid, and a CNN predicts bounding boxes and class probabilities for each grid cell. As a result, YOLO performs object detection in one pass and simultaneously operates on the entire image, making it highly efficient. Figure 1.9 is a simple representation of how YOLO architecture works.

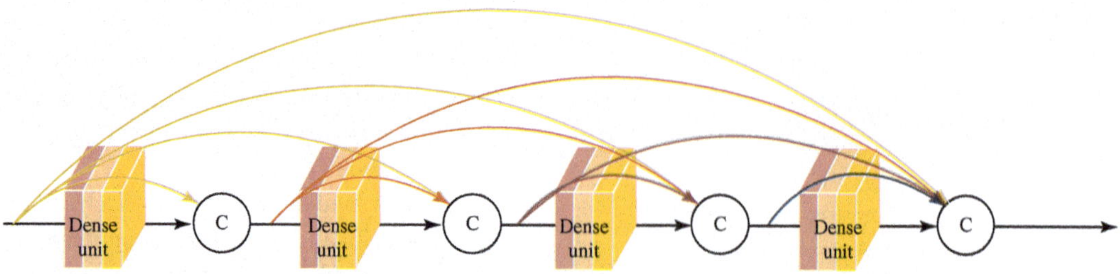

Fig. 1.5 A dense connection mode [25]. (Image source: https://www.hindawi.com/journals/bmri/2022/2384830/fig7/)

1.2.3 Selected Metrics Used for the Evaluation of Deep Learning Models

The performance of object detection and segmentation models is commonly assessed using the average precision (AP) metric [19], which is defined as the area under the precision-recall curve. Precision, which corresponds to the positive predictive value, is the ratio of true positives (TP) to the sum of TP and false positives (FP), while recall (sensitivity) is the ratio of TP to the sum of TP and false negatives (FN).

$$\text{Precision} = \frac{\text{TP}}{\text{TP} + \text{FP}}$$

$$\text{Recall} = \frac{\text{TP}}{\text{TP} + \text{FN}}$$

For a prediction to be considered as TP, the predicted class must be correct and the intersection over union (IoU) between the ground truth and the prediction must exceed a certain threshold. If the predicted class is inaccurate or if IoU drops below the threshold, the prediction is categorized as FP. On the other hand, FN predictions mean that an object was not identified despite being present in the image. With these defined, AP can be calculated using the following equation:

$$\text{AP} = \sum_{n} \left(R_n - R_{n-1} \right) P_n$$

where P_n is the precision at the nth threshold, while R_n and R_{n-1} are the recall values at the nth and $(n-1)^{\text{th}}$ threshold, respectively.

Other common metrics include accuracy, the F1 score, which is the harmonic mean of precision and recall, and the Dice score, also known as the Dice similarity coefficient.

$$\text{Accuracy} = \frac{\text{TP} + \text{TN}}{\text{TP} + \text{TN} + \text{FP} + \text{FN}}$$

$$\text{F1 score} = \frac{2 \times \text{Precision} \times \text{Recall}}{\text{Precision} + \text{Recall}}$$

$$\text{Dice score} = \frac{2\text{TP}}{2\text{TP} + \text{FP} + \text{FN}}$$

1.2.4 Privacy Considerations and Adversarial Attacks

Along with the benefits posed, AI comes with privacy challenges and ethical considerations. Understanding these concerns and potential malicious events as well as developing robust safeguards is crucial for harnessing the full potential of AI while protecting patient rights and maintaining trust in oral healthcare systems.

ML relies upon vast data, including sensitive personal information, and respecting individuals' privacy rights and obtaining proper consent for data usage is paramount. The ethical aspects are discussed in Chap. 10, so this section will focus on the robustness and safety of ML models in terms of privacy and adversarial attacks, which are often not sufficiently considered. Existing works on privacy protection can be classified into three groups, based on the role of ML in privacy [29]:

1. **Privacy of data for ML models**. This includes making both the input and output data, as well as ML model parameters private throughout the process, as the privacy threat

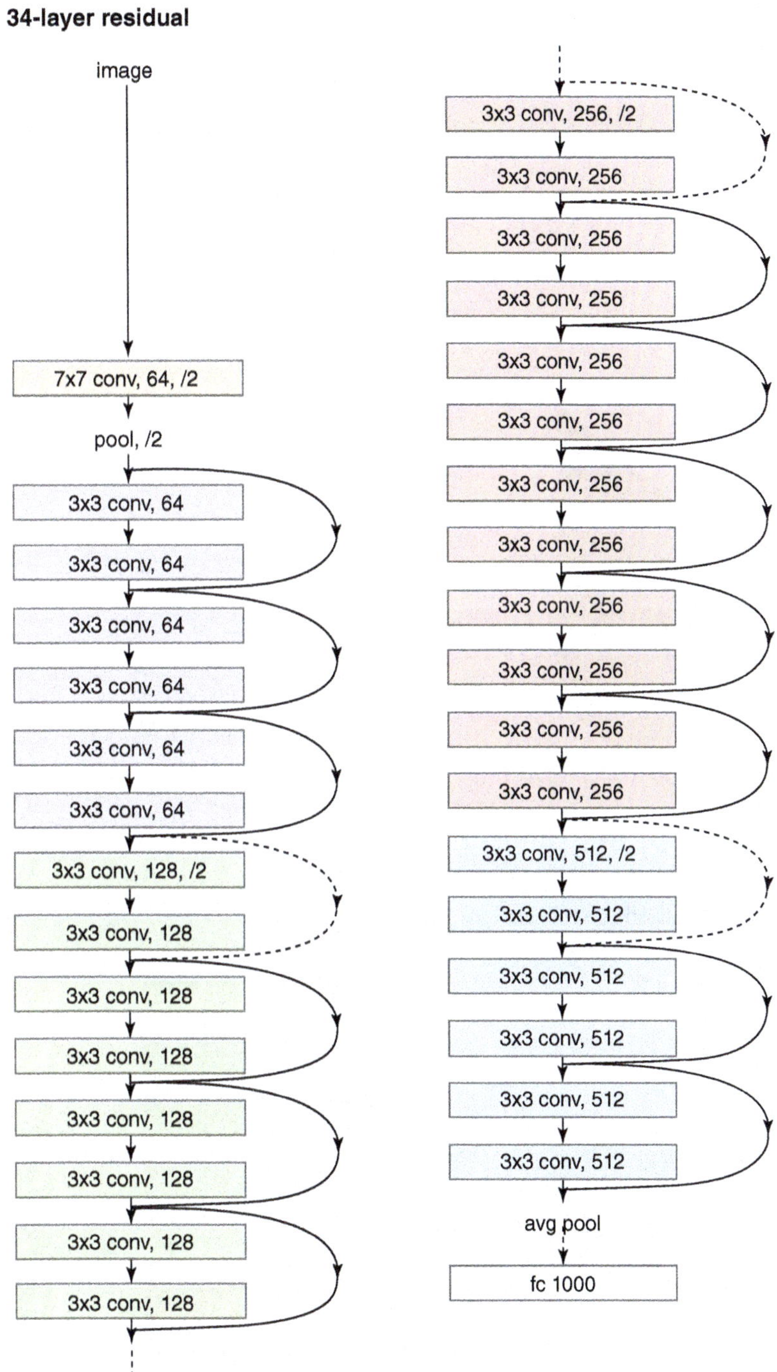

Fig. 1.6 ResNet architecture [26]

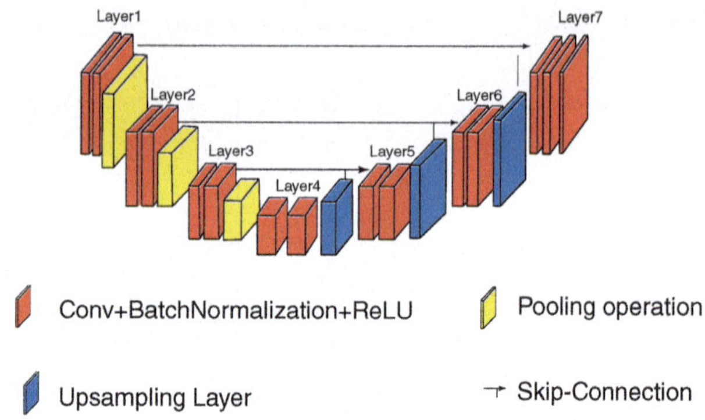

Fig. 1.7 Structure of U-Net architecture [27]

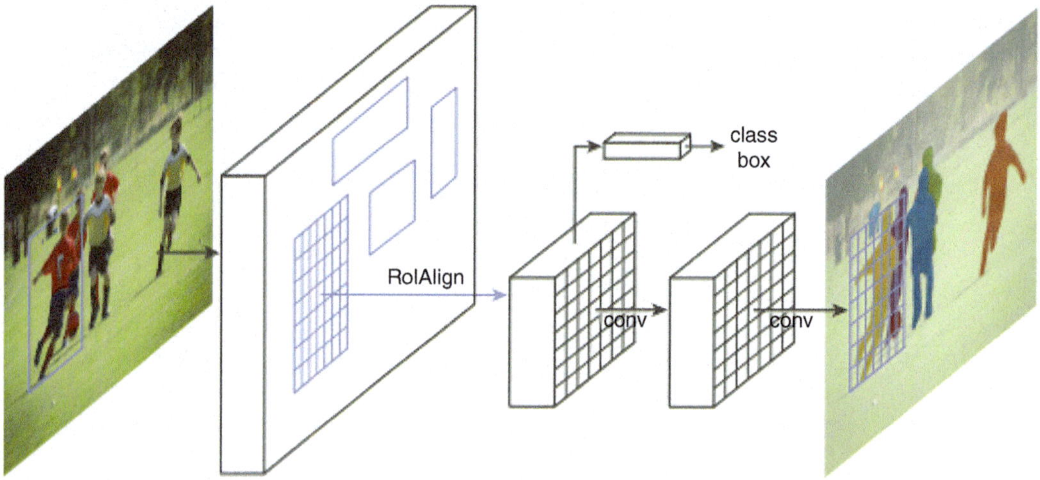

Fig. 1.8 Mask R-CNN framework [17]

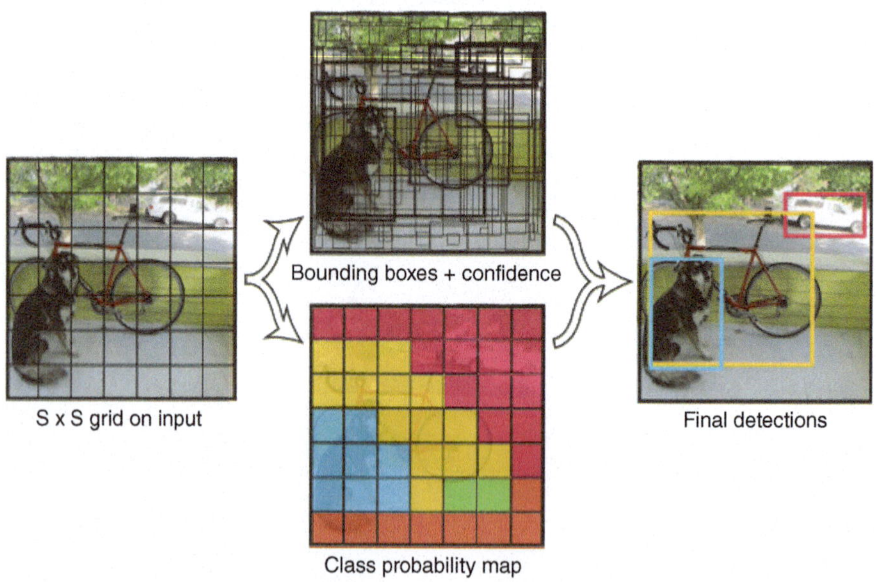

Fig. 1.9 YOLO architecture [28]

may appear at any stage. Most of the research investigated the use of differential privacy in ML and DL models.

2. **ML-enhanced privacy protection**. Works in this group employ ML models as a tool for improving privacy protection.
3. **ML-based privacy attack**. In contrast to the previous group, ML can also be used as an attacking tool. Especially DL systems may surpass conventional privacy-preserving methods, necessitating a discussion of such new threats and corresponding solutions [30].

The classification is further expanded in Fig. 1.10.

Adversarial attacks involve deliberately crafting subtle input perturbations to deceive ML models into making incorrect predictions, highlighting their vulnerability in robustness. Figure 1.11 shows how perturbations can confuse the AI model and affect its final output.

The success of adversarial attacks is due to the lack of generalization in the low probability space of data [33]. Some popular adversarial attacks proposed for natural images and applied to medical images include the *fast gradient sign method* (FGSM), *basic iterative method* (BIM), *projected gradient descent* (PGD), *Jacobian-based saliency map attack* (JSMA), and *universal adversarial perturbation* (UAP). In some studies, however, these adversarial models are

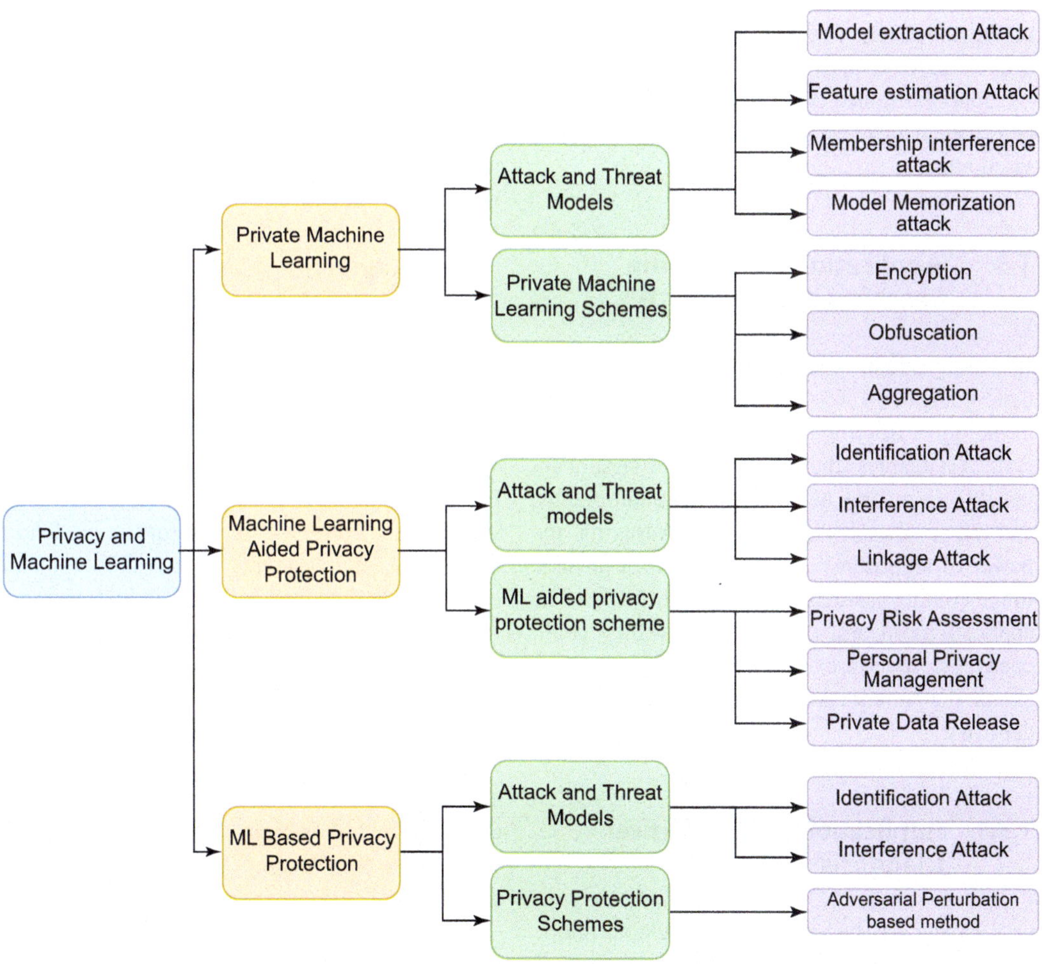

Fig. 1.10 The proposed taxonomy of privacy and ML [31]

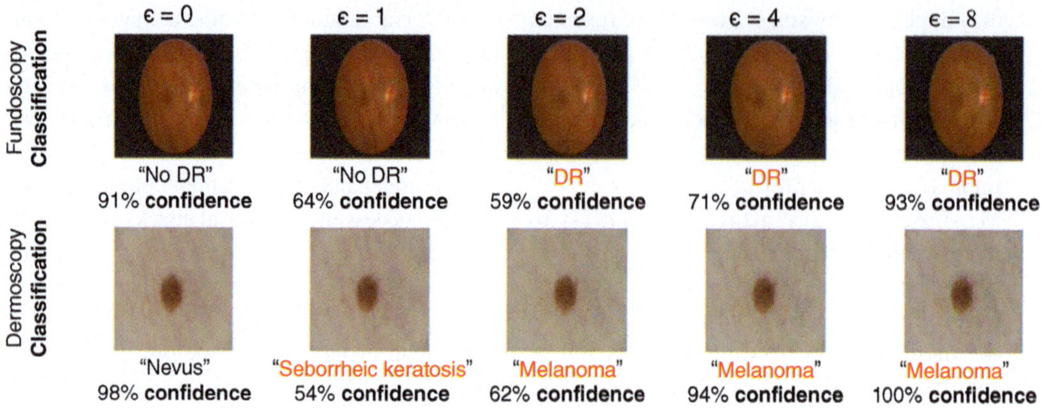

Fig. 1.11 Visualizing a medical adversarial example with predictions under different perturbations sizes ϵ. Predictions labelled in red indicate incorrect predictions [32]

intentionally incorporated into the trained DL models [31], because adversarial training is one of the most effective approaches to defending against adversarial attacks [34]. As a result, the DL models trained on a mixture of clean and perturbed data become more resistant to adversarial attacks.

1.3 Applications of Machine Learning in Oral Health

Just like medicine and other fields, oral health is undergoing a revolutionary transformation thanks to the quick development of ML and AI in general. AI enables the extraction of significant insights from oral health records, photographs, and other relevant sources by leveraging the power of algorithms and large volumes of data. In the coming sections, we will review a few ML applications in oral health and how they could contribute to improving oral health outcomes, enhancing patient care, and shaping the future of dentistry.

1.3.1 Applications in Oral Cancer Diagnosis

Oral cancer has become a serious global public health concern. Squamous cell carcinomas (SCCs), which are aggressive malignancies with a high propensity to spread locally and distantly, account for most oral cancers. It has also been observed that oral SCC (OSCC) has considerable implications on patients' posttreatment quality of life due to its location and the disease's aggressive attitude. Considering the commonly delayed diagnosis of oral cancer, the 5-year overall survival rate is roughly 51.7% [31].

Cancer treatment is mainly dependent on tumor staging. However, discrepancies in staging methods have contributed to inaccurate prognoses in OSCC patients. ML algorithms can offer valuable support to clinicians by providing them with more precise and comprehensive diagnostic and prognostic information. A paper by Huang et al. [32] proposed a new optimized CNN model for the diagnosis of oral cancer. Another recent study presented an ML model for the prediction of oral cancer in patients with oral leukoplakia and oral lichenoid mucositis [33], which accounts for age, sex, tobacco usage, alcohol consumption, diabetes status, and ten other parameters. This proves that by leveraging large data sets and analyzing complex patterns and features within histopathological images and patient data, ML can assist clinicians in making early informed decisions regarding appropriate treatment strategies, ultimately leading to improved survival rates for oral cancer patients.

AI not only changes the scope of screening and enhances accessibility to early cancer detection but may further enhance diagnosis due to its accelerated workflow and accuracy compared to traditional human screening techniques. For instance, AI does not suffer from observational fatigue, and compared to the naked eye, it is able to notice minute changes in the range of a single pixel at a higher rate [34].

1.3.1.1 Classification of Oral Lesions

Oral cancer is frequently preceded by visible oral lesions known as *oral potentially malignant disorders* (OPMDs) that can be recognized during a clinical oral examination. The likelihood of malignant transformation associated with OPMDs makes their early identification crucial for lowering oral cancer morbidity and mortality. Oral lesions have a very heterogeneous appearance, which makes it difficult for healthcare practitioners to identify them and that can delay patient referrals to oral cancer experts.

Recent advancements in computer vision have opened new possibilities for developing technologies that can automate the screening of the oral cavity. These technologies can provide real-time feedback to healthcare professionals during patient examinations and enable individuals to perform self-examinations. The existing literature on image-based automated diagnosis of oral cancer has primarily emphasized using specialized imaging techniques like *optical coherence tomography*, *hyperspectral imaging*, and *autofluorescence imaging*. These advanced imaging modalities offer unique capabilities for capturing detailed information about the oral tissues and detecting potential abnormalities or early signs of cancer. There are also attempts to detect and classify OPMDs using ML in photographs [22]. This problem can be formulated as a classification, object detection, as well as segmentation task (Fig. 1.12), and various DL architectures have been tested, including *ResNet-152*, *DenseNet-161*, *Inception-v4*, and *EfficientNet-b4* [35]. Regardless of the modality, image analysis using DL algorithms can provide a useful second opinion for non-expert clinicians, assisting them in making timely and informed decisions regarding patient care [36].

1.3.1.2 Cancer Detection Using Breath Samples

Exhaled breath analysis is another interesting field of research. The method assesses exhaled breath for volatile organic compounds (VOCs), which serve as biomarkers for many diseases and metabolic conditions. Gas chromatography combined with mass spectrometry is used to analyze VOCs, but other methods, such as proton transfer reaction mass spectrometry, have been tested as well [37]. The advantages of this method for disease identification and monitoring include non-invasiveness, cost-effectiveness, and real-time point-of-care disease diagnosis.

In relation to OSCC, electronic nose technologies, such as *near-infrared optical nose* (NIRON), have been able to distinguish OSCC, lung cancer, and a control group based on VOCs in breath samples [38]. A recent study investigated the possibilities of ML techniques, such as *multilayer perceptron* (MLP) and *probabilistic neural networks* (PNN), in electronic nose technologies for the detection of oral cancer [39]. ML techniques

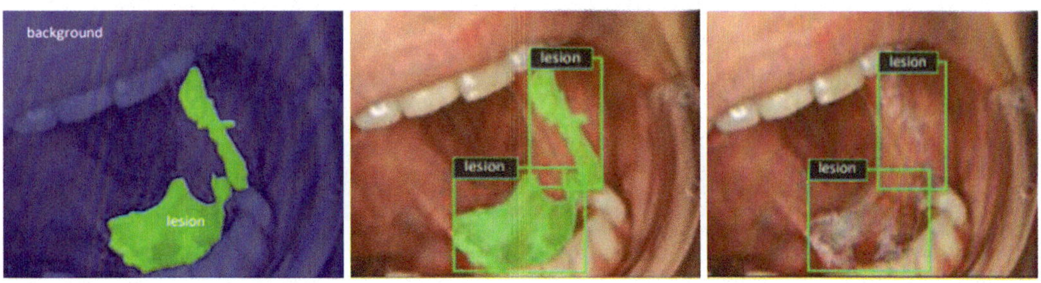

Fig. 1.12 Different types of image recognition tasks showing semantic segmentation (left), instance segmentation (center) and object detection (right) [34]

were also used for the identification of signature biomarkers of OSCC among compounds detected using gas chromatography and mass spectrometry to distinguish OSCC patients from healthy smokers [40].

1.3.1.3 Tumor Classification Based on Genetic Data

Prior to cancer treatment, the histopathological analysis is performed to confirm the diagnosis, as well as for staging and grading. However, some tumors with the same histopathological classification can exhibit varying responses to the proposed therapy. This discrepancy can be attributed to genetic variations and environmental factors that lead to alterations in the biological behavior of cancer cells. Therefore, there is a growing need for diagnostic models that incorporate genetic characteristics alongside morphological features, enabling the prediction of the biological behavior of the cancer and hence enhancing treatment selection [41]. A recent study examined such models to improve the efficiency of personalized cancer treatment [42]. The ML diagnostic tool performed exceptionally well in the diagnosis of OSCC, and it also showed that gene expression is a more important element in classifying cancer types than its histological traits. Figure 1.13 shows the workflow of the study [42], and Table 1.2 summarizes relevant research papers on the use of ML in oral cancer and OPMDs.

1.3.2 Diagnosis of Dental Caries

Dental caries is one of the most prevalent diseases in the world. Caries is characterized by the localized destruction of dental hard tissues by acidic by-products of bacterial fermentation of dietary carbohydrates. Both the crown and the root of teeth can be affected by caries [43], and if not treated, caries can ultimately result in tooth loss and a decline in quality of life [44]. On the other hand, timely detection of caries can reduce the invasiveness of the treatment or avoid it entirely [45]. ML can be used either for the detection of caries in images or to predict its development from demographic data [46]. Table 1.3 shows some recent works related to the diagnosis and treatment of dental caries, and the topic is further addressed in Chap. 7 dedicated to the use of AI in cariology.

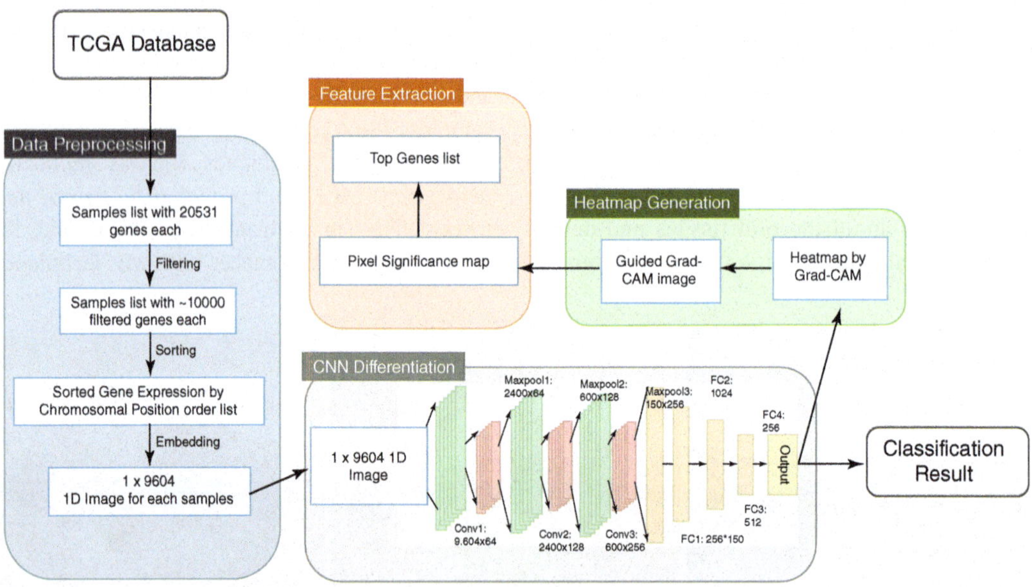

Fig. 1.13 Workflow of the study by Pratama et al. [42]

Table 1.2 Overview of papers regarding oral cancer

Year	Author	Summary	ML architecture used
2020	Kowalski et al. [31]	Survivability of oral cancer	
2020	Kar et al. [34]	AI and oral cancer screening	DCNN, CNN, SVM, DBN
2020	Tanriver et al. [36]	Detection of oral lesion with DL	U-net, R-CNN, YOLO
2020	Welikala et al. [23]	Classification of oral lesions	R-CNN, ResNet, RPN
2020	Das et al. [37]	Viability of breath analysis	
2021	Mentel et al. [40]	Breath analysis for oral cancer diagnosis	kNN, LR, RF
2021	Pratama et al. [42]	Oral cancer and gene expression with ML	CNN
2023	Adeoye et al. [33]	Prediction of oral cancer with ML	SVM, MLP, LDA
2023	Bhatt et al. [41]	Cancer detection from genomic data	SVM, kNN, CNN
2023	Huang et al. [32]	Diagnosing oral cancer with DL	CNN

Table 1.3 Recent works on dental caries using ML models

Year	Author	Summary	ML models used
2021	Lian et al. [45]	DL in caries detection and classification	DenseNet, nnU-net
2021	Lee et al. [47]	Early caries detection using radiographs	U-net, R-CNN, YOLO
2022	Reyes et al. [44]	ML in diagnosis and prognosis of dental caries	–
2022	Kang et al. [48]	Prediction of caries using ML and personalized medicine	ANN, CNN, LSTM
2022	Talpur et al. [49]	ML algorithms in diagnosis of caries	–
2023	Martins et al. [50]	ML in X-ray diagnosis for oral health	–
2023	Toledo Reyes et al. [51]	Early childhood predictors for dental caries	LR, RF, XGBoost, DT
2023	Kang et al. [52]	Dental caries prediction model using ML for DSS	GBDT, RF, LR, SVM, LSTM

1.3.2.1 Detection of Dental Caries in Radiographs

Radiographs are crucial especially in approximal caries detection, as proximal tooth surfaces can hardly be visualized otherwise [53], and a growing number of studies using AI to identify caries have been recently published [50]. For example, Lee et al. developed a U-Net model for identifying dental caries from bitewing radiographs [47]. Without any preprocessing, the bitewing radiographs were used to train the CNN model, and it was confirmed that the proposed model could aid dental professionals in making more accurate diagnoses of dental caries in real-world clinical situations. In another study, Lian et al. [45] developed a model employing nnU-Net and DenseNet121, which was used to classify lesion progression after the nnU-Net technique had segmented the carious lesions. Finally, the authors introduced a dropout mechanism and label softening to address the overfitting phenomena during model training, ensuring that it achieves the greatest potential performance. While there were many other studies on caries detection in radiographs and other images, e.g., photographs, it is beyond the scope of this chapter to examine them in detail.

1.3.2.2 Prediction of Dental Caries from Demographic Data

As dental caries is a highly prevalent oral disease, its prediction is a crucial aspect of preventive dentistry. Clinical evaluation and risk assessment are the mainstays of conventional procedures. However, the use of demographic data to forecast the risk of dental caries has become more popular with the development of ML.

Kang et al. used the data obtained from the 2018 Korean Children's Oral Health Survey and analyzed them using various models including *gradient boosted decision tree* (GBDT), *random forest* (RF), *logistic regression* (LR), *support vector machine* (SVM), and LSTM [52]. The models performed well and could be used as a diagnostic tool to find individuals affected by caries. Additionally, the models can offer helpful guidance for creating a plan to prevent and treat caries, which can significantly decrease the time required for patient diagnosis and expenditures associated with caries.

Toledo et al. proposed to use ML and predictors gathered from a 10-year prospective cohort study performed in children aged 1–5 years in southern Brazil to construct a caries prognosis models in primary and permanent teeth [51]. The development of caries was initially investigated in 2010 and then again in 2012 and 2020. As a part of the study, information on behavioral, clinical, psychological, psychosocial, and demographic aspects were collected. LR was used along with the DT, RF and extreme gradient boosting (XGBoost). All models exhibited an area under the ROC curve (AUC) above 0.70 in predicting primary tooth caries after a 2-year follow-up, with baseline caries severity being the best predictor [51].

1.3.3 Other Applications

The applications of ML in oral health encompass a diverse array of topics, showcasing the versatility and adaptability of ML algorithms in addressing numerous challenges faced by dental professionals and researchers. By harnessing the power of AI, these applications aim to augment traditional dental practices, improve clinical decision-making, optimize treatment strategies, and enable more personalized and effective patient care. In this section, we will explore AI applications in other dental fields, and as in previous sections, Table 1.4 shows an overview of selected studies in these fields.

1.3.3.1 Periodontitis

Periodontitis is another highly prevalent oral condition caused by bacterial biofilm, but it is also affected by genetic and environmental factors, particularly cigarette smoking [77]. Periodontitis is a common cause of tooth loss in adult and elderly patients, because it gradually destroys the periodontal connective tissue and bone support. Furthermore, periodontitis is associated with various systemic diseases and an increased risk of cancer [46], making its prevention, timely diagnosis, and adequate management highly important not only for oral health.

In 2020, Chang et al. [57] created a DL hybrid method for automatic periodontitis staging based on bone loss in panoramic radiographs. The proposed hybrid framework combined a DL architecture for bone level detection and traditional *computer-aided diagnosis* (CAD) processing for classification. The overall intraclass correlation coefficient value between the generated model and radiologists' diagnosis surpassed 0.9, indicating very accurate automatic periodontal bone loss diagnoses.

Other studies used ML techniques for predictive modelling. Bashir et al. [55] used American and Taiwanese national survey data and explored potential periodontitis predictors shared between the two datasets. Ten machine learning models were trained to predict the presence of periodontitis, which included AdaBoost, *artificial neural networks* (ANNs), DT, Gaussian process, k-NN, linear support vector classification, linear discriminant analysis, LR, RF, and Naïve Bayes. The obtained results concluded that the ANN model had a high accuracy. In another study, Troiano et al. [54] designed and validated models for the prognostic prediction of molar survival after periodontitis treatment. Along with LR, they also built models based on SVM, k-NN, DT, RF, ANN, gradient boosting, and Naïve Bayes. All the models showed promising results with an AUC value over 0.7. An ensemble method combining LR with neural networks reached an AUC of 0.759, making it the most reliable algorithm in the three validation cohorts.

Kim et al. [58] proposed an alternative approach, developing an ML model for chronic periodontitis prediction based on salivary bacterial copy number, which was measured in healthy individuals and patients with chronic periodontitis using PCR. Based on the severity of periodontitis, they used ANN, SVM, LR, and RF to identify bacterial combinations that could serve as a biomarker for periodontitis diagnosis and staging. Figure 1.14 depicts the ML workflow of this study. Further information on the use of AI in periodontology can be found in Chap. 4.

Table 1.4 Selected works related to ML in the other dental fields

Year	Author	Summary	ML model used
2020	Sun et al. [46]	ML applications in stomatology	–
Periodontitis			
2023	Troiano et al. [54]	LR and ML model for prediction of molar loss	LR, SVM, ANN, RF, DT, Naïve Bayes
2022	Bashir et al. [55]	Comparison of ML models for periodontitis prediction	–
2022	Chang et al. [56]	DL for radiographic diagnosis of periodontitis	CNN
2020	Chang et al. [57]	DL hybrid method for PBL	CNN
2020	Kim et al. [58]	Prediction of periodontitis from bacterial copy number	RF, SVM, LR
Endodontics			
2023	Ver Berne et al. [59]	Classification of radicular cysts and periapical granulomas	MobileNet, YOLO
2020	Orhan et al. [60]	Detecting periapical pathosis on cone-beam CT scans	CNN
2020	Mallishery et al. [61]	Difficulty assessment using ML	SVM
2019	Hiraiwa et al. [62]	Recognition of dental root structure from radiographs	AlexNet, GoogleNet
2015	Okada et al. [63]	Diagnose dental periapical lesions in cone beam CT scans	LDA-AdaBoost classifier
Orthodontics			
2023	Leavitt et al. [64]	Prediction of orthodontic extraction patterns	RF, LR, SVM
2019	Rao et al. [65]	Facial landmark recognition model	ASM, YOLO
2019	Juodzbalys et al. [66]	Automatic labelling teeth using dental surfaces from 3D intra oral scanner	MeshSegNet
2019	Tian et al. [67]	Automatic classification and segmentation of 3D dental model	CNN
2018	Xu et al. [68]	3D tooth segmentation and labelling	CNN
2016	Pei et al. [69]	Segmenting come-beam CT images	Random walk
2016	Jung and Kim [70]	Model for diagnosis of extraction	Back propagation neural network
Dental implantology			
2020	Kwak et al. [71]	Mandibular Canal detection	CNN
2019	Sorkhabi et al. [72]	Classification of alveolar bone density	DT, AdaBoost
2018	Liu et al. [73]	Predicting failure of dental implants	CNN
2018	Ha et al. [74]	Factors influencing prognosis of dental implants	KLMS, FEM
Dental age estimation			
2023	Aljameel et al. [75]	Dental age estimation using AI	CNN
2021	Shen et al. [76]	ML-assisted Cameriere method	LR, RF, SVM

1.3.3.2 Endodontics

In endodontics, pulpitis, pulp necrosis, and apical periodontitis represent the main causes for root canal treatment. Applications of ML in this field include examination of teeth anatomy, evaluation of the treatment difficulty, or the detection and classification of periapical radiolucencies.

As an example of root anatomy examination, Hiraiwa et al. [62] successfully used a DL system to determine if a second distal root is present in mandibular first molars. The analysis was done on apical radiographs, and cone-beam computed tomography (CBCT) was used as a gold standard. The analysis of root anatomy is also a part of the treatment difficulty assessment, which is usually done following the Endodontic Case Difficulty Assessment Form by the American Association of Endodontists [46]. Mallishery

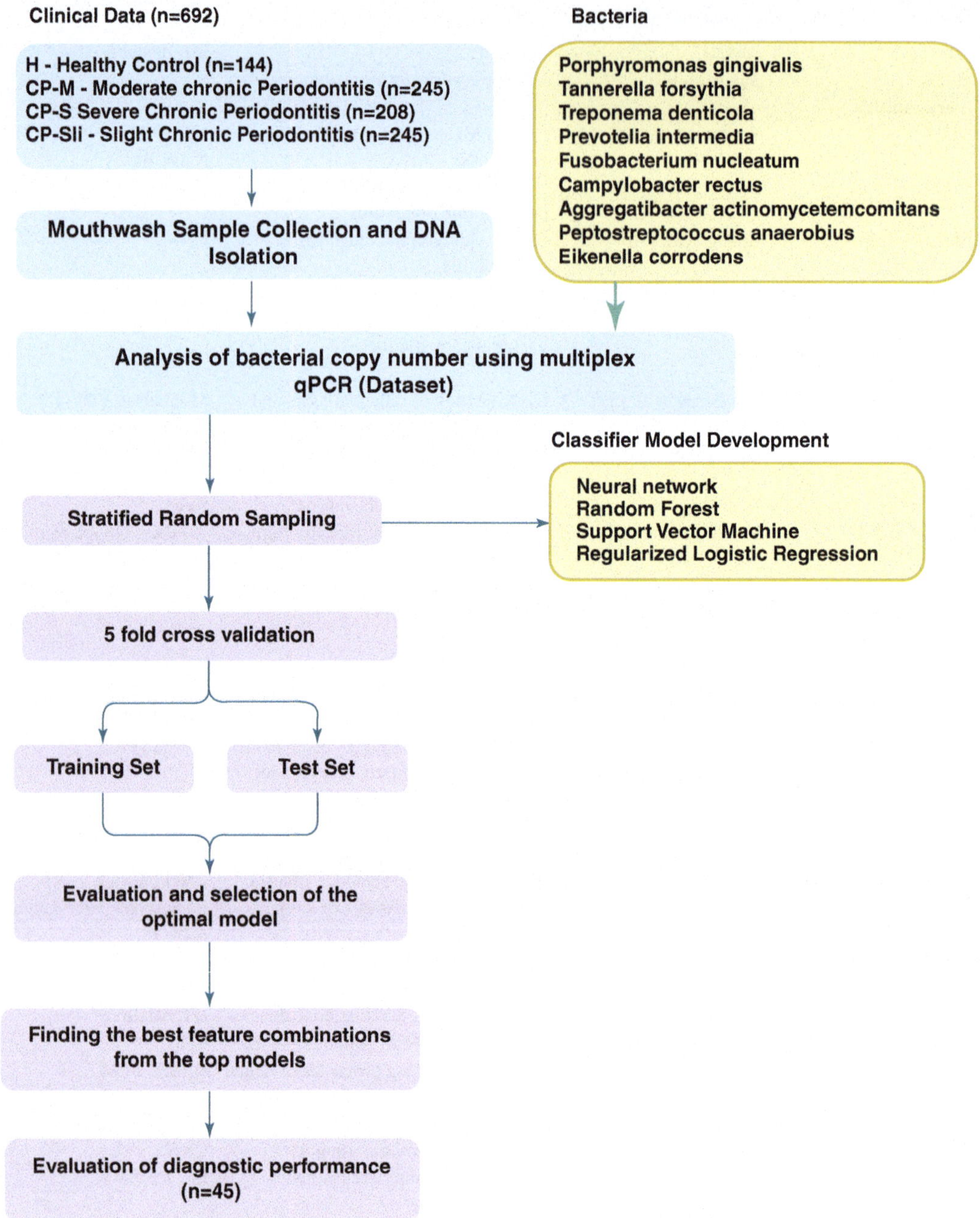

Fig. 1.14 ML workflow for the prediction of chronic periodontitis severity using qPCR data [58]

et al. [61] built an SVM model to assess the treatment difficulty using this form. The model had a sensitivity of almost 95%, and it was concluded that the automated difficulty assessment could increasing the speed of decision-making and referrals if necessary.

Other studies focused on periapical lesions in radiographs and CBCTs. For instance, Orhan et al. [60] employed a deep CNN to locate periapical lesions in CBCT scans and calculate the lesion volume, achieving promising results. Some researchers aimed at a clinically difficult task of differentiating periapical granulomas from radicular cysts in CBCTs [63] and panoramic radiographs [59]. Both the referenced studies showed excellent results, which could lead to a more efficient referral strategy and subsequent treatment efficacy. A thorough overview of AI applications in endodontics is available in Chap. 8.

1.3.3.3 Orthodontics

Orthodontic treatment involves straightening or repositioning teeth in order to improve occlusal function as well as aesthetic appearance. Applications of AI in orthodontics can improve the efficiency of treatment planning, and some of them are outlined in this section. For more details, please refer to Chap. 6.

Prior to the treatment, orthodontist thoroughly analyze the clinical situation and radiographs to compile a suitable treatment plan. Several studies used DL architectures for landmark detection in cephalometric analyses. However, there were also studies which focused on the analysis of soft tissues in facial images. Rao et al. [65] developed a facial landmark recognition model based on the *active shape model* (ASM) model and the YOLO architecture, which was more accurate in facial landmark detection and measurement compared to their manual assessment.

ML techniques may also help in choosing whether to extract premolars in cases with malocclusion that includes severe tooth crowding. Jung and Kim [70] developed a back-propagation neural network-based model for diagnosing extractions, which had a success rate of 93% in distinguishing extraction and non-extraction cases. In another study, Leavitt et al. [64] attempted to develop a generalizable ML algorithm from a large sample of orthodontic providers to accurately predict orthodontic extraction patterns in a racially and ethnically diverse populations. In total, 55 cephalometric and demographic data were provided to the ML models based on RF, LR, and SVM. The results differed for various extraction patterns, so were successful while some were rather inaccurate.

With the expansion of digital dentistry, tooth segmentation in 3D models has become increasingly important in orthodontic treatment planning and outcome prediction. Tian et al. [67] suggested a method that makes use of sparse voxel octree and 3D CNNs, which offered segmentation accuracy of 89.8%. In a similar task, Xu et al. [68] created a two-level hierarchical CNN framework that labels the teeth, gingiva, and spaces between the teeth. The boundary was then fine-tuned using improved fuzzy clustering. For the segmentation of CBCT scans, Pei et al. [69] successfully applied the 3D exemplar-based random walk, as its results agreed with manual segmentation, while Juodzbalys et al. [66] developed a novel DL method for tooth labelling in 3D intraoral scans.

1.3.3.4 Dental Implantology

Dental implants serve as a support for restorations of missing teeth, thereby playing a crucial role in restoring function, aesthetics, and oral health in general. The placement of a dental implant is influenced by various factors such as bone density and anatomical structures, as well as oral and general health. All these factors must be carefully assessed to ensure optimal outcomes, in which advanced AI technologies can assist by analyzing imaging data, predicting potential complications, and providing precise treatment planning tailored to the patient's unique conditions.

In image analysis, several studies investigated the localization of anatomical structures, e.g., the mandibular canal. Its position is important during implant placement as it contains the inferior alveolar nerve and any damage to it could have long-term or permanent impact on the patient. In one of the studies, Kwak et al. successfully detected and segmented the mandibular canal on CBCT images using U-Net [71]. Image analysis can also be used to determine the amount and quality of the available bone and its mineral density. For example, Sorkhabi et al. suggested using a CNN to assess alveolar bone density in 2019 [72].

Based on the provided data, ML can be also used to model treatment outcomes. Liu et al. [73] created an ML model that estimates the implant failure rate using the DT, SVM, LR, and classifier ensembles based on bagging and AdaBoost. It

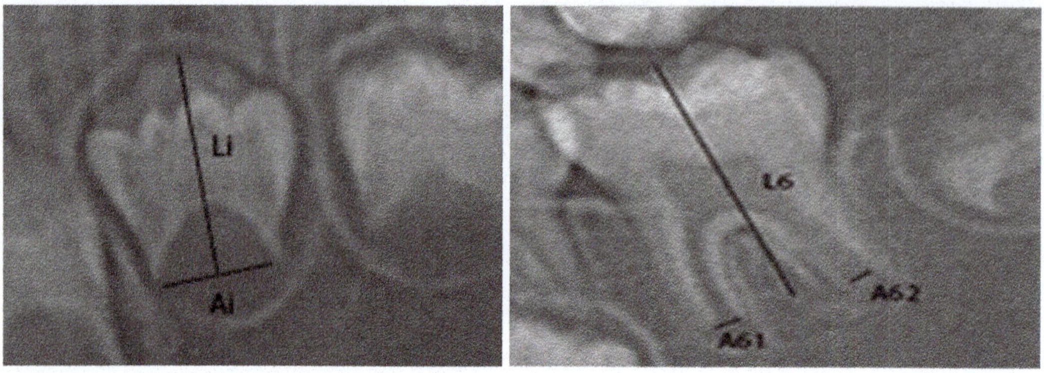

Fig. 1.15 Example of single and multiple root teeth measurement [79]

was concluded that the model can help surgeons by choosing the optimal implant system and prosthodontics treatments for their patients [73]. Another insight was brought in the study by Ha et al., which indicated that the mesiodistal position of the inserted implant is the most significant factor determining its prognosis [74]. Further studies on the topic, as well as other uses of AI in dental implantology, are presented in Chap. 5.

1.3.3.5 Dental Age Estimation

Dental age is thought to be a quick, precise, and trustworthy method of age determination in growing children. In orthodontics, planning the treatment of various malocclusions is closely related to the stage of maxillofacial growth. In pediatric dentistry, dental age may be also important in certain cases, e.g., related to irregular tooth eruption. And skeletal growth is also relevant for prosthodontics and implant planning in adolescent patients. Besides dental applications, dental age estimation is also important in forensic medicine, anthropology and bioarcheology, as it may provide information about earlier populations [78].

Over the years, several radiographic techniques for estimating dental age have been developed. These methods essentially identify the stages of tooth development in radiographs (Fig. 1.15) and code them in accordance with the readily available tables created by various authors. The best-known of these are the Willems method, the Nolla method, the Haavikko method, and the Demirjian method. Recently, Cameriere's novel strategy has received a lot of attention and favor [78].

Researchers have used the help of AI in estimating the dental age. One such study was conducted by Aljameel et al. [75] who used four CNN architectures and observed that the further they reduced the age range of the experiment, the finer the models learned and functioned. Shen et al. [76] constructed three ML models, namely, LR, RF, and SVM, to estimate children's dental age using the Cameriere's method and to compare them with the Cameriere's formula. The results showed that the SVM, LR, and RF models were more accurate than the conventional approach represented by the Cameriere's formula. This outcome encourages the use of ML techniques for dental age estimation.

1.4 Conclusion

ML has emerged as a powerful tool in oral health, offering significant potential in various aspects of diagnosis, personalized treatment planning, and prediction of outcomes. This is achieved using various ML techniques, which can analyze clinical records and patient data, as well as DL models frequently used for image analysis and other tasks. However, the widespread adoption of AI in oral health also raises significant concerns in terms of ethics and privacy, and attention also must be paid to adversarial attacks. Addressing these challenges requires collaborative efforts of all stakeholders to develop robust safeguards for the responsible use of AI in dentistry.

References

1. Qayyum A, Qadir J, Bilal M, Al-Fuqaha A. Secure and robust machine learning for healthcare: a survey. IEEE Rev Biomed Eng. 2021;14:156–80. https://doi.org/10.1109/RBME.2020.3013489.
2. Arsiwala-Scheppach LT, Chaurasia A, Müller A, Krois J, Schwendicke F. Machine learning in dentistry: a scoping review. J Clin Med. 2023;12(3):937.
3. Leite AF, Vasconcelos KF, Willems H, Jacobs R. Radiomics and machine learning in oral healthcare. Proteomics Clin Appl. 2020;14(3):1900040.
4. Yan Z, Zhan Y, Peng Z, Liao S, Shinagawa Y, Zhang S, Metaxas DN, Zhou XS. Multi-instance deep learning: discover discriminative local anatomies for body part recognition. IEEE Trans Med Imaging. 2016;35(5):1332–43.
5. Anthimopoulos M, Christodoulidis S, Ebner L, Christe A, Mougiakakou S. Lung pattern classification for interstitial lung diseases using a deep convolutional neural network. IEEE Trans Med Imaging. 2016;35(5):1207–16. https://doi.org/10.1109/TMI.2016.2535865.
6. Shen W, Zhou M, Yang F, Yang C, Tian J. Multi-scale convolutional neural networks for lung nodule classification. In: Information processing in medical imaging: 24th international conference, IPMI 2015, Sabhal Mor Ostaig, Isle of Skye, UK, June 28–July 3, 2015, proceedings 24. Cham: Springer; 2015. p. 588–99.
7. Ahishakiye E, Bastiaan Van Gijzen M, Tumwiine J, Wario R, Obungoloch J. A survey on deep learning in medical image reconstruction. Intell Med. 2021;1(3):118–27.
8. Mehta J, Majumdar A. Rodeo: robust de-aliasing autoencoder for real-time medical image reconstruction. Pattern Recogn. 2017;63:499–510.
9. Alrashedy HHN, Almansour AF, Ibrahim DM, Hammoudeh MAA. Braingan: brain MRI image generation and classification framework using GAN architectures and CNN models. Sensors. 2022;22(11):4297.
10. Lyu Q, You C, Shan H, Wang G. Super-resolution MRI through deep learning. arXiv preprint arXiv:1810.06776. 2018. https://doi.org/10.48550/arXiv.1810.06776.
11. Kumar VB, Kumar SS, Saboo V. Dermatological disease detection using image processing and machine learning. In: 2016 Third International Conference on Artificial Intelligence and Pattern Recognition (AIPR); 2016. p. 1–6. https://doi.org/10.1109/ICAIPR.2016.7585217.
12. Ravishankar H, Sudhakar P, Venkataramani R, Thiruvenkadam S, Annangi P, Babu N, Vaidya V. Understanding the mechanisms of deep transfer learning for medical images. In: Deep learning and data labeling for medical applications: first international workshop, LABELS 2016, and second international workshop, DLMIA 2016, held in conjunction with MICCAI 2016, Athens, Greece, October 21, 2016, proceedings 1. Cham: Springer; 2016. p. 188–96.
13. Zhang J, Xie Y, Wu Q, Xia Y. Medical image classification using synergic deep learning. Med Image Anal. 2019;54:10–9.
14. Cai L, Gao J, Zhao D. A review of the application of deep learning in medical image classification and segmentation. Ann Trans Med. 2020;8(11):713.
15. Sarraf S, Tofighi G. Classification of Alzheimer's disease using fMRI data and deep learning convolutional neural networks. arXiv preprint arXiv:1603.08631. 2016.
16. Minaee S, Boykov Y, Porikli F, Plaza A, Kehtarnavaz N, Terzopoulos D. Image segmentation using deep learning: a survey. IEEE Trans Pattern Anal Mach Intell. 2022;44(7):3523–42. https://doi.org/10.1109/TPAMI.2021.3059968.
17. Hafiz AM, Bhat GM. A survey on instance segmentation: state of the art. Int J Multimed Inf Retr. 2020;9(3):171–89.
18. Usman M, Latif S, Asim M, Lee B-D, Qadir J. Retrospective motion correction in multishot MRI using generative adversarial network. Sci Rep. 2020;10(1):4786.
19. Everingham M, Van Gool L, Williams CK, Winn J, Zisserman A. The Pascal visual object classes (VOC) challenge. Int J Comput Vis. 2010;88:303–38.
20. Jing B, Xie P, Xing E. On the automatic generation of medical imaging reports. arXiv preprint arXiv:1711.08195. 2017.
21. Messina P, Pino P, Parra D, Soto A, Besa C, Uribe S, Andía M, Tejos C, Prieto C, Capurro D. A survey on deep learning and explainability for automatic report generation from medical images. ACM Comput Surv (CSUR). 2022;54(10s):1–40.
22. Hao S, Zhou Y, Guo Y. A brief survey on semantic segmentation with deep learning. Neurocomputing. 2020;406:302–21.
23. Welikala RA, Remagnino P, Lim JH, Chan CS, Rajendran S, Kallarakkal TG, Zain RB, Jayasinghe RD, Rimal J, Kerr AR, et al. Automated detection and classification of oral lesions using deep learning for early detection of oral cancer. IEEE Access. 2020;8:132677–93.
24. He K, Gkioxari G, Dollár P, Girshick R. Mask R-CNN. In: Proceedings of the IEEE international conference on computer vision; 2017. p. 2961–9.
25. Zhou T, Ye X, Lu H, Zheng X, Qiu S, Liu Y, et al. Dense convolutional network and its application in medical image analysis. Biomed Res Int. 2022;2022:2384830. https://doi.org/10.1155/2022/2384830.
26. He K, Zhang X, Ren S, Sun J. Deep residual learning for image recognition. In: Proceedings of the IEEE conference on computer vision and pattern recognition; 2016. p. 770–8.
27. Cai S, Wu Y, Chen G. A novel elastomeric U-net for medical image segmentation. Front Aging Neurosci. 2022;14:31.

28. Redmon J, Divvala S, Girshick R, Farhadi A. You only look once: unified, real-time object detection. In: Proceedings of the IEEE conference on computer vision and pattern recognition; 2016. p. 779–88.
29. Liu B, Ding M, Shaham S, Rahayu W, Farokhi F, Lin Z. When machine learning meets privacy: a survey and outlook. ACM Comput Surv (CSUR). 2021;54(2):1–36.
30. Al-Rubaie M, Chang JM. Privacy-preserving machine learning: threats and solutions. IEEE Security Privacy. 2019;17(2):49–58.
31. Kowalski LP, Oliveira MM, Lopez RVM, Silva DRME, Ikeda MK, Curado MP. Survival trends of patients with oral and oropharyngeal cancer treated at a cancer center in São Paulo, Brazil. Clinics (Sao Paulo). 2020;75:e1507. https://doi.org/10.6061/clinics/2020/e1507.
32. Huang Q, Ding H, Razmjooy N. Optimal deep learning neural network using ISSA for diagnosing the oral cancer. Biomed Signal Process Control. 2023;84:104749.
33. Adeoye J, Koohi-Moghadam M, Choi S-W, Zheng L-W, Lo AWI, Tsang RK-Y, Chow VLY, Akinshipo A, Thomson P, Su Y-X. Predicting oral cancer risk in patients with oral leukoplakia and oral lichenoid mucositis using machine learning. J Big Data. 2023;10(1):1–24.
34. Kar A, Wreesmann VB, Shwetha V, Thakur S, Rao VU, Arakeri G, Brennan PA. Improvement of oral cancer screening quality and reach: the promise of artificial intelligence. J Oral Pathol Med. 2020;49(8):727–30.
35. Huang G, Liu Z, Van Der Maaten L, Weinberger KQ. Densely connected convolutional networks. In: 2017 IEEE conference on computer vision and pattern recognition (CVPR); 2017. p. 2261–9. https://doi.org/10.1109/CVPR.2017.243.
36. Tanriver G, Soluk Tekkesin M, Ergen O. Automated detection and classification of oral lesions using deep learning to detect oral potentially malignant disorders. Cancers. 2021;13(11):2766.
37. Das S, Pal M. Non-invasive monitoring of human health by exhaled breath analysis: a comprehensive review. J Electrochem Soc. 2020;167(3):037562.
38. Shumeiko V, Paltiel Y, Bisker G, Hayouka Z, Shoseyov O. A nanoscale paper-based near-infrared optical nose (NIRON). Biosens Bioelectron. 2021;172:112763.
39. Rangarajan M, Pandya HJ. Breath VOC analysis and machine learning approaches for disease screening: a review. J Breath Res. 2023;17(2):024001. https://doi.org/10.1088/1752-7163/acb283.
40. Mentel S, Gallo K, Wagendorf O, Preissner R, Nahles S, Heiland M, Preissner S. Prediction of oral squamous cell carcinoma based on machine learning of breath samples: a prospective controlled study. BMC Oral Health. 2021;21:1–12.
41. Bhatt M, Shende P. Advancement in machine learning: a strategic lookout from cancer identification to treatment. Arch Comput Methods Eng. 2023;30(4):1–16. https://doi.org/10.1007/s11831-023-09886-0.
42. Pratama R, Hwang JJ, Lee JH, Song G, Park HR. Authentication of differential gene expression in oral squamous cell carcinoma using machine learning applications. BMC Oral Health. 2021;21(1):1–8.
43. Hung M, Voss MW, Rosales MN, Li W, Su W, Xu J, Bounsanga J, Ruiz-Negrón B, Lauren E, Licari FW. Application of machine learning for diagnostic prediction of root caries. Gerodontology. 2019;36(4):395–404.
44. Reyes LT, Knorst JK, Ortiz FR, Ardenghi TM. Machine learning in the diagnosis and prognostic prediction of dental caries: a systematic review. Caries Res. 2022;56(3):161–70. https://doi.org/10.1159/000524167.
45. Lian L, Zhu T, Zhu F, Zhu H. Deep learning for caries detection and classification. Diagnostics. 2021;11(9):1672.
46. Sun M-L, Liu Y, Liu G, Cui D, Heidari AA, Jia W-Y, Ji X, Chen H, Luo Y. Application of machine learning to stomatology: a comprehensive review. IEEE Access. 2020;8:184360–74.
47. Lee S, Oh S-I, Jo J, Kang S, Shin Y, Park J-w. Deep learning for early dental caries detection in bitewing radiographs. Sci Rep. 2021;11(1):16807.
48. Kang I-A, Ngnamsie Njimbouom S, Lee K-O, Kim J-D. DCP: prediction of dental caries using machine learning in personalized medicine. Appl Sci. 2022;12(6):3043.
49. Talpur S, Azim F, Rashid M, Syed SA, Talpur BA, Khan SJ. Uses of different machine learning algorithms for diagnosis of dental caries. J Healthc Eng. 2022;2022:5032435. https://doi.org/10.1155/2022/5032435.
50. Martins MV, Baptista L, Luís H, Assunção V, Araújo M-R, Realinho V. Machine learning in X-ray diagnosis for oral health: a review of recent progress. Computation. 2023;11(6):115.
51. Toledo Reyes L, Knorst J, Ortiz F, Brondani B, Emmanuelli B, Saraiva Guedes R, Mendes F, Ardenghi T. Early childhood predictors for dental caries: a machine learning approach. J Dent Res. 2023;102(9):999–1006. https://doi.org/10.1177/00220345231170535.
52. Kang I-A, Njimbouom SN, Kim J-D. Optimal feature selection-based dental caries prediction model using machine learning for decision support system. Bioengineering. 2023;10(2):245. https://doi.org/10.3390/bioengineering10020245.
53. Ali RB, Ejbali R, Zaied M. Detection and classification of dental caries in X-ray images using deep neural networks. In: International conference on software engineering advances (ICSEA); 2016. p. 236.
54. Troiano G, Nibali L, Petsos H, Eickholz P, Saleh MH, Santamaria P, Jian J, Shi S, Meng H, Zhurakivska K, et al. Development and international validation of logistic regression and machine-learning models for the prediction of 10-year molar loss. J Clin Periodontol. 2023;50(3):348–57.
55. Bashir NZ, Rahman Z, Chen SL-S. Systematic comparison of machine learning algorithms to develop

and validate predictive models for periodontitis. J Clin Periodontol. 2022;49(10):958–69.
56. Chang J, Chang M-F, Angelov N, Hsu C-Y, Meng H-W, Sheng S, Glick A, Chang K, He Y-R, Lin Y-B, et al. Application of deep machine learning for the radiographic diagnosis of periodontitis. Clin Oral Investig. 2022;26(11):6629–37.
57. Chang H-J, Lee S-J, Yong T-H, Shin N-Y, Jang B-G, Kim J-E, Huh K-H, Lee S-S, Heo M-S, Choi S-C, et al. Deep learning hybrid method to automatically diagnose periodontal bone loss and stage periodontitis. Sci Rep. 2020;10(1):7531.
58. Kim E-H, Kim S, Kim H-J, Jeong H-O, Lee J, Jang J, Joo J-Y, Shin Y, Kang J, Park AK, et al. Prediction of chronic periodontitis severity using machine learning models based on salivary bacterial copy number. Front Cell Infect Microbiol. 2020;10:571515.
59. Ver Berne J, Saadi SB, Politis C, Jacobs R. A deep learning approach for radiological detection and classification of radicular cysts and periapical granulomas. J Dent. 2023;135:104581. https://doi.org/10.1016/j.jdent.2023.104581.
60. Orhan K, Bayrakdar I, Ezhov M, Kravtsov A, Özyürek T. Evaluation of artificial intelligence for detecting periapical pathosis on cone-beam computed tomography scans. Int Endod J. 2020;53(5):680–9.
61. Mallishery S, Chhatpar P, Banga K, Shah T, Gupta P. The precision of case difficulty and referral decisions: an innovative automated approach. Clin Oral Investig. 2020;24:1909–15.
62. Hiraiwa T, Ariji Y, Fukuda M, Kise Y, Nakata K, Katsumata A, Fujita H, Ariji E. A deep-learning artificial intelligence system for assessment of root morphology of the mandibular first molar on panoramic radiography. Dentomaxillofac Radiol. 2019;48(3):20180218.
63. Okada K, Rysavy S, Flores A, Linguraru MG. Noninvasive differential diagnosis of dental periapical lesions in cone-beam CT scans. Med Phys. 2015;42(4):1653–65.
64. Leavitt L, Volovic J, Steinhauer L, Mason T, Eckert G, Dean JA, Dundar MM, Turkkahraman H. Can we predict orthodontic extraction patterns by using machine learning? Orthod Craniofac Res. 2023;26(4):552–9. https://doi.org/10.1111/ocr.12641.
65. Rao GKL, Srinivasa AC, Iskandar YHP, Mokhtar N. Identification and analysis of photometric points on 2D facial images: a machine learning approach in orthodontics. Heal Technol. 2019;9:715–24.
66. Juodzbalys G, Stumbras A, Goyushov S, Duruel O, Tözüm TF. Morphological classification of extraction sockets and clinical decision tree for socket preservation/augmentation after tooth extraction: a systematic review. J Oral Maxillofac Res. 2019;10(3):e3. https://doi.org/10.5037/jomr.2019.10303.
67. Tian S, Dai N, Zhang B, Yuan F, Yu Q, Cheng X. Automatic classification and segmentation of teeth on 3D dental model using hierarchical deep learning networks. IEEE Access. 2019;7:84817–28.
68. Xu X, Liu C, Zheng Y. 3D tooth segmentation and labelling using deep convolutional neural networks. IEEE Trans Vis Comput Graph. 2018;25(7):2336–48.
69. Pei Y, Ai X, Zha H, Xu T, Ma G. 3D exemplar-based random walks for tooth segmentation from cone-beam computed tomography images. Med Phys. 2016;43(9):5040–50.
70. Jung S-K, Kim T-W. New approach for the diagnosis of extractions with neural network machine learning. Am J Orthod Dentofac Orthop. 2016;149(1):127–33.
71. Kwak GH, Kwak E-J, Song JM, Park HR, Jung Y-H, Cho B-H, Hui P, Hwang JJ. Automatic mandibular canal detection using a deep convolutional neural network. Sci Rep. 2020;10(1):5711.
72. Sorkhabi MM, Khajeh MS. Classification of alveolar bone density using 3-D deep convolutional neural network in the cone-beam CT images: a 6-month clinical study. Measurement. 2019;148:106945.
73. Liu C-H, Lin C-J, Hu Y-H, You Z-H. Predicting the failure of dental implants using supervised learning techniques. Appl Sci. 2018;8(5):698.
74. Ha S-R, Park HS, Kim E-H, Kim H-K, Yang J-Y, Heo J, Yeo I-SL. A pilot study using machine learning methods about factors influencing prognosis of dental implants. J Adv Prosthodont. 2018;10(6):395–400.
75. Aljameel SS, Althumairy L, Albassam B, Alsheikh G, Albluwi L, Althukair R, Alhareky M, Alamri A, Alabdan A, Shahin SY. Predictive artificial intelligence model for detecting dental age using panoramic radiograph images. Big Data Cogn Comput. 2023;7(1):8.
76. Shen S, Liu Z, Wang J, Fan L, Ji F, Tao J. Machine learning assisted Cameriere method for dental age estimation. BMC Oral Health. 2021;21(1):1–10.
77. Pihlstrom BL, Michalowicz BS, Johnson NW. Periodontal diseases. Lancet. 2005;366(9499):1809–20.
78. Kumaresan R, Cugati N, Chandrasekaran B, Karthikeyan P. Reliability and validity of five radiographic dental-age estimation methods in a population of Malaysian children. J Investig Clin Dent. 2016;7(1):102–9.
79. Cameriere R, De Angelis D, Ferrante L, Scarpino F, Cingolani M. Age estimation in children by measurement of open apices in teeth: a European formula. Int J Legal Med. 2007;121:449–53.

2 Artificial Intelligence Applications in Oral Health Imaging

Manal Hamdan, Zaid Badr, and Sergio E. Uribe

2.1 Introduction

Artificial intelligence is conventionally defined as a computer system's ability to perform tasks that typically require human intelligence [1]. In the field of oral imaging, this definition mostly pertains to the computer's capacity to analyze, detect, and classify various findings within radiographs. Other areas include image enhancement, charting findings, generating reports, and providing recommendations based on the data. While these tasks may seem straightforward to a seasoned dentist, the complexities become clear when one delves into the details [2].

Consider, for instance, the task of identifying proximal caries on bitewing radiographs. This routine but intricate process involves recognizing tooth numbers, thoroughly examining tooth surfaces, determining the presence and extent of caries, and navigating through diagnostic dilemmas posed by caries mimics, artifacts, and variations between human visual systems. In essence, it is not always a straightforward endeavor [3]. Then, there is the task of communicating the findings so that the clinician can make the best decision for the patient's health.

Furthermore, radiographs are made up of numerous tiny elements—pixels in 2D radiographs and voxels in 3D volumes. These elements exhibit varying shades of gray, corresponding to tissue density. When combined, they form an image representing a specific dental structure. The slightest hiccup during image acquisition, the introduction of artifacts, or processing errors can drastically alter these values and by extension, the resulting images. These artifacts present challenges not only to the human eye but also to AI models trained on "limited" datasets [4].

Consequently, you may wonder if AI can ever exceed the limits of human cognitive abilities when even highly skilled human diagnosticians struggle with certain diagnostic dilemmas. In our modest view, AI is not a magical fix! Dentists and radiologists remain the experts in interpreting AI-generated results, using their clinical acumen and judgment [5, 6]. However, AI offers transformational potential, promising significant improvements in diagnostic accuracy and efficiency. The fusion of human expertise with AI's

M. Hamdan (✉)
Department of Surgical and Diagnostic Sciences, Marquette University School of Dentistry, Milwaukee, WI, USA
e-mail: Manal.hamdan@marquette.edu

Z. Badr
Technological Innovation Center, Department of General Dental Sciences, Marquette University School of Dentistry, Milwaukee, WI, USA

S. E. Uribe
Department of Conservative Dentistry and Oral Health, Riga Stradins University, Latvia/Conservative Dentistry and Periodontology, LMU Klinikum, LMU Munich, Munich, Germany
e-mail: sergio.uribe@rsu.lv

F. Schwendicke et al. (eds.), *Artificial Intelligence for Oral Health Care*,
https://doi.org/10.1007/978-3-031-84047-0_2

computational ability is the cornerstone for redefining the landscape of dental diagnostics and treatment planning.

2.2 Artificial Intelligence, Machine Learning, and Deep Learning

Let's journey back to the inception of artificial intelligence, a defining moment in 1956 at Dartmouth College. Here visionaries like John McCarthy, Marvin Minsky, Nathaniel Rochester, and Claude Shannon laid the groundwork for a groundbreaking summer research project. Their aim? To make machines exhibit human-like intelligence by learning from experience, similar to human "trial and error" [7].

Fast forward to the present, thanks to the availability of vast digital datasets and ever-increasing computational power, AI has surged. The term "big data" became synonymous with AI's growth. AI's practical applications, especially in domains like radiology, have sparked a surge of enthusiasm, evident in the increasing volume of AI-related publications and the numerous AI conferences held [8].

Within AI, there is a distinction between conventional machine learning and deep learning. Machine learning, while effective, demands expertise in crafting "feature extractors" to transform raw data into understandable patterns. This requires careful engineering and domain knowledge [1].

Deep learning is a form of representation learning that allows machines to automatically uncover patterns within raw data. It is distinguished by its multilayered approach, in which nonlinear modules progressively transform raw data into abstract representations. These deep layers are capable of learning complex functions, making them ideal for tasks such as image and speech recognition [9].

What truly sets deep learning apart is that it does not rely on manual engineering to design these layers of features. Instead, it lets data dictate how the layers should be structured. This autonomous feature extraction process is a game changer, allowing machines to interpret new data without human intervention [1]. The advancement of deep learning is expected to make significant advances in various fields, including image recognition, speech recognition, drug molecule activity prediction, particle accelerator data analysis, brain circuit mapping, and natural language processing. Figure 2.1 shows the various types of learning.

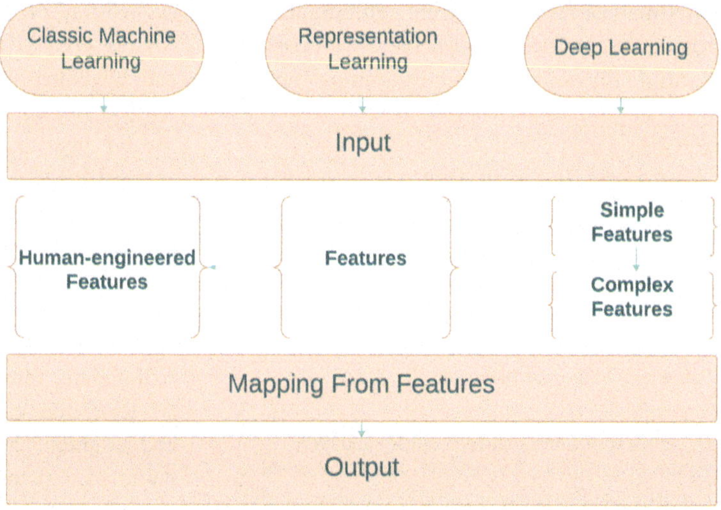

Fig. 2.1 Traditional machine learning relies on intricate feature engineering, which demands human expertise and complex, task-specific optimization. In contrast, deep learning eliminates the need for feature engineering by leveraging extensive data and flexible hierarchical models

2.3 Artificial and Convolutional Neural Networks in Imaging

Artificial neural networks are inspired by biological nervous systems and consist of interconnected nodes. These networks are composed of artificial neurons that encode features using an architecture. Each artificial neuron acts as a simple classifier, producing a decision signal based on a weighted sum of evidence. The network's weights are adjusted through a learning algorithm, which involves presenting pairs of input signals and desired output decisions [9].

In addition to the weighted sum of evidence, an activation function integrates signals from previous neurons, resulting in a decision signal. An artificial neural network comprises numerous basic computing units.

A type of deep learning algorithm, particularly relevant in radiology, known as convolutional neural networks (CNNs), is widely used for its effectiveness in tasks like image segmentation and classification.

In CNNs, lower-level information inputs are analogous to cutaneous sensory nerves and establish synaptic connections with the next layer of neurons. Each neuron in the subsequent layer can combine inputs from lower-level neurons to generate a more complex output. Increasing the number of intermediate or hidden layers enhances the accuracy of the highest layer's output. CNNs excel in capturing spatial features from an image, such as the arrangement of pixels, aiding in precise object identification, localization, and understanding of its relationships with other objects in the image akin to the workings of the human brain [10].

2.4 Prospects and Challenges of AI in Oral Radiology

The potential use of AI in oral radiology is vast, as demonstrated by diverse studies exploring its application for localizing cephalometric landmarks, classifying or segmenting maxillofacial cysts and tumors, identifying periodontitis or periapical disease, and detecting dental caries. Furthermore, AI models have been developed to diagnose maxillary sinusitis, classify stages of lower third molar development and tooth types, and identify root canal orifices, dental plaque, inflamed gingiva, and multiple dental diseases. This illustrates the broadening landscape of AI applications in dental and maxillofacial radiology.

However, concerns regarding the generalizability of these models have arisen due to issues in study subject selection. Some studies lack detailed descriptions of their datasets, leading to potential applicability issues. While most studies present a low risk concerning the selection of the reference standard, there is a considerable risk of bias in the domain of the index test. Nearly half of the included studies did not test their AI models on independent images. This calls into question the robustness, clinical validity, and practical applicability of these AI models [11].

2.5 AI Tasks in Oral Radiology

In the case of oral radiology, an AI system can assist in three areas [12]: quantification, triage, and image enhancement. For quantification, an AI model can perform segmentation functions and measure structures, such as defining the outline of a radiolucent lesion in a radiograph and making the corresponding measurements or marking normal anatomical structures, leaving the clinician to address the remaining unidentified and potentially malignant structures. For triage, an AI system can aid in detection and classification, identifying whether an image contains a lesion and determining the most probable pathologies from a group, marking those images that require verification by a specialist. Notably, there is the potential to increase detection by cross-referencing the information from images with other data, such as genomics or biomarkers, allowing AI systems to detect image patterns that are difficult or impossible for a human to evaluate. Figure 2.2 illustrates the key tasks performed by AI in oral radiology.

Lastly, AI can assist with *image processing* through image enhancement, where an image is automatically preprocessed until it reaches ideal conditions for a specialist to view, or to improve some technically deficient images, thereby reducing the repetition of tests, particularly

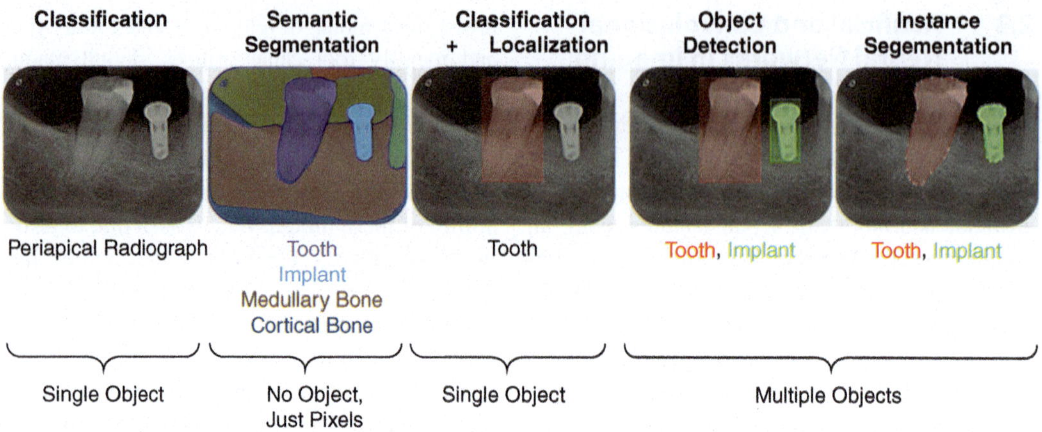

Fig. 2.2 AI detection, classification, and segmentation tasks in oral radiology

Table 2.1 Overview of AI functions in radiology applications

Specific AI function	Associated AI terms	Applications in radiology
Quantification	Segmentation, measurements	AI can define and measure the contour of radiolucent lesions in a radiograph and highlight normal anatomical structures, allowing clinicians to concentrate on unidentified, potentially malignant structures
Triage	Detection, classification	AI can determine whether an image contains a lesion, classify the most probable pathologies, and highlight images that warrant specialist review
Image enhancement	Image processing	AI can preprocess an image to reach optimal viewing conditions for specialists and enhance technically deficient images, thereby reducing the need for test repetitions

those that expose the patient to ionizing radiation. Table 2.1 summarizes these tasks.

A systematic review [13] about using AI to detect and segment anatomical and pathological images in CBCT images showed that AI performs similarly to trained dentists. The DICE/DSC score, which assesses the agreement between AI predictions and actual outcomes, was 0.85. Additionally, precision reflected the AI's success in correctly identifying positive cases, which scored 0.88. Recall, a measure of the AI's ability to capture positive cases, reached a notable 0.93. Finally, accuracy was measured, demonstrating the AI's overall correct identification of cases, achieving a score of 0.83.

While the performance of AI models varied across different algorithms, the review found that AI was consistently successful across various algorithms regarding detection and segmentation tasks. Such tasks included detecting periapical lesions, temporomandibular joint (TMJ) osteoarthritis, and impacted third molars. However, most of these studies did not compare AI performance with human intelligence or an objective gold standard.

The segmentation tasks included identifying pulp, teeth, jaws, and maxillae in cleft patients, the mandibular canal, the sinonasal cavity, and the pharyngeal airway. While the average DICE score for human performance on these tasks ranges between 0.97 and 0.98, AI could match this performance. Notably, AI accomplished these tasks with less manual labor and in a shorter time frame, demonstrating the efficiency of AI in these applications.

2.6 Role of AI Preventing Errors and Supporting the Radiologist

Artificial intelligence (AI) in dental radiology could enhance the precision of radiologists and reduce their error rate [14]. Cognitive biases such

Table 2.2 Common diagnostic errors and AI's role in overcoming them

Diagnostic error	Explanation	How AI can help
Satisfaction of search (SOS) error	This error occurs when a radiologist, after finding an initial abnormality, ceases to search for additional abnormalities, resulting in prematurely ending the case report	AI can help by thoroughly scanning the entire image without getting "satisfied" with the initial findings. It can highlight areas of concern that the radiologist may have missed during their initial scan
Confirmation bias	This is a type of cognitive bias where clinicians may look for evidence that supports their initial hypothesis while ignoring contradictory evidence	AI can provide an unbiased analysis of the data, not influenced by any preconceived hypotheses or ideas, thus mitigating confirmation bias
Anchoring bias	This bias occurs when clinicians rely too heavily on an initial piece of information (the "anchor") when making decisions	AI algorithms, not susceptible to psychological biases, can evaluate all available information independently, thus avoiding anchoring bias
Availability bias	This bias occurs when clinicians diagnose based on their memory of past cases, leading to overdiagnosis of common conditions and underdiagnosis of rarer ones	AI can provide evidence-based diagnostics based on vast amounts of data and not just memory of past cases, reducing the risk of availability bias
Premature closure	This error is common in emergency medicine and occurs when a diagnosis is made before all the relevant data has been considered	AI can help avoid premature closure by comprehensively analyzing all data before forming a diagnosis

as satisfaction of search (missing a second abnormality after finding the first), confirmation bias (interpreting ambiguous information to confirm our beliefs), anchoring bias (relying heavily on the first piece of information), availability bias (relying on immediate examples), and premature closure (settling with a diagnosis before it has been fully verified) could be mitigated through the use of AI.

AI may assist in combating these biases by providing objective analyses and second opinions, thereby ensuring that diagnoses are based on comprehensive data evaluation rather than subjective judgment. Furthermore, it can automate certain repetitive tasks, minimizing the chances of oversight due to cognitive fatigue.

Moreover, AI can potentially address radiologists' significant challenges: visual and decision fatigue. Long hours and constant screen interaction can induce visual fatigue in radiologists, affecting diagnostic precision, especially at the end of the day. AI assistance can mitigate the heightened error rate, which increases with the volume of daily studies and can peak at 13.8% for head/neck imaging exams [15]. AI can mitigate this by automating initial analysis and prioritizing essential images. Similarly, decision fatigue due to constant, prolonged decision making can cause poor judgments and errors, particularly in high-volume or complex tasks. AI can counter this by automating routine decisions and offering support for complex ones, thus reducing cognitive load.

In essence, AI can enhance diagnostic accuracy and efficiency in dental radiology and improve radiologists' work conditions.

Table 2.2 summarizes how AI can effectively mitigate dental and maxillofacial imaging diagnostic errors.

2.7 Navigating the Data Maze: Ground Truthing, Training, Validation, and Testing Data Sets

Ground truthing forms the basis of data reliability. The term "ground truth" pertains to the labels given to datasets used for training a machine learning model. These labels serve the purpose of establishing connections between new inputs and outputs and assessing the model's performance. In oral radiology, many studies admit their limitations regarding acquiring a definitive gold standard for ground truth. As an alternative, the Delphi method has often been employed as a means to establish a silver standard.

A training dataset serves as the data used to "teach" a model. This dataset encompasses input data (features) and the corresponding output values (labels or ground truth). During the training phase, the machine learning model dissects this dataset to acquire an understanding of patterns, relationships, and pertinent features. Through iterative adjustments to its parameters, the model attempts to minimize the discord between its predictions and the actual labels within the training data. The aim of training is to enable the model to extrapolate this knowledge for precise predictions or categorizations on new, previously unseen data. The quality and quantity of the training dataset play a significant role in the model's performance. A diverse and representative training dataset with sufficient data samples is essential for effective model training.

Next, the validation stage involves a thorough assessment of a model's performance, employing a separate dataset referred to as the validation set. Notably, this dataset remains unseen by the model during the training phase. The primary aim of this phase is to determine the model's ability to generalize effectively to new data by evaluating the model's predictions on this labeled dataset. Models frequently require the adjustment of hyperparameters to enhance their effectiveness. The validation dataset serves as a testing ground for exploring various hyperparameter settings and ultimately selecting the optimal ones based on performance. In addition, in the process of evaluating several models, you can effectively identify the model best suited for the specific task by considering their performances on the validation set.

Finally, the testing set is employed to conduct a rigorous assessment with complete separation from the training and validation data. This phase serves as the final step of the evaluation where models undergo exhaustive assessment with data that is entirely new, enabling us to quantitatively measure their precision, reliability, and accuracy for the chosen task [16].

2.8 Applications and Uses

2.8.1 Image Enhancement

When using ionizing radiation, the guiding principle is to keep radiation exposure "as low as reasonably achievable" (ALARA). To align with this principle, extensive efforts have been dedicated to minimizing retakes and decreasing radiation doses [17]. Leveraging AI models for enhancing the image quality of low-dose radiographs, boosting image resolution, and mitigating artifacts stands as a promising approach in achieving this goal.

Hatvani et al. implemented two convolutional neural network models to reconstruct dental cone-beam computed tomography with the aim of enhancing their resolution [18]. These CNN models exhibited notably superior results compared with conventional reconstruction methods. Hu et al. introduced a deep learning-based artifact correction technique tailored for improving the image quality of low-dose dental CBCTs. This innovative approach succeeded in elevating the image quality of low-dose scans to match that of standard-dose images [4].

Liang et al. demonstrated the efficiency of a deep learning tool in reducing metal artifacts in CBCT scans compared with traditional metal artifact reduction techniques [19]. Similarly, Du et al. explored the potential of a CNN-based model designed to mitigate the impact of positioning errors in panoramic radiographs. The model was effective in providing reconstructed images of diagnostically acceptable quality [20].

2.8.2 Teeth Detection and Labeling

Recently, AI-driven tools focused on tooth detection and labeling have emerged. These tools are primarily motivated by the potential to save time and streamline workflows, especially when dealing with large datasets. The accuracy of tooth detection and labeling varies depending on the imaging method used. For instance, Miki et al. examined tooth detection on CBCT volumes using a CNN model and achieved 77.4% sensitivity and 77.1% specificity [21].

On the other hand, Tuzoff et al. investigated tooth detection and labeling using a CNN model for the same task but on 2D radiographs, achieving a higher accuracy with 98.7% sensitivity and 99.5% precision [22]. Zhang et al. explored tooth recognition using the Fast Regions with CNN features (Fast R-CNN) approach [23]. Their method incorporated a label tree and cascade network structure to handle cases involving tooth loss, decayed teeth, and restorations, achieving a precision of 95.8% and recall of 96.1%.

In a separate study, Chen et al. applied Faster Regions with Convolutional Neural Network features (Faster R-CNN) to detect and label teeth in 1250 digitized dental periapical films [24]. Their model achieved detection precisions of 90% and 71.5% in tooth numbering when compared to evaluations by seven human experts. These studies collectively highlight the potential of deep learning technologies as efficient and automated tools to help dentists create their patients' dental charts.

2.8.3 Caries Lesion Detection

Several AI tools have been developed to assist dentists in caries lesion detection in the last couple decades. These tools can improve the accuracy and consistency of diagnoses when compared to conventional methods [3]. Some studies have shown that deep learning models can match expert dentists in identifying caries lesions on oral radiographs, whereas others have indicated that AI can outperform human accuracy by up to 20% [25–28]. When histological sectioning was used as a reference standard, an AI-powered tool detected 97% of dentinal lesions but only 60% of enamel lesions [29]. The primary limitation of AI in detecting enamel caries lesions is understandable, as these lesions are often not radiographically visible until approximately 30–40% of the enamel is affected [30].

On a different note, the combination of AI with other tools for caries lesion detection has shown promising results. A pilot study demonstrated the effectiveness of CNN for detecting caries lesions in near-infrared light transillumination images [31]. Furthermore, innovative approaches such as mobile phone-based diagnostic tools that leverage deep learning have also offered promising results in caries lesion detection [32]. However, it is important to note that while AI can enhance diagnostic precision, it may potentially lead to more aggressive treatment decisions. Therefore, dentists should carefully interpret AI-generated data to ensure well-balanced treatment choices [5].

2.8.4 Periodontal Disease

AI applications in periodontal assessment extend beyond identifying bone loss [33]. AI-powered tools have been specifically designed for various tasks, including detecting compromised periodontal teeth, measuring bone loss, and classifying the stage of periodontitis [34–37]. In the realm of bone loss detection, Kim et al. demonstrated that an AI-powered model outperformed the diagnostic abilities of dentists [36]. When it came to identify periodontally compromised teeth using AI, the results were promising. However, the accuracy of predicting extractions for severely periodontally compromised teeth varied by tooth type, achieving 76.7% accuracy for molars and 82.8% for premolars [34].

While periodontal diagnosis traditionally relies on radiographic and clinical examination, AI-driven tools can provide provisional diagnoses based on radiographic assessment. Chang et al. explored the use of a deep CNN to measure radiographic alveolar bone levels to aid in periodontal diagnosis [35]. The model demonstrated impressive accuracy in measuring alveolar bone levels and delivering provisional diagnoses based on periapical radiographs. It achieved 91% accuracy in detecting Stage 1 radiographic bone loss, 88% for Stage 2, and 99% for Stage 3, compared with assessments by a panel of experts. Notably, the model completed these tasks 15 times faster than the clinicians!

2.8.5 Dental Implantology

The use of AI in the field of dental implants has many applications that can aid in the treatment planning for dental implants and in the detection of implant disease [38–41]. For instance, AI tools can automatically detect the necessary landmarks on a dental radiograph prior to implant placement, such as the location of the mandibular canal, maxillary sinus, and nasal fossa. It can also detect edentulous sites and measure the height and width of available alveolar bone at the anticipated implant site [38]. Additionally, AI models are designed to assist in classifying dental implant systems based on radiographic data, with an impressive accuracy rate ranging from 90% to 97% [42]. This classification is invaluable, particularly when there is a need to repair or replace an existing dental implant system without complete information. Moreover, AI solutions are instrumental in identifying implant issues and diseases, including the detection of implant fractures, measurement of peri-implant bone loss ratios, and classification of bone loss severity [39, 40, 43].

2.8.6 Endodontics

AI has various applications in endodontics [39], including the detection of periapical pathology, assessment of root morphology, identification of vertical root fractures, determination of working length and apical foramen location, and predicting the need for retreatment [44–48].

Multiple studies have investigated AI models for detecting apical lesions in dental radiographs [44, 46, 49, 50]. For instance, one study used a moderately deep CNN, trained on a limited dataset of panoramic images, achieving an AUC of 85%, with a sensitivity of 65% and specificity of 87% [44]. Molars had higher sensitivity but lower specificity. In another study, a deep learning algorithm applied to CBCT images resulted in a lesion detection accuracy of 93% and specificity of 88% [46]. Orhan et al. assessed a CNN on CBCT images with 153 periapical lesions, achieving a sensitivity of 92.8% [49]. Hamdan et al. evaluated the impact of a deep learning tool on dentists' performance in detecting apical radiolucencies on periapical radiographs, confirmed by CBCTs, demonstrating improved accuracy, specificity, and sensitivity, particularly for small radiolucencies and teeth near endodontic treatment [50].

AI has also been applied to assess general root canal morphology, segmentation and classification of C-shaped canals, and detection of teeth with taurodontism [45, 51, 52]. It has been used to evaluate the number of canals, canal curvatures, and root canal morphology from 2D and 3D radiographs. In the segmentation and classification of C-shaped canals on CBCTs, three different AI platforms achieved mean sensitivity ranging from 72% to 78.6% [45, 51]. Duman et al. developed a CNN-based AI model to diagnose teeth with taurodontism on 434 panoramic radiographs, with sensitivity and precision values of 86.5% and 79.0%, respectively [52].

Detection of vertical root fractures using AI has been explored in panoramic radiography and CBCT. A CNN-based deep learning model for detecting vertical root fractures in panoramic radiography achieved promising results, with a recall of 75%, precision of 93%, and an F-measure of 0.83 in detecting 267 of 330 vertical root fractures from 300 panoramic radiographs [53]. In contrast, deep learning models developed to diagnose vertical root fractures in CBCT images demonstrated better performance, with accuracy, sensitivity, specificity, and AUC of 91.4%, 92.1%, 90.7%, and 0.96, respectively [54]. The improved performance of CBCT can be attributed to the availability of more data in 3D imaging modalities.

In addition, AI-assisted models accurately determine the location of the minor apical foramen to measure the working length. Studies by Saghiri et al. using artificial neural networks (ANN) demonstrated remarkable accuracy, correctly identifying the minor apical foramen's location between 93% and 96% of the time, outperforming endodontists with a 76% correct identification rate [47, 55].

2.8.7 Orthodontic Applications

AI advances have been applied in the field of orthodontics for deciding if extractions are necessary prior to the orthodontic treatment as well as determining if a surgical or nonsurgical approach is needed, automatic identification of cephalometric landmarks, classification of skeletal malocclusion, and in determining growth and development by cervical vertebrae stages [51, 52]. ANN can achieve 80–96% accuracy in determining whether extraction or non-extraction treatment are best for cases of malocclusion [56, 57]. Identification of cephalometric landmarks showed promising results, as a few studies concluded that there were no statistically significant differences between human experts' and the AI's predictions in identification of cephalometric landmarks [58, 59].

Shin et al. introduced a deep learning network designed to autonomously classify skeletal malocclusion and predict the need for orthodontic surgery based on cephalograms. The model achieved an impressive accuracy of 95.4% in the classification of skeletal malocclusion and prediction of orthognathic surgery requirements [60]. Similarly, Kim et al. assessed the performance of two AI models in the classification of skeletal malocclusion using CBCT cross-sections. These models delivered similar results, with accuracy ranging from 78.5% to 90.6%, depending on the location of the cross-section [61]. Another notable study by Lin et al. trained and tested a CNN algorithm to evaluate facial symmetry before and after orthognathic surgery based on CBCT scans. The model exhibited a commendable accuracy of 90% [62]. These findings strongly indicate that AI solutions can serve as valuable tools in the diagnosis and planning of orthodontic and orthognathic surgeries.

2.8.8 Third Molars

AI algorithms have progressed beyond basic labeling, with some models capable of assisting in cases of lower third molar impaction by detecting and classifying impaction while accurately predicting extraction difficulty [63–65]. Furthermore, an AI model has been developed and tested to predict the likelihood of paresthesia after extraction, yielding promising results [66]. All of these advancements can provide valuable support to both surgeons and patients in making informed decisions regarding treatment options for third molar impaction.

2.8.9 Oral Pathology and Oral Medicine

Deep learning object detection techniques can detect and classify radiolucent lesions in the jaws on various dental radiographs [67]. A model trained and tested by Lee et al. was able to differentiate Stafne's bone cavity from mandibular radiolucent lesions with an accuracy of 99.3% [68]. Deep learning algorithms have also been created to segment the cervical lymph nodes of oral cancer patients and determine whether they are metastatic or non-metastatic based on contrast-enhanced computed tomography (CT) images. A study conducted by Ariji et al. demonstrated that the performance metrics for diagnosing metastasis in segmented lymph nodes using an AI algorithm were high enough to surpass the capabilities of experienced radiologists [69]. Additionally, AI platforms can be employed for diagnosing and predicting osteoporosis [70, 71], diagnosing Sjögren's syndrome [72], detecting and classifying fractures [73], detection of maxillary sinus lesions [74], identifying sialoliths [75], diagnosing temporomandibular joint disease [76], and detecting condyle fractures [77].

2.8.10 Forensics

The combination of AI and oral radiology holds great potential in forensics. This approach proves to be less invasive and significantly more time-efficient for postmortem identification and age estimation compared with conventional techniques [73]. Automated dental identification systems that rely on CNN for postmortem identification through dental radiography exist [23]. Furthermore, alternative algorithms for age estimation utilizing dental radiology, such as those based on the pulp-to-tooth ratio in canines or specific gender-related facial features, have demonstrated superior accuracy in predicting age compared with manual age estimation methods [78–80].

2.9 Code-Free Computer Vision

The era of AI has brought numerous advantages, but many dentists and researchers lack the coding skills and computational knowledge required to train and implement their computer vision models. However, a recent breakthrough in AI, often referred to as "no-code," "low-code," or "code-free" computer vision, offers a potential solution to this coding knowledge limitation [81–84].

No-code computer vision, exemplified by platforms like LandingLens (Landing AI, Palo Alto, CA, USA), empowers regular users to create, train, and evaluate AI models without the need for extensive software engineering expertise [85]. Here's the typical process:

(a) Users upload a dataset of images onto the online platform.
(b) They select the specific task, whether it is object detection, image segmentation, or classification.
(c) After labeling the dataset, the images are divided into training, validation, and testing subsets. Users can choose to either have the platform automatically split them or manually assign them to specific subsets.
(d) Automated training proceeds, resulting in the creation of an algorithm, which is achieved without traditional coding. Users can also apply data augmentation techniques such as horizontal and vertical flips to enhance the diversity of training samples and set the number of epochs.
(e) The developed algorithm can then be used and deployed, simplifying the process of building computer vision models.

While this approach broadens the accessibility of machine learning for diverse applications, it particularly excels in semantic segmentation tasks. Nevertheless, some of these platforms may come with restrictions concerning cross-validation support and the availability of extensive customization options for models [86]. It's crucial to emphasize that the computer vision platforms developed through this method should not be employed for diagnostic purposes (e.g., as medical devices) without obtaining FDA clearance [5, 6].

Additionally, even though the allure of easily implementing technology is evident, there is an obligation to gain a comprehensive understanding of the technology, encompassing both its advantages and potential limitations. Most AI algorithms operate in an "black box" manner, concealing the internal mechanics of their analysis, and there's a risk associated with perpetuating this lack of transparency. The challenge of achieving a profound comprehension in the midst of rapidly evolving AI technology presents a significant ethical dilemma [5].

2.10 Balancing Privacy and Collaboration: Data Sharing and Federated Learning

Oral and Maxillofacial Radiology primarily focuses on the generation and interpretation of diagnostic images for the purpose of diagnosing and managing conditions and diseases that affect the craniofacial complex. A variety of imaging techniques are employed in maxillofacial imaging, including bitewings, periapicals, panoramic radiographs, dental tomosynthesis, cone beam computed tomography (CBCT), magnetic resonance imaging (MRI), nuclear imaging, and ultrasonography [8].

While these imaging modalities offer various diagnostic capabilities, not all of them are commonly encountered in the daily practices of oral radiologists and dentists. For instance, modalities like nuclear imaging are less frequently used in the field of oral radiology [2]. Furthermore, the accessibility and proficiency in ultrasonography can vary among oral radiologists. The most commonly used and encountered imaging modalities for both dentists and radiologists include bitewings, periapicals, panoramic radiographs, and CBCT scans. Consequently, a significant portion of research in this field has been dedicated to harnessing the potential of these imaging techniques for detecting oral and maxillofacial conditions [2].

The process of assembling an imaging dataset is a crucial step in the development of artificial intelligence systems for radiology. These datasets serve various purposes, including training and evaluating algorithms. Large datasets containing thousands of images are often used to train convolutional neural networks for image recognition. However, smaller datasets also have value, particularly in tasks such as texture analysis. Access to comprehensive and diverse datasets has the potential to enhance the effectiveness of predictive models across different data types [8].

Nevertheless, obtaining such data presents challenges due to the considerable investments in time, effort, and financial resources required for their collection and protection. In oral radiology, which frequently involves complex tasks like segmentation and detection, the labor-intensive process of establishing accurate ground truth data limits dataset expansion. Additionally, this is compounded by universal regulations and privacy barriers, which hinder the smooth exchange of raw data [87].

One potential solution to address the challenges of data sharing is federated learning. Federated learning allows multiple participants to collaboratively train AI models, expanding access to knowledge from a more diverse set of data sources without the need for direct data sharing. In this approach, knowledge is shared in the form of trained AI models or their outputs. This innovative technique enables the generalization of AI models while preserving the privacy of the underlying training data, which is particularly critical in the context of sensitive medical data analysis tasks. Typically, a central server, often a trusted service provider, oversees the entire federated learning process based on predefined protocols [8].

2.11 Assessing Commercially Available AI Solutions for Oral Health Imaging: A Roadmap

The swift progress of AI has significantly impacted various sectors, including medical imaging. Radiologists and dentists are increasingly open to AI techniques to handle growing workloads and improve patient outcomes. In the quest to aid radiologists and physicians in evaluating commercial AI solutions for medical imaging, a set of guidelines known as the ECLAIR guidelines has been created [88]. These guidelines (Table 2.3) are designed to simplify the selection process for the most appropriate AI solution, offering a comprehensive checklist of essential considerations.

These guidelines may act as a roadmap for navigating commercial AI solutions in the field of imaging. By adhering to these guidelines, you can ensure that the AI technology you are interested in is in harmony with your clinical prerequisites and regulatory standards.

Table 2.3 ECLAIR guidelines—a checklist to assist radiologists and physicians in selecting AI solutions that meet clinical and regulatory requirements

Relevance	Before adopting an AI solution, it's crucial to define the specific problem it aims to solve, the intended users, and its principles of operation. These considerations include the medical conditions to be addressed, the target end-users, the intended use (research or clinical), and the application's potential benefits
Benefits and risks	Assess the benefits and potential risks associated with the AI system. Benefits can be categorized for patients, radiologists, institutions, and society. Risks, such as misdiagnosis, legal exposure, and workflow disruption, should be thoroughly evaluated
Performance and validation	Evaluate the AI algorithm's design specifications, data used for training and validation, labeling methods, and performance metrics. This includes assessing the algorithm's robustness to technical variations in medical images

(continued)

Table 2.3 (continued)

Bias detection	Determine if the AI system has been evaluated for bias and inquire about the steps taken to mitigate potential biases, which are especially crucial in healthcare
Adaptability	Understand whether the AI system is capable of continuous adaptation to new data and improvements over time. This adaptability might be important as AI technology evolves
Usability and integration	Examine how the AI application can be integrated into the clinical workflow, considering factors like manual interaction, processing speed, and impact on the workflow, including potential reallocation of resources
IT infrastructure	Assess the requirements for information technology infrastructure, considering hardware and network specifications, particularly for on-premises deployment
Interoperability	Determine how data can be exported for research purposes and check if the AI system complies with interoperability standards such as DICOM (Digital Imaging and Communications in Medicine)
Accessibility	Explore whether the AI system makes data accessible to non-radiologists, such as referring physicians and patients
Interpretability	Examine the interpretability of the AI model's results and whether it can explain its reasoning to physicians
Regulatory and legal compliance	Ensure that the AI application complies with local medical device regulations, including CE marking in Europe and FDA clearance in the United States. Additionally, verify compliance with data protection regulations, such as GDPR or HIPAA
Financial and support services	Consider the licensing model, cost structure, training, maintenance, and support services associated with the AI solution
Handling malfunctions	Develop a clear understanding of how malfunctions and errors will be addressed, including repair procedures, reaction times, and adverse event reporting

2.12 Ethical Challenges in Integrating AI

As we've explored thus far, AI has shown remarkable potential in disease detection, clinical diagnosis, workflow improvement, and image enhancement. However, its integration into oral imaging presents a set of ethical dilemmas. Transparency emerges as a crucial element, emphasizing the need for comprehensive documentation of AI models. This documentation must transparently outline the criteria for data inclusion and exclusion of data and allow for reproducibility. Furthermore, there is a paramount need to ensure diversity in datasets, preventing biases related to ethnicity, age, gender, or health conditions. This approach ensures inclusivity, thereby promoting fairness within the healthcare system [6].

It's also essential to underscore that AI should not supersede the autonomy of patients but rather empower them to actively engage in the decision-making process.

The protection of privacy is a critical concern that demands strict adherence to data protection regulations. In terms of accountability, a shared responsibility model prevails, with both clinicians and patients jointly navigating the realm of AI-driven decisions. The principle of equity seeks to address disparities and actively prevent the exacerbation of existing inequalities. Additionally, fostering digital literacy among clinicians is essential to enable them to effectively interpret AI outcomes [5].

Promoting solidarity and mutual support among healthcare stakeholders is also imperative. AI's development and implementation should diligently adhere to existing regulations and oversight, ensuring an ethical and responsible path forward in dentistry.

2.13 Practical Aspects of Using AI in Oral Radiology

In today's healthcare landscape, radiologists play a pivotal role in patient care, serving as a key link between different medical specialties and the patients themselves. Their day-to-day responsibilities cover a wide range of activities, from administrative tasks to in-depth consultations with other specialists. Radiologists play a crucial role in guiding the selection and sequencing of diagnostic imaging procedures, ensuring that each test contributes effectively to a comprehensive diagnosis. Beyond these interactions, they are also heavily involved in the analysis of imaging results, interpreting studies thoroughly and producing detailed reports that are essential for clinicians and patients to make informed healthcare decisions. The integration of artificial intelligence (AI) into radiology has the potential to significantly enhance some of these radiologist tasks. AI's capabilities, particularly in image management and interpretation, offer promising ways to improve the radiologist workflow. In addition, AI's advanced analytical tools can assist radiologists in the triage process and enhance their ability to detect abnormalities, as discussed in this chapter. This synergy of AI and radiologist expertise is unlocking a transformative era of diagnostic precision and patient-centered care.

This gradual integration of AI into radiology must be approached with careful consideration of practical aspects, particularly in the development, purchase, implementation, and monitoring of AI tools [89].

Development The focus should be on clinical utility and improving existing workflows, with clinician insights incorporated early in the design process. When developing AI for dental radiology, the focus is not only on developing hardware and software but also on data quality and relevance. Radiologists must be actively involved in the testing and evaluating AI models to ensure that the datasets used for training accurately represent the patient population. This process helps identify patient demographics where AI can improve diagnosis and highlights scenarios, where AI may be ineffective or harmful. This collaborative approach ensures that AI tools are fine-tuned for accuracy and safety in clinical settings.

Purchasing Evaluate AI tools based on their integration into clinical workflows, user training requirements, performance on local data, and potential psychological impact on users. When purchasing AI tools for dental radiology, it's important to consider both radiologist and patient outcomes. This includes assessing ROI and time savings for radiologists, as well as patient-centered benefits such as reduced need for repeat examinations, more efficient use of resources, and overall improved patient outcomes. Such a balanced approach ensures that the AI tool truly improves the quality and efficiency of dental care.

Implementation Ensure seamless integration with existing IT infrastructure and workflows, and address user training for effective use and bias mitigation. This includes not only technical compatibility but also training users—dentists, hygienists, and technicians—in effective use and understanding potential biases in AI analysis. For example, incorporating AI into systems used to diagnose periodontal disease requires not only technical setup but also training the dental team to interpret AI-generated insights and understand their limitations in different patient scenarios.

Monitoring Continuously monitor AI tools for long-term stability and safety, adapting to changes in patient demographics, equipment, and protocols. Regularly reassess the tool's performance and ensure readiness for any necessary updates or adjustments. This includes adapting to changes in patient demographics, updating equipment compatibility, and adapting to new protocols. Regular performance assessments are essential to identify and address any problems early on. For example, an AI tool used to detect oral pathology needs to be routinely assessed for accuracy and relevance, especially as new imaging technologies emerge and patient profiles evolve. This ongoing process ensures that the AI tool remains a reliable asset in the dynamic field of dental radiology.

Each step involves a balance of technical, ethical, and practical considerations to ensure that AI tools are effective, safe, and beneficial in radiology practice. In 2016, a pioneer in deep learning predicted that radiologists would be obsolete within 5 years because machines could handle all their tasks [90]. This prediction underestimated the multifaceted nature of clinical tasks, where image assessment is just one component of a diagnostic process that includes reviewing patient history, consulting with colleagues, and more. In reality, AI aids but is unlikely to replace human judgment in decision-making entirely. For example, in airports, machines still require human confirmation to detect dangerous objects in luggage. Diagnosing a tumor in a CBCT volume is exponentially more complex. AI serves as an augmentative tool, fine-tuning a clinician's sensitivity and specificity, almost like corrective lenses. It can also act as a second set of eyes, reducing error rates, and even improve diagnostic capabilities by discerning image patterns undetectable to the human eye. Therefore, while AI has transformative potential, it is more an enabler and enhancer rather than a replacement for skilled clinical judgment.

2.14 Key Takeaways

Artificial intelligence is reshaping the landscape of oral health imaging, offering solutions to challenges in dental diagnostics. A key aspect to ensure its effectiveness is the need for high-quality datasets with well-structured ground truth information, serving as the backbone for AI model training. AI's versatility is evident as it finds applications across various domains within oral health imaging, from detecting teeth and caries lesions to evaluating periodontal health and assisting in endodontics. Remarkably, AI is reported to surpass human diagnosticians in tasks like identifying root fractures. The advent of "no-code" computer vision platforms democratizes AI, making its power accessible to nonexperts. Ethical considerations, particularly concerning privacy and data sharing, are central to responsible AI implementation. Practical frameworks for assessing AI solutions in dentistry provide valuable guidance. In conclusion, AI, when guided by evidence-based research, ethical principles, and proper implementation, is transforming the field of oral health imaging. The involvement of radiologists in the development and evaluation of these AI tools is critical, given their multiple roles in patient care. Their expertise in understanding patient demographics and specific diagnostic scenarios will ensure that AI models are not only technically proficient but also clinically relevant and safe for patient use. Importantly, AI has the potential to assist in some of these roles, particularly in image interpretation and workflow optimization. This collaborative approach between technology and medical expertise is key to realizing the full potential of AI in oral health imaging.

References

1. Mupparapu M, Wu C-W, Chen Y-C. Artificial intelligence, machine learning, neural networks, and deep learning: futuristic concepts for new dental diagnosis. Quintessence Int. 2018;49:687–8.
2. Rieke N, et al. The future of digital health with federated learning. NPJ Digit Med. 2020;3:119.
3. Mohammad-Rahimi H, et al. Deep learning for caries detection: a systematic review. J Dent. 2022;122:104115.
4. Hu Z, et al. Artifact correction in low-dose dental CT imaging using wasserstein generative adversarial networks. Med Phys. 2019;46:1686–96.
5. Rokhshad R, Ducret M, Chaurasia A, Karteva T, Radenkovic M, Roganovic J, Hamdan M, Mohammad-Rahimi H, Krois J, Lahoud P, Schwendicke F. Ethical considerations on artificial intelligence in dentistry: a framework and checklist. J Dent. 2023;135:104593. https://doi.org/10.1016/j.jdent.2023.104593.
6. Currie G, Hawk KE, Rohren EM. Ethical principles for the application of artificial intelligence (AI) in nuclear medicine. Eur J Nucl Med Mol Imaging. 2020;47(4):748–52. https://doi.org/10.1007/s00259-020-04678-1.
7. McCarthy J, Minsky ML, Rochester N, Shannon CE. A proposal for the Dartmouth summer research project on artificial intelligence, August 31, 1955. AI Mag. 2006;27:12.
8. Rischke R, et al. Federated learning in dentistry: chances and challenges. J Dent Res. 2022;101:1269–73.
9. Chartrand G, et al. Deep learning: a primer for radiologists. Radiographics. 2017;37:2113–31.
10. Pai A. CNN vs. RNN vs. ANN—analyzing 3 types of neural networks in deep learning. Analytics Vidhya, Feb 17, 2020.

11. Hung K, Montalvao C, Tanaka R, Kawai T, Bornstein MM. The use and performance of artificial intelligence applications in dental and maxillofacial radiology: a systematic review. Dentomaxillofac Radiol. 2019;49:20190107D.
12. Rajpurkar P, Lungren MP. The current and future state of AI interpretation of medical images. N Engl J Med. 2023;388:1981–90.
13. Badr FF, Jadu FM. Performance of artificial intelligence using oral and maxillofacial CBCT images: a systematic review and meta-analysis. Niger J Clin Pract. 2022;25:1918–27.
14. Lee CS, Nagy PG, Weaver SJ, Newman-Toker DE. Cognitive and system factors contributing to diagnostic errors in radiology. AJR Am J Roentgenol. 2013;201:611–7.
15. Ivanovic V, Paydar A, Chang Y-M, Broadhead K, Smullen D, Klein A, Hacein-Bey L. Impact of shift volume on neuroradiology diagnostic errors at a large tertiary academic center. Acad Radiol. 2023;30:1584–8.
16. Lebovitz S, Levina N, Lifshitz-Assaf H. Is AI ground truth really true? The dangers of training and evaluating AI tools based on experts' know-what. MIS Q. 2021;45(3):1501–26. https://doi.org/10.25300/MISQ/2021/16564.
17. Carter L, et al. American Academy of Oral and maxillofacial radiology executive opinion statement on performing and interpreting diagnostic cone beam computed tomography. Oral Surg Oral Med Oral Pathol Oral Radiol Endod. 2008;106:561–2.
18. Hatvani J, et al. Deep learning-based super-resolution applied to dental computed tomography. IEEE Trans Radiat Plasma Med Sci. 2018;3:120–8.
19. Liang K, et al. Metal artifact reduction for practical dental computed tomography by improving interpolation-based reconstruction with deep learning. Med Phys. 2019;46:e823–34.
20. Du X, Chen Y, Zhao J, Xi Y. A convolutional neural network based auto-positioning method for dental arch in rotational panoramic radiography. In: 2018 40th annual international conference of the IEEE engineering in medicine and biology society (EMBC); 2018. p. 2615–8.
21. Miki Y, et al. Tooth labeling in cone-beam CT using deep convolutional neural network for forensic identification. In: Medical imaging 2017: computer-aided diagnosis, vol. 10134; 2017. p. 874–9. https://doi.org/10.1117/12.2254332.
22. Tuzoff DV, et al. Tooth detection and numbering in panoramic radiographs using convolutional neural networks. Dentomaxillofac Radiol. 2019;48:20180051.
23. Zhang K, Wu J, Chen H, Lyu P. An effective teeth recognition method using label tree with cascade network structure. Comput Med Imaging Graph. 2018;68:61–70.
24. Chen H, et al. A deep learning approach to automatic teeth detection and numbering based on object detection in dental periapical films. Sci Rep. 2019;9:3840.
25. Wenzel A, Hintze H, Kold LM, Kold S. Accuracy of computer-automated caries detection in digital radiographs compared with human observers. Eur J Oral Sci. 2002;110:199–203.
26. Araki K, Matsuda Y, Seki K, Okano T. Effect of computer assistance on observer performance of approximal caries diagnosis using intraoral digital radiography. Clin Oral Investig. 2010;14:319–25.
27. Gakenheimer DC. The efficacy of a computerized caries detector in intraoral digital radiography. J Am Dent Assoc. 2002;133:883–90.
28. Tracy KD, et al. Utility and effectiveness of computer-aided diagnosis of dental caries. Gen Dent. 2011;59:136–44.
29. Valizadeh S, Goodini M, Ehsani S, Mohseni H, Azimi F, Bakhshandeh H. Designing of a computer software for detection of approximal caries in posterior teeth. Iran J Radiol. 2015;12(4):e16242. https://doi.org/10.5812/iranjradiol.12(2)2015.16242.
30. Krick R, et al. Piecemeal microautophagy of the nucleus: genetic and morphological traits. Autophagy. 2009;5:270–2.
31. Schwendicke F, Elhennawy K, Paris S, Friebertshäuser P, Krois J. Deep learning for caries lesion detection in near-infrared light transillumination images: a pilot study. J Dent. 2020;92:103260.
32. Thanh MTG, et al. Deep learning application in dental caries detection using intraoral photos taken by smartphones. Appl Sci. 2022;12:5504.
33. Krois J, et al. Deep learning for the radiographic detection of periodontal bone loss. Sci Rep. 2019;9:8495.
34. Lee J-H, Kim D, Jeong S-N, Choi S-H. Diagnosis and prediction of periodontally compromised teeth using a deep learning-based convolutional neural network algorithm. J Periodontal Implant Sci. 2018;48:114–23.
35. Chang H-J, et al. Deep learning hybrid method to automatically diagnose periodontal bone loss and stage periodontitis. Sci Rep. 2020;10:7531.
36. Kim J, Lee H-S, Song I-S, Jung K-H. DeNTNet: deep neural transfer network for the detection of periodontal bone loss using panoramic dental radiographs. Sci Rep. 2019;9:17615.
37. Revilla-León M, Gómez-Polo M, Barmak AB, Inam W, Kan JYK, Kois JC, Akal O. Artificial intelligence models for diagnosing gingivitis and periodontal disease: a systematic review. J Prosthet Dent. 2023;130(6):816–24. https://doi.org/10.1016/j.prosdent.2022.01.026.
38. Kurt Bayrakdar S, et al. A deep learning approach for dental implant planning in cone-beam computed tomography images. BMC Med Imaging. 2021;21:86.
39. Cha J-Y, Yoon H-I, Yeo I-S, Huh K-H, Han J-S. Peri-implant bone loss measurement using a region-based convolutional neural network on dental periapical radiographs. J Clin Med. 2021;10:1009.
40. Liu M, Wang S, Chen H, Liu Y. A pilot study of a deep learning approach to detect marginal bone loss around implants. BMC Oral Health. 2022;22:11.

41. Revilla-León M, Gómez-Polo M, Vyas S, Barmak BA, Galluci GO, Att W, Krishnamurthy VR. Artificial intelligence applications in implant dentistry: a systematic review. J Prosthet Dent. 2023;129(2):293–300. https://doi.org/10.1016/j.prosdent.2021.05.008.
42. Kim J-E, et al. Transfer learning via deep neural networks for implant fixture system classification using periapical radiographs. J Clin Med. 2020;9:1117.
43. Lee D-W, Kim S-Y, Jeong S-N, Lee J-H. Artificial intelligence in fractured dental implant detection and classification: evaluation using dataset from two dental hospitals. Diagnostics. 2021;11:233.
44. Ekert T, et al. Deep learning for the radiographic detection of apical lesions. J Endod. 2019;45:917–22.
45. Sherwood AA, et al. A deep learning approach to segment and classify C-shaped canal morphologies in mandibular second molars using cone-beam computed tomography. J Endod. 2021;47:1907–16.
46. Setzer FC, et al. Artificial intelligence for the computer-aided detection of periapical lesions in cone-beam computed tomographic images. J Endod. 2020;46:987–93.
47. Saghiri MA, et al. A new approach for locating the minor apical foramen using an artificial neural network. Int Endod J. 2012;45:257–65.
48. Campo L, et al. Retreatment predictions in odontology by means of CBR systems. Comput Intell Neurosci. 2016;2016:39.
49. Orhan K, Bayrakdar IS, Ezhov M, Kravtsov A, Özyürek T. Evaluation of artificial intelligence for detecting periapical pathosis on cone-beam computed tomography scans. Int Endod J. 2020;53:680–9.
50. Hamdan MH, et al. The effect of a deep-learning tool on dentists' performances in detecting apical radiolucencies on periapical radiographs. Dentomaxillofac Radiol. 2022;51:20220122.
51. Yang S, et al. Development and validation of a visually explainable deep learning model for classification of C-shaped canals of the mandibular second molars in periapical and panoramic dental radiographs. J Endod. 2022;48:914–21.
52. Duman S, et al. Detecting the presence of taurodont teeth on panoramic radiographs using a deep learning-based convolutional neural network algorithm. Oral Radiol. 2023;39:207–14.
53. Fukuda M, et al. Evaluation of an artificial intelligence system for detecting vertical root fracture on panoramic radiography. Oral Radiol. 2020;36:337–43.
54. Hu Z, et al. Diagnosis of in vivo vertical root fracture using deep learning on cone-beam CT images. BMC Oral Health. 2022;22:382.
55. Saghiri MA, Garcia-Godoy F, Gutmann JL, Lotfi M, Asgar K. The reliability of artificial neural network in locating minor apical foramen: a cadaver study. J Endod. 2012;38:1130–4.
56. Xie X, Wang L, Wang A. Artificial neural network modeling for deciding if extractions are necessary prior to orthodontic treatment. Angle Orthod. 2010;80:262–6.
57. Jung S-K, Kim T-W. New approach for the diagnosis of extractions with neural network machine learning. Am J Orthod Dentofacial Orthop. 2016;149:127–33.
58. Park J-H, et al. Automated identification of cephalometric landmarks: part 1—comparisons between the latest deep-learning methods YOLOV3 and SSD. Angle Orthod. 2019;89:903–9.
59. Hwang H-W, et al. Automated identification of cephalometric landmarks: part 2-might it be better than human? Angle Orthod. 2020;90:69–76.
60. Shin W, et al. Deep learning based prediction of necessity for orthognathic surgery of skeletal malocclusion using cephalogram in Korean individuals. BMC Oral Health. 2021;21:1–7.
61. Kim I, et al. Malocclusion classification on 3D cone-beam CT craniofacial images using multi-channel deep learning models. In: 2020 42nd annual international conference of the IEEE engineering in medicine & biology society (EMBC); 2020. p. 1294–8.
62. Lin H-H, et al. On construction of transfer learning for facial symmetry assessment before and after orthognathic surgery. Comput Methods Prog Biomed. 2021;200:105928.
63. Yoo J-H, et al. Deep learning based prediction of extraction difficulty for mandibular third molars. Sci Rep. 2021;11:1954.
64. Choi E, et al. Artificial intelligence in positioning between mandibular third molar and inferior alveolar nerve on panoramic radiography. Sci Rep. 2022;12:2456.
65. Liu MQ, Xu ZN, Mao WY, Li Y, Zhang XH, Bai HL, Ding P, Fu KY. Deep learning-based evaluation of the relationship between mandibular third molar and mandibular canal on CBCT. Clin Oral Investig. 2022;26(1):981–91. https://doi.org/10.1007/s00784-021-04082-5.
66. Kim BS, et al. Deep learning-based prediction of paresthesia after third molar extraction: a preliminary study. Diagnostics. 2021;11:1572.
67. Ariji Y, et al. Automatic detection and classification of radiolucent lesions in the mandible on panoramic radiographs using a deep learning object detection technique. Oral Surg Oral Med Oral Pathol Oral Radiol. 2019;128:424–30.
68. Lee A, et al. Deep learning neural networks to differentiate Stafne's bone cavity from pathological radiolucent lesions of the mandible in heterogeneous panoramic radiography. PLoS One. 2021;16:e0254997.
69. Ariji Y, Kise Y, Fukuda M, Kuwada C, Ariji E. Segmentation of metastatic cervical lymph nodes from CT images of oral cancers using deep-learning technology. Dentomaxillofac Radiol. 2022;51:20210515.
70. Sukegawa S, et al. Identification of osteoporosis using ensemble deep learning model with panoramic radiographs and clinical covariates. Sci Rep. 2022;12:6088.
71. Tassoker M, Öziç MÜ, Yuce F. Comparison of five convolutional neural networks for predicting osteoporosis based on mandibular cortical index on

panoramic radiographs. Dentomaxillofac Radiol. 2022;51:20220108.
72. Kise Y, et al. Preliminary study on the application of deep learning system to diagnosis of Sjögren's syndrome on CT images. Dentomaxillofac Radiol. 2019;48:20190019.
73. Wang X, et al. Detection and classification of mandibular fracture on CT scan using deep convolutional neural network. Clin Oral Investig. 2022;26:4593–601.
74. Jung S-K, Lim H-K, Lee S, Cho Y, Song I-S. Deep active learning for automatic segmentation of maxillary sinus lesions using a convolutional neural network. Diagnostics. 2021;11:688.
75. Ishibashi K, et al. Efficacy of a deep learning model created with the transfer learning method in detecting sialoliths of the submandibular gland on panoramic radiography. Oral Surg Oral Med Oral Pathol Oral Radiol. 2022;133:238–44.
76. Jung W, Lee K-E, Suh B-J, Seok H, Lee D-W. Deep learning for osteoarthritis classification in temporomandibular joint. Oral Dis. 2023;29:1050–9.
77. Nishiyama M, et al. Performance of deep learning models constructed using panoramic radiographs from two hospitals to diagnose fractures of the mandibular condyle. Dentomaxillofac Radiol. 2021;50:20200611.
78. Farhadian M, Salemi F, Saati S, Nafisi N. Dental age estimation using the pulp-to-tooth ratio in canines by neural networks. Imaging Sci Dent. 2019;49:19–26.
79. De Tobel J, Radesh P, Vandermeulen D, Thevissen PW. An automated technique to stage lower third molar development on panoramic radiographs for age estimation: a pilot study. J Forensic Odontostomatol. 2017;35:42.
80. Patil V, et al. Artificial neural network for gender determination using mandibular morphometric parameters: a comparative retrospective study. Cogent Eng. 2020;7:1723783.
81. Rokis K, Kirikova M. Challenges of low-code/no-code software development: a literature review. International conference on business informatics research; 2022. p. 3–17.
82. Korot E, et al. Code-free deep learning for multimodality medical image classification. Nat Mach Intell. 2021;3:288–98.
83. Touma S, Antaki F, Duval R. Development of a code-free machine learning model for the classification of cataract surgery phases. Sci Rep. 2022;12:2398.
84. Pettersen HS, et al. Code-free development and deployment of deep segmentation models for digital pathology. Front Med (Lausanne). 2022;8:816281.
85. Rossi D, Zhang L. Landing AI on networks: an equipment vendor viewpoint on autonomous driving networks. IEEE Trans Netw Serv Manag. 2022;19:3670–84.
86. Santomartino SM, Hafezi-Nejad N, Parekh VS, Yi PH. Performance and usability of code-free deep learning for chest radiograph classification, object detection, and segmentation. Radiol Artif Intell. 2023;5:e220062.
87. Kairouz P, et al. Advances and open problems in federated learning. Found Trends Mach Learn. 2021;14:1–210.
88. Omoumi P, et al. To buy or not to buy—evaluating commercial AI solutions in radiology (the ECLAIR guidelines). Eur Radiol. 2021;31:3786–96.
89. Brady AP, Allen B, Chong J, Kotter E, Kottler N, Mongan J, Oakden-Rayner L, Dos Santos DP, Tang A, Wald C, Slavotinek J. Developing, purchasing, implementing and monitoring AI tools in radiology: practical considerations. A multi-society statement from the ACR, CAR, ESR, RANZCR & RSNA. Can Assoc Radiol J. 2024;75(2):226–44. https://doi.org/10.1177/08465371231222229.
90. Geoff Hinton: on radiology. 2016. https://www.youtube.com/watch?v=2HMPRXstSvQ. Accessed 19 May 2021.

Artificial Intelligence Applications in Oral and Maxillofacial Medicine

3

Sergio E. Uribe

3.1 Introduction

Artificial intelligence (AI) represents a field of computer science that focuses on developing algorithms and systems capable of performing tasks that usually require human intelligence. These tasks include learning from experiences, understanding complex concepts, reasoning through problems, recognizing patterns, interpreting oral and visual information, and making decisions. In dentistry, AI has the potential to enhance diagnostic precision, automate repetitive tasks, and eventually improve patient outcomes. For instance, AI algorithms have been developed to analyze radiographic images for early detection of oral cancer, interpreting patterns the human eye might overlook. In oral pathology, machine learning models can learn from vast amounts of data, enabling classification of dental diseases based on the patterns identified in radiographs or tissue samples. AI applications in dentistry for individual patient care include image analysis, data synthesis, evidence-supported treatment planning, and enhanced patient interaction. AI can also enhance community and public dental health services by expanding access to care and facilitating better information and decision-making. Also, AI in dentistry has the potential to transform the traditional focus of dentistry from a technical-surgical to a biological-medical profession. However, AI's risks and limitations in dentistry include biases in algorithms, limited generalizability of AI applications, data accessibility and interoperability issues, and challenges in implementation and maintenance.

3.1.1 Uses of AI in Dentistry

Artificial intelligence (AI) applied to dentistry offers potential as a complementary tool to enhance detection, diagnosis, therapeutic decision-making, and prognosis. Oral medicine can benefit from AI as it predominantly works with images (radiographic or histological), where AI can assist in pattern detection, including some that may only be identifiable after years of training. This could prove beneficial in areas with few specialists. These specialties also work with structured data, such as laboratory tests, genomic data, or electronic records, which algorithms can read to generate a model that allows cross-referencing this information. In this case, these multimodal AI systems, which feed on different data types (e.g., images, electronic records, genomics), can enhance a clinician's capacity to manage information.

S. E. Uribe (✉)
Department of Conservative Dentistry and Oral Health, Riga Stradins University, Latvia/
Conservative Dentistry and Periodontology, LMU Klinikum, LMU Munich, Munich, Germany
e-mail: sergio.uribe@rsu.lv

F. Schwendicke et al. (eds.), *Artificial Intelligence for Oral Health Care*,
https://doi.org/10.1007/978-3-031-84047-0_3

3.1.1.1 AI in Dental Image Analysis

AI systems can augment image analysis in dentistry through quantification, triage, and image enhancement. They can define and measure structures, identify lesions, classify pathologies, and improve image quality, potentially reducing unnecessary exposure to ionizing radiation [1]. Integrating additional data, such as genomics and biomarkers, can enable these systems to identify patterns unrecognizable by humans. We will explore these applications further in the Oral Radiology chapter.

3.1.1.2 AI Treatment Decision Support System

An AI system can process all available information, including a patient's clinical history, to present treatment options. This system could also integrate with biomedical databases to allow the clinician to visualize all treatment alternatives and the available evidence to assist decision-making. Furthermore, the same system could translate the different choices into patient-accessible language.

3.1.1.3 AI-Enabled Prognostic Integration

Finally, dentistry lacks robust prognostic evidence due to the scarcity of well-designed, long-term prospective studies. AI systems can help mitigate this by aggregating real-time information from federated servers. These federated servers allow the AI model to interact with and learn from the data while ensuring the data never leaves the clinical center. This provides a balance between preserving data privacy and utilizing data for improved healthcare outcomes. This approach enables the incorporation of information from various centers, thereby expanding the diversity of the dataset. This enriched dataset allows the AI model to learn from the outcomes of a wide range of patients, enhancing its prediction and recommendation capabilities. These systems could also integrate personal information from patients contained in wearable devices, such as daily activity, exercise patterns, and diet, to offer a personalized plan with a personalized prognostic estimate.

3.1.1.4 Administrative Tasks and Enhancing Patient Care

While AI's direct clinical applications often receive significant attention, its potential indirect impact on dental care is even more substantial. Healthcare expenses have risen sharply in developed countries in recent years, partly due to increased administrative work from patient care to professional interaction. AI can take care of these administrative tasks, reducing costs and improving dental care coverage. Furthermore, AI systems can directly assist dentists by taking over some of the administrative responsibilities, such as maintaining clinical records and compiling insurance or health system information. Consequently, dentists can allocate more time to their primary role in patient care.

In addition, a specialized language model for dentistry could be developed to provide patients and dentists with natural language answers to their questions. This tool would provide patients with personalized information, providing them with real-time, advice whenever needed.

For dentists, these AI systems could respond to natural language queries by filtering the best available evidence. This capability allows clinicians to have the highest quality evidence at their disposal, assisting them in making well-informed decisions to enhance the quality of patient care. A summary of AI improvement areas in Dentistry is presented in Table 3.1.

3.1.2 Challenges of AI Implementation in Dentistry

To date, most research has shown that good results or precision are demonstrated under controlled conditions and testing using datasets or samples similar to those used for training artificial intelligence systems. There is almost no research showing the clinical utility of these systems applied in real clinical or hospital environ-

Table 3.1 AI applications in dentistry

Application of AI in dentistry	Specific function	Associated AI terms	Applications in dentistry
Clinical			
Image processing	Quantification, segmentation, triage, enhancement	Measurements, detection, classification, segmentation, detection, image processing	AI can identify, categorize, and measure lesions across various dental imagery such as radiographs, histological slides, and intraoral scans. It enhances image quality, minimizes repeat tests, and improves diagnostic accuracy
Decision-making	Clinical decision support	Natural language processing (NLP), decision trees	AI can analyze a patient's full clinical history to suggest treatment alternatives and translate these into comprehensible language, simplifying decision-making by improving patient understanding of their options and the corresponding evidence
Prognosis	Predictive modeling	Data integration, federated learning, wearable technology	AI can aggregate real-time data from diverse health centers and wearable devices, considering treatments, patient traits, outcomes, and lifestyle habits. It utilizes this information to offer personalized prognoses and care plans
Administrative and other			
Administrative efficiency	Automating administrative tasks	Natural language processing, large language models, robotic process automation	Maintaining clinical records, filling and compiling insurance information/electronic health records (EHR), answering patient queries
Patient education	Providing tailored information and advice	Large language models	Answering questions in natural language, providing real-time advice to patients
Evidence synthesis	Generating summaries of dental research findings	Large language models	Supporting dentists in staying updated with the latest evidence, providing evidence-based advice for patient care

ments, with *prospective testing*, that is, data to which neither the model nor the researchers have had access, or with *geographical testing*, that is, from different centers, which possibly use different equipment, annotations, or diagnostic thresholds. Moreover, research has primarily focused on the development and internal testing of AI. However, there is insufficient evidence to determine the extent to which AI applications change diagnostic or treatment decisions or impact patient outcomes and society.

However, new developments in AI may bridge the gap between the promising results seen in research and actual clinical practice. Firstly, the development of generalist AI models allows the incorporation of multimodal data, which are processed by the second major advancement, foundation models. These foundation models, trained on extensive unlabeled datasets, emerge as a promising solution. They include generative AI systems such as OpenAI's ChatGPT and Google's Gemini capable of creating contextually relevant, human-like text responses. These models can enhance numerous aspects of dental practice, including patient communication, professional learning, and information synthesis. For example, they can sift through voluminous dental health records and research studies, delivering synthesized information for patient diagnostics and care.

However, despite their potential, these models also present certain challenges. They may occasionally produce convincing yet unreliable outputs, referred to as "hallucinations," can only consider a finite amount of information at a given time and cannot learn from past interactions.

Therefore, using these models with caution is essential, especially in contexts where high reliability is crucial.

While AI can improve dental healthcare by complementing diagnostics, decision-making, and prognosis, it is equally important to consider the associated risks. These include:

1. *Data Privacy and Security*: AI systems require extensive, sensitive patient data, presenting potential data breaches or unauthorized access risks.
2. *Overreliance and Misdiagnosis*: Clinicians might overly depend on AI for decision-making (automation bias), leading to incorrect diagnoses or treatment plans if the AI system is erroneous.
3. *False Perception of Clinical Efficacy:* Existing studies often focus on technical metrics that may not translate to clinical impact or could even pose risks such as overdiagnosis and overtreatment.
4. *Bias and Fairness*: If AI systems are trained on biased data, they can perpetuate healthcare disparities.
5. *Reduced Human Interaction*: Overreliance on AI may reduce personal connections between patients and providers, impacting patient satisfaction and adherence to treatment.
6. *Lack of Transparency*: AI algorithms, often termed "black boxes," can make it hard for clinicians to understand the reasoning behind the AI's recommendations, impacting trust in the technology.
7. *Post-deployment Monitoring*: Once an AI system is deployed, continuous monitoring is necessary to track its performance and potential drift over time.

3.1.3 Dental AI Research: Technical Vs. Clinical Application

When reading an article on AI within any domain of dentistry, it is key to identify whether the research focuses on *technical* and developmental aspects or *clinical* application. For instance, internal development and testing—the testing undertaken by the same research team using a dataset similar to the one for system training—yield preliminary findings. For instance, an AI model trained to detect apical lesions in radiographs from patients in Germany with good diagnostic pefromance. But when used in a different population may significantly decrease its diagnostic performance [2]. So, when reading AI research, you should be ritical with information about the composition of the dataset (are they similar to my patients?), who annotated the data (do they have similar diagnostic criteria to me?), and how they did it (is it an accepted diagnostic criterion with recognized clinical utility?).

Taking diagnostic studies as an example, an AI system that identifies a larger number of tumors might not hold clinical relevance. Essentially, we categorize tumors into four types: benign tumors that don't necessitate treatment; slow-progressing malignant tumors, where patients often succumb to other causes rather than cancer; malignant tumors, where treatments are either non-existent or the stage renders available treatments ineffective; and malignant tumors detected early, where effective treatments are at our disposal. An optimal cancer detection system should provide us with information that influences our diagnostic or treatment decisions, impacts patient-centered outcome measures, or resonates at a societal level. You will find more information about the diverse queries and metrics detailing the utility of AI in dentistry in the chapter "A Primer on Artificial Intelligence Research in Dentistry."

Also, it's essential to assess the literature by adhering to available reporting guidelines, which allow us to evaluate the validity of the research and its applicability. By validity, we mean whether the study has a defined question, if its design can adequately answer it, and if it provides enough information to replicate the results. Applicability refers to whether the report provides sufficient information to estimate if applying the study's findings will yield similar outcomes in our patients. This usually requires a detailed description of the dataset on which the AI model was trained and the annotation criteria that enabled the model to establish its diagnostic, prognostic, or treatment decision-making criteria. The ITU/WHO group has developed a specific reporting guideline for AI in dentistry [3]. The reference is freely available and discussed in greater detail in the chapter "A Primer on Artificial Intelligence Research in Dentistry."

3.1.4 Differences Between Generative AI and Traditional AI in Dentistry Applications

Recently, a new set of AIs has become available, known as Generative AI. While Traditional AI requires labelled data for training and focuses on a specific task, Generative AI is trained on unlabelled data using a reinforcement learning where a human correct and tune the learning of the algorithm. So GenAI can not only perform one task (identifying a type of radiograph), but also do things for which it has not been specifically trained (creating a poem from the element of the radiograph). Figure 3.1 provides a comparative overview that summarizes the essential definitions, key characteristics, and examples of both AI categories, setting the stage for their application in the dental field.

Traditional or discriminative AI in dentistry: Traditional AI, often seen in traditional AI applications, focuses primarily on analysis and interpretation. In dentistry, this includes analyzing images, electronic health records, and genomic data to diagnose, plan treatments, and predict outcomes. For example, traditional AI systems in oral radiology analyze X-ray images to identify lesions or classify pathologies. Based on pattern recognition and statistical analysis, these systems are adept at interpreting existing data and supporting decision-making. In addition, traditional AI has the potential to design novel dental materials or drug compounds, based on existing data. An example of this is the achievement of using explainable deep learning to discover a new class of antibiotics that target drug-resistant bacteria [4].

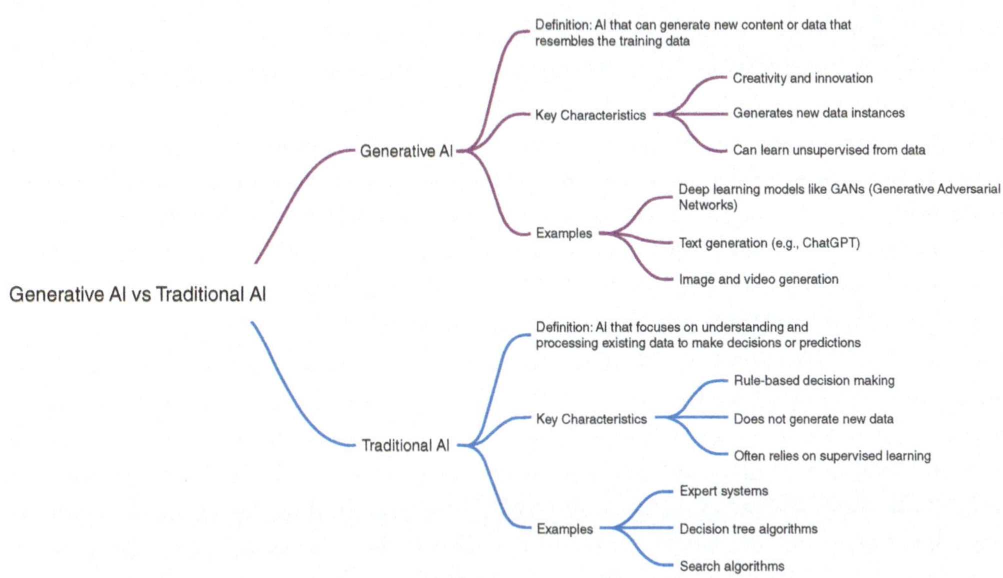

Fig. 3.1 Comparative overview of generative AI and traditional AI in dentistry

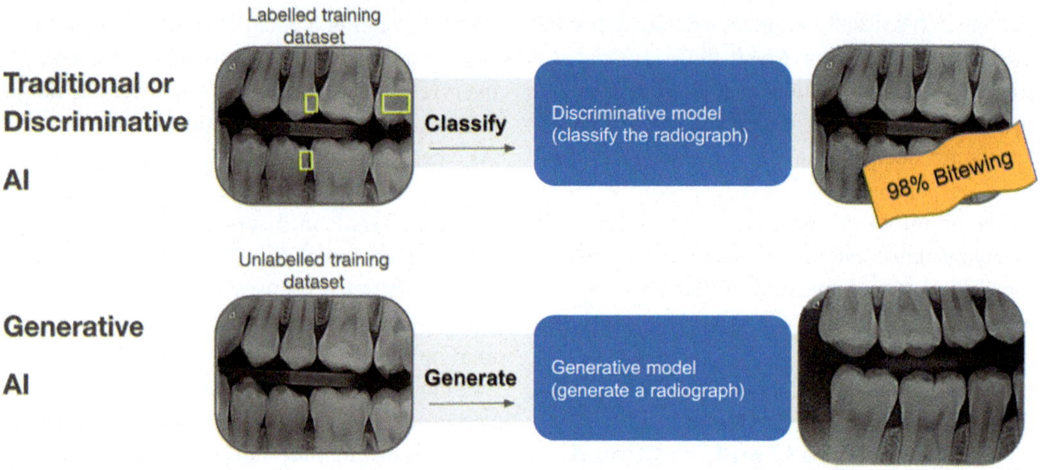

Fig. 3.2 Illustration of generative AI creating synthetic dental radiographs

Generative AI in dentistry: On the other hand, generative AI, a relatively new field, goes a step further by creating new data that is similar, but not identical, to existing data. In dentistry, generative AI could be used to simulate dental conditions or predict the progression of a disease by generating new, hypothetical patient data or images. For example, generative AI can create realistic dental images for educational purposes or simulate different treatment outcomes based on a patient's data. This aspect of AI is particularly useful in training and simulation, as it can generate different scenarios for practitioners to learn from. An illustrative example of generative AI in action is shown in Fig. 3.2, where a generative model is used to create a synthetic dental radiograph.

In summary, while traditional AI in dentistry focuses primarily on analysis, interpretation, and decision support based on existing data, generative AI introduces the ability to create new, synthetic data instances. Understanding and using these two aspects of AI can significantly enhance the practice of dentistry, from diagnosis and treatment planning to educational and research applications.

A summary is provided in Table 3.2.

3.1.5 Summary: Uses of AI in Dentistry

Despite the potential risks and constraints, with ongoing optimization and appropriate regulation, AI systems hold potential to significantly improve the efficiency and precision of dental diagnostics and patient care and enhance patient health outcomes [5]. However, to fully realize these advantages, it is crucial to employ rigorous clinical evaluations [3] and maintain continuous monitoring after deployment. Figure 3.3 presents an illustrative overview of the AI-supported dentistry workflow.

Table 3.2 Comparative overview of traditional and generative AI applications in dentistry

Aspect	Traditional or discriminative AI in dentistry	Generative AI in dentistry
Focus	Analysis and interpretation of existing data	Creation of new data similar to existing data
Dataset annotations	Dataset of labeled or annotated data	Unlabeled data
Training	Supervised	Semi or non-supervised
Learning	Learns the relationship between the features of the data points and the labels	Understand data distribution
Applications	– Analyzing images (e.g., X-rays) for lesion identification	– Simulating dental conditions for training
	– Interpreting electronic health records for treatment planning	– Generating hypothetical patient data for disease progression prediction
	– Utilizing genomic data for outcome prediction	– Creating realistic dental images for educational purposes
Capabilities	– Diagnosis based on pattern recognition	– Generating diverse scenarios for practitioner training
	– Treatment planning using statistical analysis	– Designing novel dental materials and drug compounds
	– Decision support by extracting insights from existing data	– Innovating in research and development through data synthesis
Role in dentistry	– Enhancing accuracy in diagnosis and treatment planning	– Expanding the scope for training, simulation, and innovation
	– Aiding in decision-making processes	– Providing diverse learning materials and predictive models
	– Utilizing data for improved healthcare outcomes	– Facilitating research through creative data generation

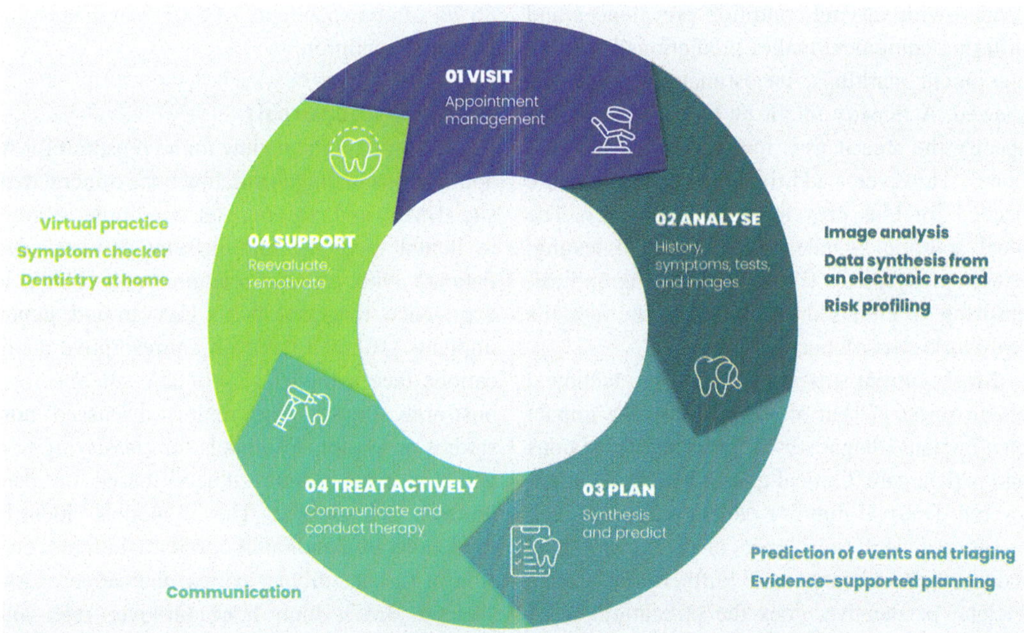

Fig. 3.3 A schematic representation of the integration of artificial intelligence in dentistry. Each stage shows specific tasks AI enhances, such as symptom checking, image analysis, risk profiling, communication, and evidence-supported planning. The figure emphasizes the continuous nature of the process, highlighting how AI can enhance every stage of the patient's experience in modern dentistry. (Modified from FDI White Paper: Artificial Intelligence for Dentistry [6]

3.2 Uses in Oral Radiology, Oral Medicine, and Maxillofacial Surgery

Next, we will explore the applications and available evidence, focusing on systematic reviews synthesizing scientific evidence, to illustrate uses in these areas. We will examine radiology's general role and utility, but please refer to the dedicated Radiology chapter in this book for a more detailed exploration.

While most research under controlled conditions presents promising results, their immediate applicability to individual clinical practice is not guaranteed due to small datasets, lack of prospective or multicenter testing, and incomplete report details, e.g., dataset composition, annotators details, or annotators criteria. Often, internal validation is used, partitioning a single dataset into training and internal testing subsets. This introduces the risk of data leakage, where training data unintentionally biases the model, potentially overestimating its real-world utility. For example, if a model trained on data from two centers with varying condition prevalences and differing equipment makes predictions based on equipment markings, its estimations might be skewed. A remedy might be to have the model specify the area it uses for probability calculations. However, additional precautions are needed for bias prevention and accuracy. The ideal solution is independent external testing, either prospective temporal or geographical, ensuring an unbiased evaluation of the model's real-world performance.

Most current research addresses technical effectiveness [7] but often overlooks the impact on clinicians' diagnostic or therapeutic decisions and patient care. Critical questions remain unanswered: Does AI improve patient outcomes such as survival rates, prevalence, or incidence? Does it decrease healthcare costs? Furthermore, from a societal perspective, does the utilization of AI result in overall healthcare savings? These areas require further exploration to understand AI's broader impacts in healthcare fully.

3.2.1 Artificial Intelligence in Oral Medicine

A systematic review [8] found that AI has been tested for disease diagnosis and prognosis in oral medicine. Multiple studies reported promising results in various areas of application [9].

3.2.1.1 Maxillary Sinusitis

For maxillary sinusitis diagnosis, various CNN models have been successfully applied on different radiographic images, displaying good diagnostic accuracy [8]. When applied to CBCT images, a three-step CNN model achieved an AUC of 91% for mucosal thickening and 84% for mucous retention cyst. Similarly, a DetectNet CNN model used on panoramic radiographs resulted in an accuracy of 90–91% for sinusitis diagnosis and an impressive 97–100% for sinus cysts. Another CNN model used with Water's view radiographs demonstrated high diagnostic accuracy for maxillary sinusitis. Applying the AlexNet model on panoramic radiographs yielded an accuracy of 87.5%, a sensitivity of 86.7%, and a specificity of 88.3% in diagnosing the same condition.

3.2.1.2 Osteoporosis

Another systematic review found potential for AI applications in diagnosing low bone mineral density (BMD) and osteoporosis, conditions relevant in dental medicine and implant dentistry [9]. Patients with osteoporosis are more likely to experience marginal bone loss around dental implants [10], and those on antiresorptive medications face a higher risk of jaw osteonecrosis post-oral surgery. The review discussed nine studies proposing AI models for classifying normal and osteoporotic subjects based on panoramic radiographs. These models identify reductions in mandibular cortical width and erosion of the mandibular cortex, indicative of low skeletal BMD, high bone turnover rate, and increased risk of osteoporotic fractures. The diagnostic performance of these models has improved over time, with recent studies achieving accuracy, sensitivity, and specificity of 95% or above under controlled non-clinical conditions. This progress suggests that these models could soon be useful in clinical practice.

3.2.1.3 Orofacial Pain

A systematic review evaluated the efficacy of machine learning in diagnosing orofacial pain [11]. Upon reviewing 34 articles, it was found that there was a substantial risk of bias and inconsistencies within the studies. Many of these studies were skewed, containing more positive cases than the true prevalence, presumably to simplify the machine learning process. It was observed that patient-reported symptoms and clinical history tended to be less reliable for training effective machine learning models compared to radiographs or histology. It was suggested that a low level of agreement among clinicians training the models might adversely affect the prediction accuracy. Comparisons drawn with the references found that clinicians with less than 3 years of experience, who are not specialized, were at a disadvantage compared to the trained models.

3.2.1.4 Temporomandibular Disorders

Several studies have utilized artificial intelligence to explore temporomandibular joint disorders (TMJ), with promising results. Specifically, machine learning algorithms like K-nearest neighbors (KNN) and random forest, when applied to magnetic resonance imaging (MRI) data, exhibited accuracies of 77% in diagnosing condylar changes and 74% for disc displacement [8]. Further, a convolutional neural network (CNN) model, ResNet, utilized on panoramic radiographs, provided an accuracy of 78% for diagnosing osteoarthritis within TMJ disorders. In another instance, applying a Bayesian Belief Network to MRI images resulted in an accuracy of 99% in determining the progression of TMJ disorders [8].

In a systematic review with meta-analysis exploring the use of AI for detecting temporomandibular joint osteoarthritis through radiographic image data [12], the quality of included studies raised concerns. While half the studies had a high risk of bias in patient selection, index test, flow, and timing, the other half were unclear. Applicability issues were low in most studies for patient selection and reference standards but were unclear or high for the index test in most cases. As for diagnostic accuracy, the sensitivity and specificity of the studies varied, with ranges from 0.54 to 0.94 and 0.50 to 0.91, respectively. The pooled sensitivity for AI models was 0.80, with severe heterogeneity of 89%, while the pooled specificity was 0.90, with moderate heterogeneity of 53%. According to the SROC curve, the AUC was 0.92, indicating good diagnostic accuracy. A meta-regression analysis identified the imaging modality, ethnicity, sex, age, AI techniques, and sample size as potential sources of heterogeneity. Despite the risk of bias and heterogeneity in the studies, AI shows potential in detecting temporomandibular joint osteoarthritis. Also, the review [12] found differences in the efficacy of different AI networks in disease detection. In particular, the convolutional neural network (CNN), outperformed the K-nearest neighbors (KNN) model in terms of accuracy. This difference in performance is likely due to their unique structures and functions, emphasizing the need to choose the appropriate AI model depending on the task at hand.

The findings in another systematic review [13] showed similar results. AI showed encouraging results despite studies displaying a high risk of bias. For studies using panoramic radiography with transfer learning models (ResNet), the pooled sensitivity (the ability to correctly identify positive cases) was 0.76 (95% CI 0.35–0.95), and the specificity (the ability to correctly identify negative cases) was 0.79 (95% CI 0.75–0.83). Studies report a blend of manual and automated methods for identifying the region of interest (ROI). For example, one study commenced with an automated tool, later followed by manual selection for ROI identification [14]. In another distinct approach, CBCT images were segmented to generate 3D surface models, then cropped to delineate the ROI [15]. None of these studies have been independently replicated.

3.2.1.5 Oral Cancer

Diagnosis

Oral cancer presents an opportune domain for the application of AI, given the high accuracy of existing diagnostic methods in imaging [16, 17] and histopathology [18]. AI algorithms can enhance the precision and reliability of these diagnostic tools.

In the first systematic review from 2020, about using AI in the diagnosis of head and neck precancerous and cancerous lesions [19], focused on whole slide images (WSI) of human tissue slides. Out of 315 studies, eleven met the criteria. These studies analyzed different types of oral disorders using AI methods: oral epithelial dysplasia (1 study), oral submucous fibrosis (5 studies), oral squamous cell carcinoma (OSCC) (4 studies), and oropharyngeal squamous cell carcinoma (1 study).

AI techniques included a mix of heuristics, supervised, and unsupervised learning methods, utilizing over ten different classification and segmentation techniques. However, as with many AI research, most studies used datasets from a single source, with images ranging from 40 to 270.

Regarding performance, one study reported 78% sensitivity and 71% specificity in classifying suspicious oral lesions. Another study achieved 88.69% accuracy in differentiating normal tissue from dysplastic or atrophic oral submucous fibrosis. For OSCC detection, one study reported 96.88% accuracy using a texture-based classification method, and another study achieved 100% accuracy in distinguishing normal from cancerous cells. Lastly, one study applied unsupervised machine learning methods for detecting oropharyngeal squamous cell carcinoma, achieving a pixel-level F1 score of 80–81% [19].

Despite these results, it is important to note that the quality of evidence is generally low. Most studies displayed a high risk of bias, which likely inflated the accuracy rates reported. Hence, while AI holds potential in oral pathology, these findings must be interpreted with caution due to the methodological limitations of the existing studies.

Another systematic review highlights AI's capability in differentiating oral cancerous lesions from normal mucosa using oral mucosal imaging [20]. AI-assisted screening showed a high diagnostic sensitivity of 0.92. When distinguishing oral cancerous lesions, the diagnostic odds ratio (DOR) was found to be 121.66 from seven studies, and for all oral precancerous lesions, the DOR was 63.02 from twelve studies. Optical coherence tomography (OCT) showed higher diagnostic accuracy upon subgroup analysis than photographic images and autofluorescence. These findings suggest that AI-based image analysis can serve as a rapid, noninvasive diagnostic tool for oral cancer, offering potential as a clinical tool for early diagnosis.

In addition to imaging, other diagnostic modalities have been explored for OSCC detection. A systematic review [21] of studies conducted between 2005 and 2021, primarily from China and India, shows the potential of AI for diagnosing OSCC across various diagnostic modalities. Ten of the 16 studies were retrospective, evaluating past samples or images, while the remaining six were prospective. The studies utilized diverse tests to diagnose OSCC, including image analysis, fluorescence spectroscopy, Raman spectroscopy, mass spectrometry, telecytology, noninvasive examination scoring, oral microbiota gene testing, and breath analyzers. Convolutional neural networks (CNN), random forest, and support vector machines (SVM) were the most commonly employed regarding AI models. These models were found to enhance the accuracy of detection under controlled conditions. The meta-analysis of available studies indicates a promising performance of AI-assisted systems. The pooled sensitivity, specificity, positive and negative likelihood ratios, and diagnostic odds ratio demonstrated accuracy rates over 90%. Beyond detection, AI has also been tested for OSCC resection, segmentation, metastasis prediction, and treatment selection. However, despite its high accuracy, AI-based tests have yet to fully replace traditional gold-standard techniques in actual medical practice. The review points the need for more prospective studies to validate the efficacy of AI systems in a real-world population, taking into account the observed publication bias toward better diagnostic accuracy in smaller studies. Therefore, while AI holds immense potential in aiding histopathological examination for early diagnosis of OSCC, further rigorous evaluation is necessary before its routine clinical deployment.

Prognosis

Machine learning (ML), a subset of AI, has also been researched for the prognosis and management of OSCC [22]; ML has been tested in evaluating key prognostic indicators, such as recurrence prognosis and lymph node metastasis (LNM), including occult LNM (OLNM). One study revealed an 86% accuracy rate when using dynamic Bayesian networks to evaluate the risk of progression [23]. Additionally, an investigation using clinical, radiological, and genomic data to train multiple models for recurrence risk assessment achieved perfect discrimination in retrospective data. In another series of studies conducted in 2019, ML was used to estimate the risk of locoregional recurrence in early-stage SCC of the tongue with impressive accuracy. Similarly, an ML model significantly reduced the risk of overtreatment while maintaining high accuracy [24]. In the most extensive study, ML was utilized to predict a 5-year overall survival in OSCC patients, with results surpassing those of the traditional TNM staging system [25]. These results shows the potential of ML as a tool for improving OCSCC prognosis prediction and management, and its efficacy is likely to increase as more data becomes available.

3.2.2 AI in Maxillofacial Surgery

3.2.2.1 Third Molar and Associated Anatomical Structures

In a narrative review investigating the use of AI in maxillofacial surgery, numerous applications of this AI in maxillofacial surgery have been highlighted [26]. Here, the role of AI includes identifying and locating anatomical structures, such as the mandibular canal. For instance, using ResNet-152, a machine learning model to identify the mandibular canal in panoramic radiographs, achieved a sensitivity of 84.09%, a specificity of 94.11%, a positive predictive value (PPV) of 92.11%, and an accuracy of 88.86% [27]. In another research, using MobileNet-V2 to assess the relationship between the mandibular canal and the mandibular third molar achieved a weighted accuracy of 0.951, precision of 0.943, sensitivity of 0.941, specificity of 0.800, negative predictive value of 0.865, and an F1-score of 0.938 [28]. Since no code or app is available, these results hardly can be replicated.

Beyond these, AI also ould play a role in predicting paresthesia of the inferior alveolar nerve following third molar extraction using panoramic radiographic images. The prediction accuracies were 78.91% for C1 (depth), 82.03% C2 (ramal relationship), and 90.23% C3 (angulation). These predictions were made using a ResNet-34 neural network pretrained on the ImageNet dataset [29]. The predictive capacity of AI demonstrates its potential for mitigating possible surgical complications.

3.2.2.2 Guided Surgery

A protocol for authentic three-dimensional (3D) planning of dental implants has been proposed [30], using both artificial intelligence (AI) and augmented reality (AR). The protocol involves five main steps, including 3D data acquisition with an intraoral scanner (IOS) and cone-beam computed tomography (CBCT), application of AI for CBCT segmentation to obtain STL models, AR system used for surgical planning, surgical guide design with open-source CAD software, and the surgery itself. This AI and AR technology evolution could replace conventional software for authentic 3D planning in guided implant surgery

3.2.2.3 Cleft Lip and Palate

According to a systematic review, AI has shown considerable promise in complementing the role of surgeons in managing lip and cleft palate [31]. AI in lip and cleft palate management covers five areas: genetic risk assessment, dental and jaw relationship analysis, hypernasality detection, surgery, and diagnosis and prediction. AI investigates genetic variations to predict and diagnose lip and cleft conditions and has shown high accuracy in analyzing dental traits and jaw relationships, for example, achieving 95.6% accuracy in cephalometric analysis. In diagnosis and prediction, an AI model achieved 92.6% accuracy. However, while these models show potential, their broad application needs more validation.

3.2.2.4 Segmentation of Maxillofacial Structures and Lesions

AI has shown promising results in the complex task of segmenting CBCT images. A CNN was developed for automating 3D maxillary alveolar bone segmentation on CBCT images. The study employed 141 CBCT scans to train, validate, and test the CNN model. The technical metrics of automated segmentation indicated a high degree of accuracy, albeit slightly inferior to manual methods. However, the AI-driven approach was considerably faster, 116 times quicker than manual segmentation [32].

Furthermore, there is potential using deep learning for automating mandibular canal segmentation, a crucial step in dental implantology to avoid nerve damage. After enhancing the visibility of mandibular canals with a histogram-based dynamic windowing scheme, a 3D deeply supervised attention UNet architecture localized the volumes of interest, and a Multi-Scale input Residual UNet (MSiR-UNet) architecture performed the segmentation [33].

Beyond structural analysis, AI models have been utilized for lesion segmentation. While automatic segmentation models for radicular cysts, keratocysts, and dentigerous cysts have been developed, initial lesion detection still necessitates manual intervention, indicating that fully automated cyst or tumor detection continues to be challenging [34].

3.2.3 Forensic Dentistry

Finally, a systematic review studied the application of artificial intelligence (AI) in forensic odontology (FO), focusing on identifying individuals through dental remains [35]. The research, collected from 2000 to 2020, used AI for tasks like bite-mark identification, mandibular morphology prediction, gender determination, and age estimation. Models employed primarily used artificial neural networks (ANNs) or convolutional neural networks (CNNs), assessing dental images like panoramic radiographs and digital photographs. Findings suggest that AI can match the accuracy of trained examiners in these tasks, promising victim identification in mass disasters and aiding in medicolegal situations. The potential application areas included:

1. *Bite Mark Analysis:* A study that used artificial neural networks to identify bite marks, aiming to overcome human bias. The resulting accuracy was not high, but the initial findings indicate potential, suggesting a need for further study and model improvement.
2. *Mandibular Morphology:* AI was used to predict mandibular morphology, which is critical for facial reconstruction, particularly in mass disasters. The employed AI model showed high predictability, with results similar to other studies, demonstrating potential in improving facial reconstruction techniques.
3. *Gender Determination:* AI was utilized to identify gender differences in canines, contributing to the identification process in mass disasters and medicolegal cases. Multiple AI methods were compared, with the multilayer perceptron model achieving the highest accuracy rate. Another study applied AI to gender determination using panoramic radiographs, outperforming standard techniques such as discriminant analysis and logistic regression.
4. *Age Estimation:* Multiple studies applied AI to age estimation, a critical process for legal confirmation. The studies used various images, including hand-wrist radiographs and panoramic X-rays of jawbones. Different AI models were utilized, with Deep Learning Convolutional Neural Networks showing superior performance in some scenarios. Furthermore, a model incorporating gender-specific features improved age prediction performance, particularly in young subjects with developing dentitions.

3.2.4 The Lack of Controlled Trials in Dental Medicine

Most studies primarily focus on developing AI models with single-source datasets, typically restricted to internal validation in research settings, rather than clinical real-world environments. Currently, no clinical trials evaluate effectiveness, clinical deployment—including workflow integration—or patient-centered outcomes are available. Future research will identify which patients benefit most from AI-health models, which clinicians (generalists or specialists, experts or novices) can utilize them most effectively, and which clinical settings (rural or urban, large centers or smaller practices) are most appropriate. Thus, current findings should be viewed as proof of concept rather than definitive evidence of clinical utility in dental medicine.

3.3 The Future of AI in Dentistry

Presently, AI's role in dentistry is somewhat restrictive, often limited to specific tasks built on human-annotated data. However, the trend is shifting toward a more holistic utilization of AI: foundation models (FM).

A foundation model is a particular kind of AI model that's pretrained on comprehensive datasets, which allows it to be flexible for a wide range of tasks. A FM rely on an initial training phase that uses large, mostly unlabeled datasets. The model is tuned using Reinforcement Learning from Human Feedback (RLHF), where the model annotates the data under the supervision and correction of a human.

A key architecture underpinning these models is the "transformer," a neural network design that, compared to its predecessors, excels in handling sequential data and maintaining long-term relationships within the data, making it especially adept at tasks like language processing. In healthcare, when these foundation models are customized for electronic medical records (EMRs), they are referred to as Clinical Moundation Models (CFMs). These clinical CFMs may involve two main categories [36]:

1. *Clinical Language Models (CLaMs):* These are a subset of the larger language models but where the focus is on clinical/biomedical text. They are trained on, consume, and output clinical or biomedical text.
2. *Foundation Models for Electronic Medical Records (FEMRs) or Emerging Generalist Medical AI* [37]: These models are trained on a patient's complete medical history timeline. Instead of outputting medical text, they output a machine-readable "representation' of the patient. The models can thus create detailed dental reports that combine clinical findings with patient data and previous examination data, helping in decision-making. Uniquely, these models can recognize diseases or conditions without additional guidance, a feature known as zero-shot learning.

This Zero-shot learning refers to the ability of an AI model to correctly infer or predict instances it has not seen during training. In dentistry, an example might be an AI model identifying a rare oral pathology it was not explicitly trained to recognize. Few-shot learning, meanwhile, trains the AI model on a small number of examples and then expects it to make accurate predictions on unseen data. For instance, an AI model might learn to identify a specific type of oral lesion from a limited dataset and then apply this knowledge to a larger, unseen set of images.

These CFMs are becoming capable of identifying numerous pathological or clinical findings from multimodal (radiographs, scanner data, clinical files, info, lab, and saliva test) dental examinations, providing dentists with detailed insights. They aim to generate comprehensive dental reports by interpreting findings, linking clinical context with patient data, and using previous examination data for decision-making. In Fig. 3.4, you'll see how these multimodal AI systems can integrate into the dental clinical workflow, aiding clinicians and patients in specific queries or comprehensive data analysis.

The development of medical large language models is set to accelerate this progress. For instance, the open-source model, Med-Flamingo [38], or closed as MedPaLM-2 [39]

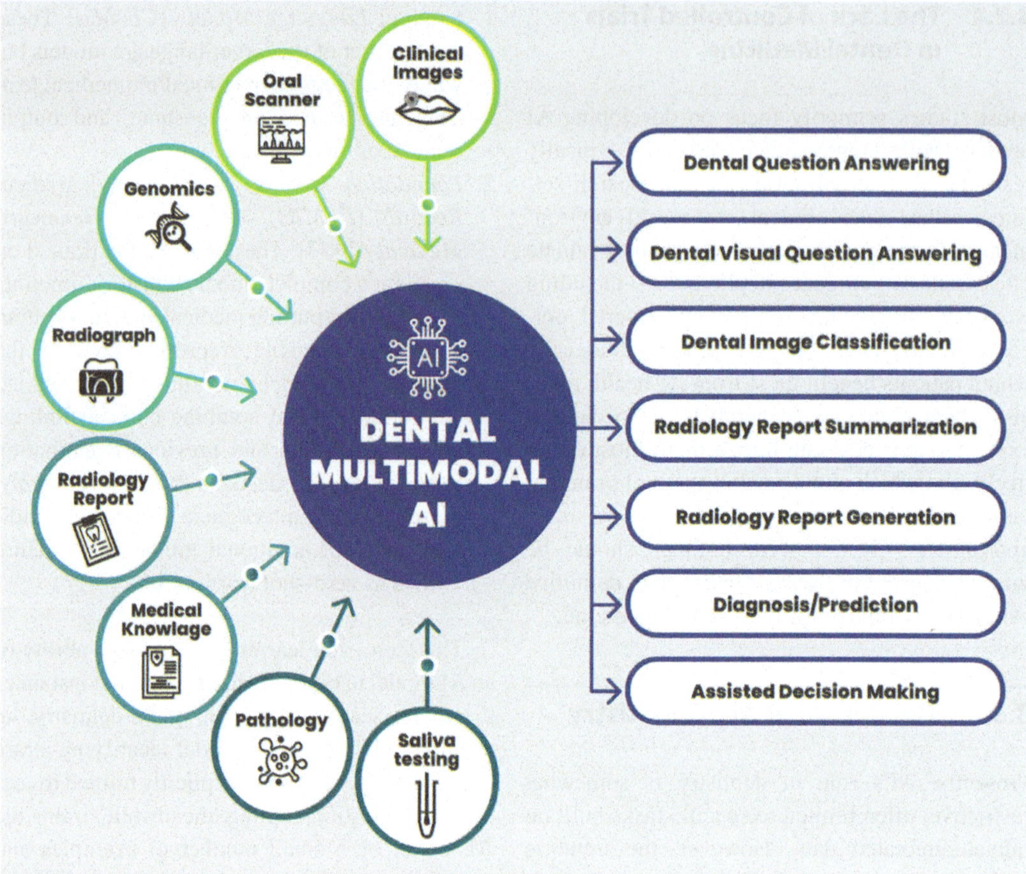

Fig. 3.4 The anatomy of a multimodal AI dental system: integrating patient data and scientific evidence for assisted decision making in dentistry

are multimodal few-shot learners specifically tailored for the medical domain. These models have the potential to be trained not only on clinical data gathered from hospitals but also on clinical images sourced from social media. For instance, the "OpenPath" project, wherein researchers curated a dataset consisting of over 208,000 pathology images, each matched with natural language descriptions collected from Twitter. This extensive dataset was used to train a multimodal artificial intelligence model named Pathology Language and Image Pretraining (PLIP). Remarkably, PLIP outperformed previous image classification benchmarks and made it possible to retrieve cases using images or text [40].

Another example is Google's Articulate Medical Intelligence Explorer (AMIE), an AI system based on a large language model (LLM) and fine-tuned for medical diagnostic reasoning and conversations [41]. AMIE aims to refine the precision of diagnostic conversations, focusing on clear and empathetic communication to improve accuracy in identifying medical conditions. It employs a self-play simulation for role-playing both doctor and patient across various medical scenarios, with automated feedback guiding iterative improvements in performance. Additionally, AMIE utilizes a real-time, chain-reasoning strategy to adjust its logical inferences dynamically during interactions (Fig. 3.5).

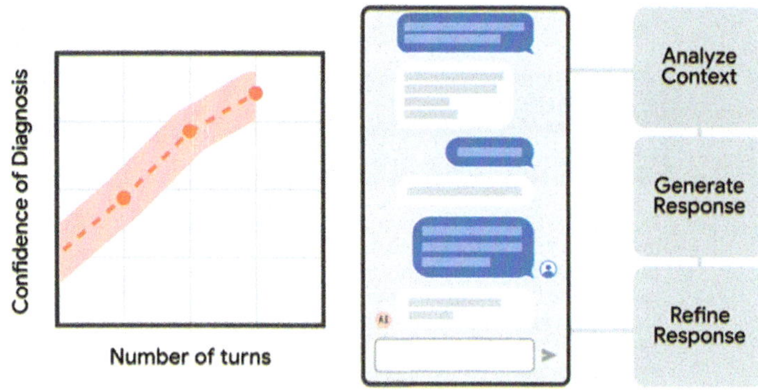

Fig. 3.5 Example of AMIE's optimization for balancing uncertainty reduction, empathy, and clear communication in diagnostic conversations. (Modified with permission from [41])

By linking logical steps based on the progress of the conversation, AMIE dynamically updates its analysis to reflect new information or clarifications provided during the dialogue [42]. This allows AMIE's responses adapt in real-time, considering both relevant information and the patient's specific context for deeper insights [41]. The development of AMIE illustrates the future of AI in medicine with training and reasoning strategies tailored to specific fields such as dentistry. It also highlights the growing potential role of AI in improving healthcare interactions and promises to augment and enhance diagnostic conversations through improved accuracy, empathy, and efficiency. An example of a simulated chat session is shown in Fig. 3.6.

A recent review of foundation models (FMs) in Medicine found that although these models show significant promise in improving patient care and hospital operations, there is a critical gap in understanding these models' true capabilities. The assessment of 84 foundation models trained on non-imaging electronic medical records (EMRs) revealed that most models are trained on small, narrowly focused clinical datasets and are evaluated on tasks that do not provide meaningful insights into their usefulness to health systems. The primary benefits of clinical FMs as identified in this review are [36]:

1. *Improved Predictive Performance*: With deeper insights into patient-oriented outcomes and a focus on safety and fairness, these models not only concentrate on technical metrics like recall (known as sensitivity) or precision (known as positive predictive value).
2. *Reduced Need for Labeled Data*: These models can automatically label datasets, effectively saving time that would otherwise be spent on manual labeling.
3. *Simplified Model Deployment:* Integration into existing clinical electronic datasets is made easier with these models, which can help reduce training costs and measure resource savings when deploying foundation models (FMs).
4. *Emerging Clinical Applications:* FMs can take care of new dental tasks, such as generating patient-friendly summaries of reports.
5. *Multimodality:* FMs enable the use of diverse data sources—including clinical records, lab tests, and imaging results—to provide predictions, like predicting potential oral disorders.
6. *Innovative Human-AI Interaction:* FMs can offer interactive tools to improve user satisfaction and engagement, such as impact metrics related to appointment scheduling, ideally suited to developing structured prompts for dental history.

To incorporate AI into dentistry successfully, it must meet the usual requirements for any new device, intervention or drug: prospective studies and randomized controlled trials, ensuring proper external and independent validation and oriented to the clinician and patient-relevant outcomes. The complexity of AI models results in a "black-box problem," making it difficult to understand their decision-making process and identify potential biases.

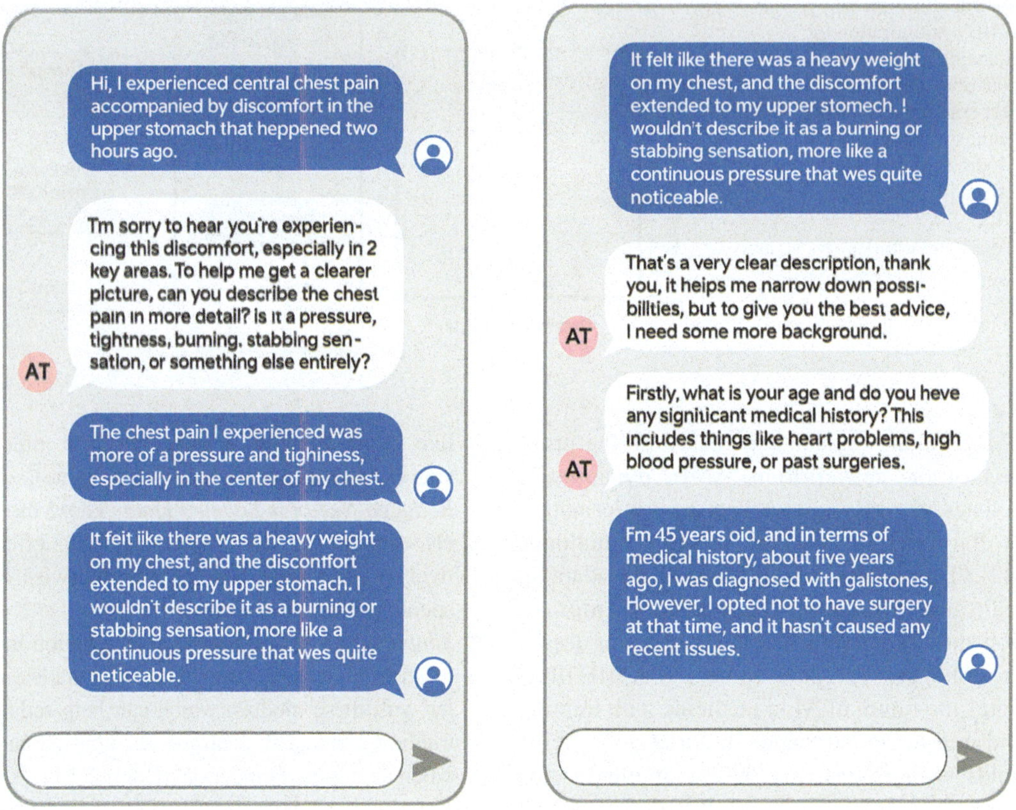

Fig. 3.6 Simulated chat session between a human patient and AMIE, showing how an AI chatbot can dynamically adapt and respond to a patient with empathy. (Modified with permission from [41])

Integrating AI with existing dental electronic health systems is challenging and requires data integrity, interoperability, and security strategies. With the increase of AI applications in dentistry, there is a growing risk of cyberattacks, making robust cybersecurity measures essential to safeguard sensitive patient information.

While AI holds the potential to revolutionize dentistry, its role remains mainly in pattern recognition and task automation. It is not an immediate solution, and issues surrounding data, bias, and security must be tackled for successful AI implementation in Dentistry.

3.4 Conclusion

AI is here to stay. Current research shows potential clinical benefit, but current research is equivalent to 'in vitro' research, tested under very controlled conditions, with retrospective data and without external and independent testing. The future of AI in dentistry, with its potential for adaptive diagnostics and comprehensive treatment planning models, is further enriched by the emerging potential of generative AI. This new branch of AI could impact dental education, patient case simulation, and even the development of new dental materials and pharmacological compounds. Generative AI will greatly enhance the capabilities of Clinical foundation models (CFMs), enabling them not only to manage multimodal data—such as clinical records, laboratory tests, and imaging results—for improved predictions and decision-making but also to create and simulate a wide range of dental scenarios and conditions. This capability opens the door to more advanced training tools, personalized treatment simulations, and research.

To realize the full potential of generative AI in combination with traditional AI models, good evidence, namely controlled clinical trials, remains essential. These clinical research should focus on patient outcomes, as well as comprehensive, unbiased post-implementation assessments using validated benchmarks. While generative AI promises to significantly enhance dental diagnostics, treatment planning, and educational resources, it complements rather than replaces the need for skilled clinical judgement.

References

1. Rajpurkar P, Lungren MP. The current and future state of AI interpretation of medical images. N Engl J Med. 2023;388:1981–90.
2. Krois J, Garcia Cantu A, Chaurasia A, Patil R, Chaudhari PK, Gaudin R, Gehrung S, Schwendicke F. Generalizability of deep learning models for dental image analysis. Sci Rep. 2021;11:6102.
3. Schwendicke F, Singh T, Lee J-H, Gaudin R, Chaurasia A, Wiegand T, Uribe S, Krois J, IADR e-oral health network and the ITU WHO focus group AI for Health. Artificial intelligence in dental research: checklist for authors, reviewers, readers. J Dent. 2021;107:103610.
4. Wong F, Zheng EJ, Valeri JA, et al. Discovery of a structural class of antibiotics with explainable deep learning. Nature. 2024;626:177–85.
5. Ahuja AS. The impact of artificial intelligence in medicine on the future role of the physician. PeerJ. 2019;7:e7702.
6. Schwendicke F, Blatz M, Uribe SECW, Verma M, Linton J, Kim YJ. Artificial intelligence for dentistry—FDI white paper. International Dental Federation; 2023.
7. Fryback DG, Thornbury JR. The efficacy of diagnostic imaging. Med Decis Mak. 1991;11:88–94.
8. Fatima A, Shafi I, Afzal H, Díez IDLT, Lourdes DR-SM, Breñosa J, Espinosa JCM, Ashraf I. Advancements in dentistry with artificial intelligence: current clinical applications and future perspectives. Healthcare (Basel). 2022;10:2188. https://doi.org/10.3390/healthcare10112188.
9. Hung K, Montalvao C, Tanaka R, Kawai T, Bornstein MM. The use and performance of artificial intelligence applications in dental and maxillofacial radiology: a systematic review. Dentomaxillofac Radiol. 2019;49:20190107.
10. Slaidina A, Springe B, Abeltins A, Uribe SE, Lejnieks A. The effect of general bone mineral density on the quantity and quality of the edentulous mandible: a cross-sectional clinical study. Dent J. 2023;11:17.
11. Farook TH, Jamayet NB, Abdullah JY, Alam MK. Machine learning and intelligent diagnostics in dental and orofacial pain management: a systematic review. Pain Res Manag. 2021;2021:6659133.
12. Xu L, Chen J, Qiu K, Yang F, Wu W. Artificial intelligence for detecting temporomandibular joint osteoarthritis using radiographic image data: a systematic review and meta-analysis of diagnostic test accuracy. PLoS One. 2023;18:e0288631.
13. Almăşan O, Leucuţa D-C, Hedeşiu M, Mureşanu S, Popa Ştefan L. Temporomandibular joint osteoarthritis diagnosis employing artificial intelligence: systematic review and meta-analysis. J Clin Med Res. 2023;12:942. https://doi.org/10.3390/jcm12030942.
14. de Dumast P, Mirabel C, Cevidanes L, et al. A web-based system for neural network based classification in temporomandibular joint osteoarthritis. Comput Med Imaging Graph. 2018;67:45–54.
15. Choi E, Kim D, Lee J-Y, Park H-K. Artificial intelligence in detecting temporomandibular joint osteoarthritis on orthopantomogram. Sci Rep. 2021;11:10246.
16. Brown JS, Crowder LP, Willcocks EJ, Bajwa MS, Schache AG. Accuracy of preoperative clinical examination and imaging for mandibular resection in oral cancer: a systematic review of diagnostic test accuracy studies. Br J Oral Maxillofac Surg. 2023;61:28–38.
17. Uribe S, Rojas LA, Rosas CF. Accuracy of imaging methods for detection of bone tissue invasion in patients with oral squamous cell carcinoma. Dentomaxillofac Radiol. 2013;42:20120346.
18. Dolens EDS, Dourado MR, Almangush A, Salo TA, Gurgel Rocha CA, da Silva SD, Brennan PA, Coletta RD. The impact of histopathological features on the prognosis of oral squamous cell carcinoma: a comprehensive review and meta-analysis. Front Oncol. 2021;11:784924.
19. Mahmood H, Shaban M, Indave BI, Santos-Silva AR, Rajpoot N, Khurram SA. Use of artificial intelligence in diagnosis of head and neck precancerous and cancerous lesions: a systematic review. Oral Oncol. 2020;110:104885.
20. Kim J-S, Kim BG, Hwang SH. Efficacy of artificial intelligence-assisted discrimination of oral cancerous lesions from normal mucosa based on the oral mucosal image: a systematic review and meta-analysis. Cancers. 2022;14:3499. https://doi.org/10.3390/cancers14143499.
21. Elmakaty I, Elmarasi M, Amarah A, Abdo R, Malki MI. Accuracy of artificial intelligence-assisted detection of oral squamous cell carcinoma: a systematic review and meta-analysis. Crit Rev Oncol Hematol. 2022;178:103777.
22. Chiesa-Estomba CM, Graña M, Medela A, et al. Machine learning algorithms as a computer-assisted decision tool for oral cancer prognosis and management decisions: a systematic review. ORL J Otorhinolaryngol Relat Spec. 2022;84:278–88.
23. Exarchos KP, Goletsis Y, Fotiadis DI. A multiscale and multiparametric approach for modeling the progression of oral cancer. BMC Med Inform Decis Mak. 2012;12:136.

24. Chang S-W, Abdul-Kareem S, Merican AF, Zain RB. Oral cancer prognosis based on clinicopathologic and genomic markers using a hybrid of feature selection and machine learning methods. BMC Bioinformatics. 2013;14:170.
25. Karadaghy OA, Shew M, New J, Bur AM. Development and assessment of a machine learning model to help predict survival among patients with oral squamous cell carcinoma. JAMA Otolaryngol Head Neck Surg. 2019;145:1115–20.
26. Rasteau S, Ernenwein D, Savoldelli C, Bouletreau P. Artificial intelligence for oral and maxillo-facial surgery: a narrative review. J Stomatol Oral Maxillofac Surg. 2022;123:276–82.
27. Lo Casto A, Spartivento G, Benfante V, Di Raimondo R, Ali M, Di Raimondo D, Tuttolomondo A, Stefano A, Yezzi A, Comelli A. Artificial intelligence for classifying the relationship between impacted third molar and mandibular canal on panoramic radiographs. Life. 2023;13:1441.
28. Kempers S, van Lierop P, Hsu T-MH, Moin DA, Bergé S, Ghaeminia H, Xi T, Vinayahalingam S. Positional assessment of lower third molar and mandibular canal using explainable artificial intelligence. J Dent. 2023;133:104519.
29. Yoo J-H, Yeom H-G, Shin W, Yun JP, Lee JH, Jeong SH, Lim HJ, Lee J, Kim BC. Deep learning based prediction of extraction difficulty for mandibular third molars. Sci Rep. 2021;11:1954.
30. Mangano FG, Admakin O, Lerner H, Mangano C. Artificial intelligence and augmented reality for guided implant surgery planning: a proof of concept. J Dent. 2023;133:104485.
31. Huqh MZU, Abdullah JY, Wong LS, et al. Clinical applications of artificial intelligence and machine learning in children with cleft lip and palate-a systematic review. Int J Environ Res Public Health. 2022;19:10860. https://doi.org/10.3390/ijerph191710860.
32. Fontenele RC, do Nascimento Gerhardt M, Picoli FF, Van Gerven A, Nomidis S, Willems H, Freitas DQ, Jacobs R. Convolutional neural network-based automated maxillary alveolar bone segmentation on cone-beam computed tomography images. Clin Oral Implants Res. 2023;34:565–74. https://doi.org/10.1111/clr.14063.
33. Usman M, Rehman A, Saleem AM, Jawaid R, Byon S-S, Kim S-H, Lee B-D, Heo M-S, Shin Y-G. Dual-stage deeply supervised attention-based convolutional neural networks for mandibular canal segmentation in CBCT scans. Sensors. 2022;22:9877.
34. Kolarkodi SH, Alotaibi KZ. Artificial intelligence in diagnosis of oral diseases: a systematic review. J Contemp Dent Pract. 2023;24:61–8.
35. Khanagar SB, Vishwanathaiah S, Naik S, Al-Kheraif AA, Devang Divakar D, Sarode SC, Bhandi S, Patil S. Application and performance of artificial intelligence technology in forensic odontology—a systematic review. Legal Med. 2020;48:101826.
36. Wornow M, Xu Y, Thapa R, Patel B, Steinberg E, Fleming S, Pfeffer MA, Fries J, Shah NH. The shaky foundations of large language models and foundation models for electronic health records. NPJ Digit Med. 2023;6:135.
37. Moor M, Banerjee O, Abad ZSH, Krumholz HM, Leskovec J, Topol EJ, Rajpurkar P. Foundation models for generalist medical artificial intelligence. Nature. 2023;616:259–65.
38. Moor M, Huang Q, Wu S, Yasunaga M, Zakka C, Dalmia Y, Reis EP, Rajpurkar P, Leskovec J. Med-Flamingo: a multimodal medical few-shot learner. arXiv [cs.CV]. 2023.
39. Singhal K, Tu T, Gottweis J, et al. Towards expert-level medical question answering with large language models. arXiv [cs.CL]. 2023.
40. Huang Z, Bianchi F, Yuksekgonul M, Montine TJ, Zou J. A visual-language foundation model for pathology image analysis using medical twitter. Nat Med. 2023;29:2307–16. https://doi.org/10.1038/s41591-023-02504-3.
41. Karthikesalingam A, Natarajan V. AMIE: a research AI system for diagnostic medical reasoning and conversations. In: Google Research. 2024. https://blog.research.google/2024/01/amie-research-ai-system-for-diagnostic_12.html. Accessed 3 Feb 2024.
42. McDuff D, Schaekermann M, Tu T, et al. Towards accurate differential diagnosis with large language models. arXiv [cs.CY]. 2023; https://doi.org/10.48550/arXiv.2312.00164.

4 Artificial Intelligence in Periodontology: Current Applications and Future Perspectives

Lata Goyal, Kunaal Dhingra, and Jaya Pandey

4.1 Introduction

Artificial intelligence (AI) in simple words is a machine performing tasks that normally need human intelligence [1]. AI is one of the significant contributions of the modern digital era and continuously growing in all fields. It can learn from human experience and can perform the tasks with humanlike intelligence [2].

With the progress of time, as the digitization of patient data and clinical records has given way in modern dentistry, this technology integrates the digital record, interprets, processes and helps clinicians in diagnosis, treatment planning, and predicting treatment outcomes. It can serve as a valuable tool to reduce the workload of healthcare professionals. It has been used in all the specialties of dentistry like periodontics, orthodontics, prosthodontics, maxillofacial surgery, oral radiology, and medicine. Periodontitis is one of the most common and prevalent diseases affecting the major portion of the global population. It is a chronic inflammatory disease mediated by altered host immune inflammatory response through host cell receptors [3]. This altered response is affected by both local and systemic factors resulting in tissue destruction [4, 5]. Early detection and treatment are necessary to prevent periodontal disease from progressing into a more advanced stage [6].

The traditional approach to diagnose and treat periodontal disease essentially relies on the clinical expertise of the dental professionals and assessment of probing pocket depth, bleeding on probing, tooth mobility, clinical attachment loss, and bone loss. But the interexaminer reliability and variability are the major drawbacks of this approach. However, modern tools based on AI can provide solutions to the challenges and limitations faced by traditional approaches. But, for machine-based tools to function effectively, the input data must be homogeneous, because they are unable to identify data quality that has a major role and could exacerbate the bias associated with it. With utilization of evidence-based decisions and employing new machine-based technology based on (AI) may offer innovative solutions to enhance the accuracy, efficiency, and effectiveness of periodontal care.

L. Goyal
Division of Periodontology, Centre for Dental Education and Research, All India Institute of Medical Sciences, Bathinda, Punjab, India

K. Dhingra (✉)
Division of Periodontology, Centre for Dental Education and Research (CDER), All India Institute of Medical Sciences, New Delhi, New Delhi, India

J. Pandey
Division of Periodontology, Centre for Dental Education and Research, All India Institute of Medical Sciences, New Delhi, India

F. Schwendicke et al. (eds.), *Artificial Intelligence for Oral Health Care*,
https://doi.org/10.1007/978-3-031-84047-0_4

4.2 Applications of AI in Periodontal Diagnosis

4.2.1 Image Analysis

AI-driven image recognition algorithm has shown the potential to analyze the clinical images (frontal and lateral photographs). They can assist in detection of dental biofilm and can diagnose the signs of inflammation, calculus, gingival overgrowth, and aberrant frenal attachments [7].

Intraoral images both frontal and lateral photographs have been used as input data in various studies with the aim to diagnose gingivitis. These machine learning-based models reported an accuracy from 47%–83% in diagnosing gingivitis. However, comparisons among the various studies are a daunting task because of heterogeneity in terms of variability in the dataset, population, and objective definitions. Some of the studies where the diagnosis of gingival diseases with the aid of machine-based learning models have been summarized in Table 4.1.

4.2.2 Radiographic Analysis

AI models can be trained to accurately diagnose the grade and severity of periodontal disease. Radiographic datasets can be used to train algorithms to recognize significant landmarks in radiographic images, such as alveolar bone loss, cementoenamel junction, and furcation involvement [10]. It will assist in predicting the progression of diseases by analyzing sequential images over a period of time and also giving valuable inputs regarding the effectiveness of therapy. Combining radiographic images with clinical data and patient electronic health records can also improve the accuracy of disease diagnosis. It can also detect anomalies and artificial and accidental findings in images that are sometimes overlooked by the human eye like pathologies, radiopaque lesions, cysts, etc.

Bone quality and quantity can also be analyzed giving valuable information for the procedures requiring regenerative periodontal surgeries and dental implants. Moreover, dental implant

Table 4.1 Diagnosis of gingival diseases with machine learning models

	Authors	Dataset	Recommendations
1.	Chau et al. [8]	Frontal view intraoral photographs	AI could discriminate oral sites with gingival inflammation with sensitivity of 0.92 and specificity of 0.94, which was at par with visual examination in the Chinese population. This AI-based system built with DeepLabv3+ may be used as a monitoring tool for plaque control effectiveness
2.	Andrade et al. [9]	Frontal and lateral photographs	Dental biofilm can be diagnosed by employing the U-Net model with an accuracy of 91.8% and specificity and sensitivity of 94.4% and 67.2%, respectively, and can be used as a valuable tool for improving oral hygiene
3.	Ertaş et al. [10]	Periodontal recordings Orthopantomography	Using the clinical data, diagnostic accuracy for staging and grading of periodontal disease was 97.2%, but this accuracy was lower when only radiographs were used. There is a need to optimize the algorithm to improve the results for grading of periodontitis
4.	Li et al. [11]	Oral photographs	CNN model was used to screen gingivitis, soft deposits, and calculus. Area under the curve (AUC) for detecting gingivitis was 87.11%, while for dental calculus and soft deposits, 80.11%, and 78.57%, respectively, which showed the potential of AI in screening oral diseases at mass level
5.	Kurt-Bayrakdar et al. [7]	Oral photographs	The AI model can be used successfully to interpret anatomical structures like gingival inflammation, frenum attachment, and gingival overgrowth with a sensitivity of 0.737, 0.894, and 0.757 and precision of 0.875, 0.775, and 0.675 respectively

systems can be identified and classified using dental imaging. AI-based models showed high accuracy in identification and classification implant systems based on radiographic images [12]. A systematic review revealed that deep learning-based implant classification had an accuracy of 70.75%. This approach can analyze vast and diverse datasets, detect and interpret patterns, understand relationships between conditions, and recognize variability among different populations, distinguishing normal ranges from diseases. It can greatly contribute to advancing knowledge in the field of periodontology [12].

AI-based analysis of radiographic images also reduces human error when used as a supportive tool and also addresses the interexaminer variability in interpreting the radiographic images. Some of the studies which depict the use of radiographic images as a dataset in diagnosing periodontitis have been summarized in Table 4.2.

These machine-based learning tools can help in diagnosing periodontal conditions by analyzing clinical records and radiographic images. But assessing the quality of records is a huge challenge for interpretation [22]. A systematic review comprising 13 articles concluded that while this

Table 4.2 Diagnosis of periodontitis based on radiographic Images using artificial intelligence tools

	Authors	Dataset	Inference
1.	Liu et al. [13]	Panoramic radiographs (PANs)	CNN model was able to diagnose periodontitis with relatively less time. The accuracy of the model was 0.800 as compared to periodontal experts, which was 0.813. The time taken to analyze the radiograph was longer in the periodontist group as compared to the model (6.042 ± 1.148 s vs. (0.027 ± 0.002 s)
2.	Chen et al. [14]	Periapical X-ray images	This deep learning model was able to diagnose periodontitis and dental caries at the same time. For the recognition of periodontitis and dental caries, AUC was 98.67% and 98.31%, respectively
3.	Mao et al. [15]	Periapical radiographs	The proposed deep learning model was able to detect furcation involvement ranging from 92.96% to 94.97% on periapical radiographs
4.	Chen et al. [6]	Periapical radiographs	Deep learning trained model has the potential for detection of periapical radiographs with an accuracy of 90%. Accuracy for detection of bone level and bone loss was 92.61% and 97.0%, respectively. AI models proved superior accuracy as compared to general dentists which was 76–78%
5.	Wang et al. [16]	Periodontal examination data and radiographs	This deep learning model predicted the site-level effectiveness of periodontal therapy. Pocket closure as a variable had an average probing depth accuracy of 92.4% For sites with baseline PD <5 mm and PD ≥ 5 mm, prediction accuracy was 94.6% and 79.9%, respectively
6.	Uzun Saylan et al. [17]	Panoramic radiograph	Using the segmentation method, AI models were evaluated to detect the presence or absence of alveolar bone loss. Alveolar bone loss was associated with the lowest sensitivity and the incisor region showed higher values
7.	Chang et al. [18]	Full mouth periapical radiographs	The model demonstrated promising results with an accuracy of 0.87 ± 0.01 in categorizing mild or severe bone loss
8.	Alotaibi et al. [19]	Periapical radiograph	CNN Algorithm was useful in detecting alveolar bone loss. Diagnostic accuracy for classification of disease based on severity of alveolar bone loss was 59% of disease as compared to 73% in normal
9.	Jiang et al. [20]	Panoramic images	A deep learning model was established for assessing the radiographic bone loss with an overall classification accuracy of 0.77
10.	Kim et al. [21]	Panoramic radiograph	DENTNet model detects bone loss and also provides the corresponding tooth number. It uses clinical knowledge and learning to overcome morphological variations

Table 4.3 Biomarker-based detection of periodontitis using machine learning models

S. no	Authors	Dataset	Inference
1.	Kim et al. [23]	Saliva sample	DNA was isolated from 692 subjects from mouthwash samples, and nine pathogens from q PCR were isolated. This study suggested salivary bacteria can be used as a biomarker for diagnosing the healthy and severe form of chronic periodontitis
2.	Eriksson et al. [24]	Salivary sample	As compared to microbes and mediators alone, the combination of these is more effective predictive biomarker for periodontitis and rheumatoid arthritis
3.	Deng et al. [25]	Oral rinse point of care activated MMP 8 test, and bleeding on brushing	On 408 samples, three nonclinical indices in the form of bleeding on brushing, oral rinse activated MMP 8, and a self-administered questionnaire was applied. Machine-based random forest analyzers were found to be an accurate screening tool for periodontal health and disease
4.	Liu et al. [26]	Tongue dorsum and saliva	AI models were validated for predicting the risk of periodontal disease, like gingival bleeding, and etiological factors, like calculus; there is dominance of polygenetic risk scores over oral microflora. Each individual has specific microbiota, and differences can be attributed to genetic differences between the individuals
5.	Kim et al. [27]	Saliva	Metabolic profiles of healthy and periodontitis groups were separated, and then metabolites were confirmed in the validation set. Machine-based learning tools based on these biomarkers had the potential for the detection and screening of periodontal diseases and also for monitoring of periodontal therapy

rapidly advancing technology is beneficial in determining and classifying disease conditions, caution should be exercised when considering its application to periodontal bone loss due to the paucity of evidence and the inconsistent performance of algorithms [22].

4.2.3 Biomarker Based

Artificial intelligence can be used to detect disease activity and diagnose periodontitis based on oral biomarkers. Some of the studies have been summarized in Table 4.3.

4.3 AI-Assisted Disease Classification and Decision-Making

AI models can be trained and validated to develop the classification of periodontal disease, which can assist the clinician in staging and grading of disease and, at the same time, serve as indispensable tools for decision-making. Ozden et al., in 2015, studied 150 patients and developed a classification system based on machine-based algorithms [28]. One hundred patients were used for training and 50 were used for validation. Periodontal clinical data, radiographic images, and risk factors were used as input data. Support vector machines and decision trees were found to be accurate and practical tools for decision-making.

Ertaş et al., in 2023, based on a machine learning algorithm, designed a decision-based system to classify the disease conditions and determine the stage and grade of periodontitis [10]. Based on the clinical data of 144 individuals, models were created and then panoramic images were processed. The accuracy was 97.2 to 98.6%. However, they concluded based on radiographic images that accuracy was comparatively lower. This system can facilitate periodontal diagnosis, but further optimization is required to increase the accuracy [10].

4.3.1 AI-Assisted Treatment Planning

Artificial intelligence-based tools can provide assistance in treatment planning for periodontal surgical procedures and dental implants. Anatomical landmarks can be detected and surgical procedures can be planned precisely. An AI-based tool that interprets radiographic images (CBCT, panoramic, periapical) can provide vital information on bone density, alveolar pattern, tooth morphology, and proximity to critical structures. By identifying these landmarks, reference points, insertion angles, and placement sites of the implant can be predicted accurately [29].

Simulation surgeries can be planned to better visualize the surgical plan in a controlled environment. During implant placement, angle, depth, and diameter can be predicted accurately. Mangano et al., in 2023, described a protocol for accurate positioning of implants using artificial intelligence and augmented reality [30].

Thanathornwong et al., in 2023, developed a clinical decision support system from retrospective data of 400 patients. A faster CNN network, when merged with clinical workflow, will be helpful for general practitioners to give expert-level care to the geriatric population [31]. Artificial intelligence-based assessment of soft tissue thickness can be measured, which is an important parameter in periodontal surgical procedures and future development of minimal invasive procedures [32].

Accuracy and overall success of surgical procedures can be enhanced using AI leading to better treatment outcomes.

4.4 AI-Assisted Prediction of Treatment Outcomes

Artificial intelligence-based models can interpret preoperative data. These models can predict the effectiveness of periodontal therapy, helping clinicians to meet patient expectations and counseling them for future intervention [16]. These models can analyze patients' demographics and clinical features and can also suggest personalized treatment plans. Wang et al., in 2023, developed a model to predict the effectiveness of periodontal therapy with an average site probing depth accuracy of 92.4% and sensitivity of 98.6% with pocket closure as variable. This accuracy varied between the patients having probing depth of more than 5 mm and also varied between molars and non-molar teeth [16].

Patient-specific data like systemic illness, frequency of oral hygiene, susceptibility to disease, genetic predilection, and risk factors can be analyzed preoperatively. Risks and complications associated with any surgical procedures can be predicted, and risk mitigation strategies can be predicted well in advance.

Huang et al., in 2022, investigated the feasibility of predicting the risk of failure of dental implants based on preoperative CBCT [33]. An integrated model based on clinical features and radiographs was able to predict the 5 years survival of implant with great accuracy. These types of models are very useful in the future for predicting the outcomes and at the same time counselling the patients to meet realistic expectations. Trionao et al., in 2023, validated a model for predictingmolar loss, which will be available for clinical use [34]. Zhang et al., in 2023, also predicted the dental implant failure with a deep learning convolutional neural network. A total of 529 IOPAs and 551 panoramic radiographs were collected and, based on an alveolar pattern model, achieved diagnostic accuracy of 78.6% and 78.7%, respectively. Both the images showed prediction accuracy of 87% with the precision of 0.85 [35]. Data analysis also showed that COPD could be predicted based on patients' data and oral health. And also found was periodontitis, which could be an important predictor of COPD [36].

Natural language processing (NLP) techniques enable the extraction of valuable information from electronic health records, patient histories, and clinical notes. AI-powered systems can automatically analyze this unstructured data, aiding in the identification of risk factors, progression of disease, and treatment outcomes.

4.5 Patient Education

Artificial intelligence can act as a valuable educational tool in enhancing the knowledge of the patient. Personalized and custom educational material pertaining to particular disease conditions and preferences can be executed, so that the patient receives exactly the piece of information, which is required [37]. 3D-based animations, 3D models, and interactive sessions can help the patients to identify the treatment needs. AI-driven language tools, visual aids, and video content can provide simpler solutions to patients of different and diverse cultural backgrounds. Patient feedback can also be collected to refine the content.

AI driven teledentistry can provide education and oral hygiene reinforcements, monitoring their progress of oral hygiene measures [38]. Models can be created so that patients can self-diagnose the conditions and take appropriate preventive measures at an early stage of disease.

Kim et al., in 2020, validated a deep learning-based mobile app to identify plaque at home. Light-induced fluorescence-based system was developed to identify plaques and then a mobile application to show the plaque on dental images. It emphasized the potential use of this application as a home product for early identification of dental plaque [39]. Chen et al., in 2020, developed intelligent brush monitoring that recognizes the posture of the toothbrush by using a smart toothbrush [40, 41]. Using artificial intelligence at home setting had a positive effect on treatment outcomes of periodontal therapy. Patients reported better treatment outcomes who received AI-assisted counseling [42].

By leveraging AI for patient education, dental healthcare professionals can empower their patients with the knowledge required to actively participate in their own oral healthcare. This leads to improved treatment adherence, motivation, desired outcomes, and enhanced overall patient satisfaction.

4.6 Incorporating AI into Clinical Practice

AI can be easily merged with clinical periodontal practice but that requires careful planning and implementation. Based on our requirements like diagnosis, treatment planning, prediction of outcome or education, we have to select the area and have to formulate clear objectives. Based on objective, we can select input data, which could be photographic images, radiographs, demographics, or clinical data. Then, select the appropriate AI tool taking into consideration the compatibility with existing systems. Then, merge that AI tool with your clinical dataset, whether images electronic records or photographic images. Then based on your practice, customize the tool based on the need. Do initial pilot testing to check the workflow, which requires training and education. Check for accuracy, sensitivity, and precision and based on indicators; monitor and evaluate the performance.

Integrating artificial intelligence (AI) into a periodontal practice involves careful planning, implementation, and ongoing training. The steps to effectively incorporate AI into a periodontology practice are shown in Fig. 4.1.

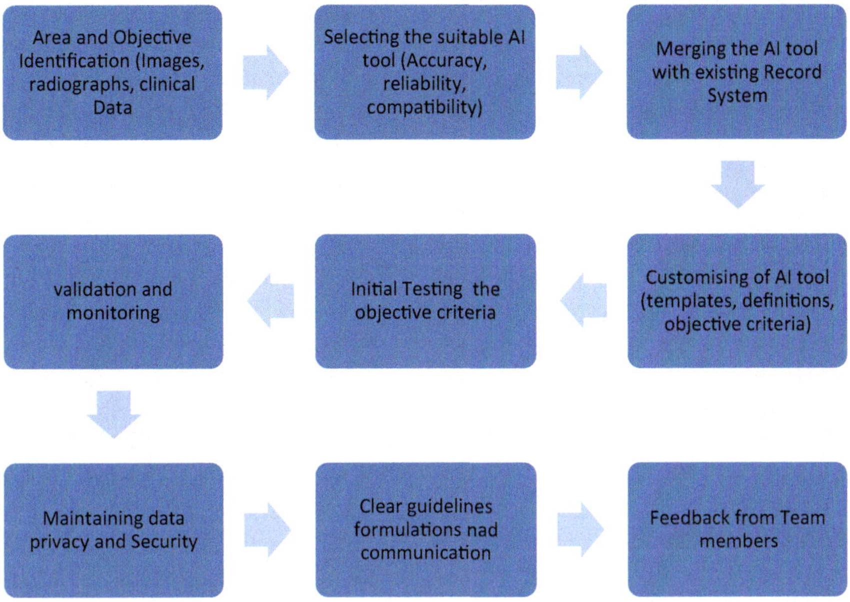

Fig. 4.1 Steps to incorporate AI into periodontology practice

4.7 Limitations

While artificial intelligence (AI) holds the potential to revolutionize periodontal practice, it is important to acknowledge its current limitations. These include:

- Dataset dependence: AI models for training and validation require a huge amount of dataset in the form of images, radio graphics, health records, etc. It may be possible that for data collection and data reporting, there may be heterogeneity and lack of standardization [43]. It can pose a challenge for accurate prediction of treatment outcomes. The periodontal practice involves a diverse range of clinical scenarios, and it will be a struggle and a challenge to account for all the possible variations for determining the diagnosis.
- Lack of emotion: Machine-based learning models can analyze the situation in a more logical and mathematical manner. AI lacks consciousness and human emotions, which limits its ability to solve the complex health-care situation, which depends on human interactions. Humans have the ability to understand complex emotions, nuances in languages, interpreting expressions, common sense, and reasoning [44].
- Lack of clinical judgment: AI has a supportive role in diagnosis and treatment planning as it has no clinical judgement of its own. There are certain aspects like doctor patient relationship, communication, clinical assessment, psychological, social, individualized expectations, which are beyond the domains of AI. There are certain domains of healthcare where human touch is irreplaceable.
- Bias amplification: Evidence suggests that there are no guidelines for reporting and comparing the models. AI models can employ and amplify the bias and can affect decision making. Ultimately, the responsibility does not lie with the machines but with the individuals who created them.
- Interdisciplinary considerations: Periodontal treatment often involves collaboration with other dental specialists, such as prosthodon-

tists or oral surgeons. AI models may not always integrate seamlessly with existing workflows and may not capture the full complexity of interdisciplinary treatment planning.

There are certain limitations while adopting the AI tools. One has to understand that AI can be used as a supportive tool. It is a machine-based learning system which lacks clinical judgment.

While incorporating AI in periodontal practice, a well-balanced approach is required to make most of the advancements.

4.8 Challenges and Considerations

While AI holds great promise in periodontology, there are several challenges that should be addressed. These include data privacy, the need for robust validation of AI models, and ensuring that AI complements, rather than replaces, the clinical expertise of periodontal professionals.

- Data privacy and security: Patient personal information is sensitive and must be handled with care. Transferring data for analysis, preventing security breaches, and ensuring secure storage are some of the major challenges associated with digital technologies [45].
- Heterogeneity of data: As the healthcare conditions are complex and often interrelated with other specialties. To make accurate predictions with precision require very large amount of data so that all the diverse scenario can be interpreted and AI models can be trained, but if the data is limited, it will result in biased decisions and inaccurate information [46]. Data has to be integrated with existing health records but merging and integrating the different data face the issue of compatibility. Models trained in one clinical setting in particular population may not be valid for a different population in another setting.
- Patient acceptance: As it is growing technologies, patients have varying levels of comfort in trusting the digital technologies. Acquiring patient acceptance and trust in these technologies is yet another concern.
- Adopting the new technology: Clinicians who lack the use of digital technologies may be hesitant in adopting the AI models.
- Legal and ethical considerations: Patient consent, security of personal information, and data breach is some of the major challenges in adopting the AI. Responsibility of machine-based errors, meeting all the regulatory standards, and following guidelines are some of the crucial factors that should be taken into account [47, 48].
- Financial considerations: Hardware and software for designing the models for data storage involve preliminary investments. These models need to be continuously updated as the new protocols are developed.
- Future outcome: Although AI is a rapidly developing technology, there are currently no long-term research to assess its efficacy.
- Training: Healthcare professionals need to be trained and educated to have hold in using AI-based tools. This includes understanding the limitations of AI, interpreting AI-generated information, and integrating it into their clinical practice which requires education and training.
- Overcoming the challenges associated with artificial intelligence requires collaboration from all stakeholders. An interdisciplinary approach is required so that AI can be used ethically and legally. With the advancements, many challenges and limitations will be addressed over a period of time by developing new integrated and hybrid models. But it is need of the hour that we integrate these advancements by taking into consideration the challenges associate with it [49].

4.9 Future Directions

Personalized treatment strategies can be developed considering patient-specific data using demographics, genotype, environmental, systemic, and psychosocial risk factors.

Long-term data is needed to validate the effectiveness of AI-based application in improving patient experiences, comfort, and outcome [50].

Artificial intelligence can be integrated with other advance modalities. More and more hybrid models are merging clinical and radiographic data and augmented and virtual reality for effective treatment planning.

4.10 Conclusion

Artificial intelligence has emerged as a powerful tool in the field of periodontics, with applications ranging from diagnosis, treatment planning, predicting the treatment outcome to remote monitoring. While challenges and limitations exist, the potential advantages of AI in improving the accuracy and efficiency of periodontal care are substantial. Continued research and collaboration between dental professionals and AI experts will be crucial in realizing the full potential of this technology in periodontology. By following these steps, periodontal practices can successfully integrate AI technology, enhancing diagnostic accuracy, treatment planning, and overall patient care. It's important to approach AI as a supportive tool that complements the expertise and clinical judgment of the periodontal professionals.

References

1. Scott J, Biancardi AM, Jones O, Andrew D. Artificial intelligence in periodontology: a scoping review. Dent J (Basel). 2023;11(2):43.
2. Patil S, Albogami S, Hosmani J, Mujoo S, Kamil MA, Mansour MA, Abdul HN, Bhandi S, Ahmed SSSJ. Artificial intelligence in the diagnosis of oral diseases: applications and pitfalls. Diagnostics (Basel). 2022;12(5):1029.
3. Goyal L, Bey A, Gupta ND, Sharma VK. Comparative evaluation of serum C-reactive protein levels in chronic and aggressive periodontitis patients and association with periodontal disease severity. Contemp Clin Dent. 2014;5(4):484–8.
4. Goyal L, Goyal T, Gupta ND. Osteoporosis and periodontitis in postmenopausal women: a systematic review. J Midlife Health. 2017;8(4):151–8.
5. Gupta N, Gupta ND, Garg S, Goyal L, Gupta A, Khan S, Moin S. The effect of type 2 diabetes mellitus and smoking on periodontal parameters and salivary matrix metalloproteinase-8 levels. J Oral Sci. 2016;58(1):1–6.
6. Chen CC, Wu YF, Aung LM, Lin JC, Ngo ST, Su JN, Lin YM, Chang WJ. Automatic recognition of teeth and periodontal bone loss measurement in digital radiographs using deep-learning artificial intelligence. J Dent Sci. 2023;18(3):1301–9.
7. Kurt-Bayrakdar S, Uğurlu M, Yavuz MB, Sali N, Bayrakdar İŞ, Çelik Ö, Köse O, Beklen A, Uzun Saylan BC, Jagtap R, Orhan K. Detection of tooth numbering, frenulum attachment, gingival overgrowth, and gingival inflammation signs on dental photographs using convolutional neural network algorithms: a retrospective study. Quintessence Int. 2023;54(8):680–93.
8. Chau RCW, Li GH, Tew IM, Thu KM, McGrath C, Lo WL, Ling WK, Hsung RT, Lam WYH. Accuracy of artificial intelligence-based photographic detection of gingivitis. Int Dent J. 2023;73(5):724–30.
9. Andrade KM, Silva BPM, de Oliveira LR, Cury PR. Automatic dental biofilm detection based on deep learning. J Clin Periodontol. 2023;50(5):571–81.
10. Ertaş K, Pence I, Cesmeli MS, Ay ZY. Determination of the stage and grade of periodontitis according to the current classification of periodontal and peri-implant diseases and conditions (2018) using machine learning algorithms. J Periodontal Implant Sci. 2023;53(1):38–53.
11. Li W, Liang Y, Zhang X, Liu C, He L, Miao L, Sun W. A deep learning approach to automatic gingivitis screening based on classification and localization in RGB photos. Sci Rep. 2021;11(1):16831.
12. Chaurasia A, Namachivayam A, Koca-Ünsal RB, Lee JH. Deep-learning performance in identifying and classifying dental implant systems from dental imaging: a systematic review and meta-analysis. J Periodontal Implant Sci. 2024;54(1):3–12.
13. Liu Q, Dai F, Zhu H, Yang H, Huang Y, Jiang L, Tang X, Deng L, Song L. Deep learning for the early identification of periodontitis: a retrospective, multicentre study. Clin Radiol. 2023;78(12):e985–92.
14. Chen IDS, Yang CM, Chen MJ, Chen MC, Weng RM, Yeh CH. Deep learning-based recognition of periodontitis and dental caries in dental X-ray images. Bioengineering (Basel). 2023;10(8):911.
15. Mao YC, Huang YC, Chen TY, Li KC, Lin YJ, Liu YL, Yan HR, Yang YJ, Chen CA, Chen SL, Li CW, Chan ML, Chuo Y, Abu PAR. Deep learning for dental diagnosis: a novel approach to furcation involvement detection on periapical radiographs. Bioengineering (Basel). 2023;10(7):802.
16. Wang R, Wang R, Yang T, Jiao J, Cao Z, Meng H, et al. Deep learning improves prediction of periodontal therapy effectiveness in Chinese patients. J Periodontal Res. 2023;58(3):520–8.
17. Uzun Saylan BC, Baydar O, Yeşilova E, Kurt Bayrakdar S, Bilgir E, Bayrakdar İŞ, Çelik Ö, Orhan

K. Assessing the effectiveness of artificial intelligence models for detecting alveolar bone loss in periodontal disease: a panoramic radiograph study. Diagnostics (Basel). 2023;13(10):1800.
18. Chang J, Chang MF, Angelov N, Hsu CY, Meng HW, Sheng S, Glick A, Chang K, He YR, Lin YB, Wang BY, Ayilavarapu S. Application of deep machine learning for the radiographic diagnosis of periodontitis. Clin Oral Investig. 2022;26(11):6629–37.
19. Alotaibi G, Awawdeh M, Farook FF, Aljohani M, Aldhafiri RM, Aldhoayan M. Artificial intelligence (AI) diagnostic tools: utilizing a convolutional neural network (CNN) to assess periodontal bone level radiographically-a retrospective study. BMC Oral Health. 2022;22(1):399.
20. Jiang L, Chen D, Cao Z, Wu F, Zhu H, Zhu F. A two-stage deep learning architecture for radiographic staging of periodontal bone loss. BMC Oral Health. 2022;22(1):106.
21. Kim J, Lee HS, Song IS, Jung KH. DeNTNet: Deep Neural Transfer Network for the detection of periodontal bone loss using panoramic dental radiographs. Sci Rep. 2019;9(1):17615.
22. Patil S, Joda T, Soffe B, Awan KH, Fageeh HN, Tovani-Palone MR, Licari FW. Efficacy of artificial intelligence in the detection of periodontal bone loss and classification of periodontal diseases: a systematic review. J Am Dent Assoc. 2023;154(9):795–804.e1.
23. Kim EH, Kim S, Kim HJ, Jeong HO, Lee J, Jang J, Joo JY, Shin Y, Kang J, Park AK, Lee JY, Lee S. Prediction of chronic periodontitis severity using machine learning models based on salivary bacterial copy number. Front Cell Infect Microbiol. 2020;10:571515.
24. Eriksson K, Lundmark A, Delgado LF, Hu YOO, Fei G, Lee L, Fei C, Catrina AI, Jansson L, Andersson AF, Yucel-Lindberg T. Salivary microbiota and host-inflammatory responses in periodontitis affected individuals with and without rheumatoid arthritis. Front Cell Infect Microbiol. 2022;12:841139.
25. Deng K, Zonta F, Yang H, Pelekos G, Tonetti MS. Development of a machine learning multiclass screening tool for periodontal health status based on non-clinical parameters and salivary biomarkers. J Clin Periodontol. 2024;51(12):1547–60.
26. Liu X, Tong X, Zhu J, Tian L, et al. Metagenome-genome-wide association studies reveal human genetic impact on the oral microbiome. Cell Discov. 2021;7(1):117.
27. Kim S, Kim HJ, Song Y, Lee HA, Kim S, Chung J. Metabolic phenotyping of saliva to identify possible biomarkers of periodontitis using proton nuclear magnetic resonance. J Clin Periodontol. 2021;48(9):1240–9.
28. Ozden FO, Özgönenel O, Özden B, Aydogdu A. Diagnosis of periodontal diseases using different classification algorithms: a preliminary study. Niger J Clin Pract. 2015;18(3):416–21.
29. Oliveira-Santos N, Jacobs R, Picoli FF, Lahoud P, Niclaes L, Groppo FC. Automated segmentation of the mandibular canal and its anterior loop by deep learning. Sci Rep. 2023;13(1):10819.
30. Mangano FG, Admakin O, Lerner H, Mangano C. Artificial intelligence and augmented reality for guided implant surgery planning: A proof of concept. J Dent. 2023;133:104485.
31. Thanathornwong B, Suebnukarn S, Ouivirach K. Clinical decision support system for geriatric dental treatment using a bayesian network and a convolutional neural network. Healthc Inform Res. 2023;29(1):23–30.
32. Yang M, Li C, Yang W, Chen C, Chung CH, Tanna N, Zheng Z. Accurate gingival segmentation from 3D images with artificial intelligence: an animal pilot study. Prog Orthod. 2023;24(1):14.
33. Huang N, Liu P, Yan Y, Xu L, Huang Y, Fu G, Lan Y, Yang S, Song J, Li Y. Predicting the risk of dental implant loss using deep learning. J Clin Periodontol. 2022;49(9):872–83.
34. Troiano G, Nibali L, Petsos H, Eickholz P, Saleh MHA, Santamaria P, Jian J, Shi S, Meng H, Zhurakivska K, Wang HL, Ravidà A. Development and international validation of logistic regression and machine-learning models for the prediction of 10-year molar loss. J Clin Periodontol. 2023;50(3):348–57.
35. Zhang C, Fan L, Zhang S, Zhao J, Gu Y. Deep learning based dental implant failure prediction from periapical and panoramic films. Quant Imaging Med Surg. 2023;13(2):935–45.
36. Vollmer A, Vollmer M, Lang G, Straub A, Shavlokhova V, Kübler A, Gubik S, Brands R, Hartmann S, Saravi B. Associations between periodontitis and COPD: an artificial intelligence-based analysis of NHANES III. J Clin Med. 2022;11(23):7210.
37. Snider V, Homsi K, Kusnoto B, Atsawasuwan P, Viana G, Allareddy V, Gajendrareddy P, Elnagar MH. Effectiveness of AI-driven remote monitoring technology in improving oral hygiene during orthodontic treatment. Orthod Craniofac Res. 2023;26 Suppl 1:102–10.
38. Batra P, Tagra H, Katyal S. Artificial intelligence in teledentistry. Discoveries (Craiova). 2022;10(3):153.
39. Kim JM, Lee WR, Kim JH, Seo JM, Im C. Light-induced fluorescence-based device and hybrid mobile app for oral hygiene management at home: development and usability study. JMIR Mhealth Uhealth. 2020;8(10):e17881.
40. Chen CH, Wang CC, Chen YZ. Intelligent brushing monitoring using a smart toothbrush with recurrent probabilistic neural network. Sensors (Basel). 2021;21(4):1–18.
41. Chen CH, Wang CC, Chen YZ. Intelligent brushing monitoring using a smart toothbrush with recurrent probabilistic neural network. Sensors (Basel). 2021;21(4):1238.
42. Shen KL, Huang CL, Lin YC, Du JK, Chen FL, Kabasawa Y, Chen CC, Huang HL. Effects of artificial intelligence-assisted dental monitoring intervention in patients with periodontitis: a

randomized controlled trial. J Clin Periodontol. 2022;49(10):988–98.
43. Ahmed N, Abbasi MS, Zuberi F, Qamar W, Halim MSB, Maqsood A, Alam MK. Artificial intelligence techniques: analysis, application, and outcome in dentistry-a systematic review. Biomed Res Int. 2021;2021:9751564.
44. Pethani F. Promises and perils of artificial intelligence in dentistry. Aust Dent J. 2021;66(2):124–35.
45. Mörch CM, Atsu S, Cai W, Li X, Madathil SA, Liu X, Mai V, Tamimi F, Dilhac MA, Ducret M. Artificial intelligence and ethics in dentistry: a scoping review. J Dent Res. 2021;100(13):1452–60.
46. Reyes LT, Knorst JK, Ortiz FR, Ardenghi TM. Scope and challenges of machine learning-based diagnosis and prognosis in clinical dentistry: a literature review. J Clin Transl Res. 2021;7(4):523–39.
47. Satapathy P, Hermis AH, Rustagi S, Pradhan KB, Padhi BK, Sah R. Artificial intelligence in surgical education and training: opportunities, challenges, and ethical considerations - correspondence. Int J Surg. 2023;109(5):1543–4.
48. Rokhshad R, Ducret M, Chaurasia A, Karteva T, Radenkovic M, Roganovic J, Hamdan M, Mohammad-Rahimi H, Krois J, Lahoud P, Schwendicke F. Ethical considerations on artificial intelligence in dentistry: a framework and checklist. J Dent. 2023;135:104593.
49. Schwendicke F, Samek W, Krois J. Artificial intelligence in dentistry: chances and challenges. J Dent Res. 2020;99(7):769–74.
50. Chen YW, Stanley K, Att W. Artificial intelligence in dentistry: current applications and future perspectives. Quintessence Int. 2020;51(3):248–57.

5 Artificial Intelligence for Prosthetic and Implant Dentistry

Rata Rokhshad, Faleh Tamimi, Pauline Blinvignac, Raphael Richert, and Maxime Ducret

5.1 Introduction

Prosthetic and implant dentistry have been pioneers in the integration of digital dentistry within the clinical setting. The advent of cone-beam computed tomography (CBCT) and intraoral scanners, which were adopted several decades ago, revolutionized treatment planning in implantology. Additionally, the fields have seen significant advancements with the introduction of computer-aided design and manufacturing (CAD-CAM) for the creation of dental prostheses [1].

R. Rokhshad
Pediatric Dentistry Resident, Department of Pediatric Dentistry, Loma Linda School of Dentistry, Loma Linda, CA, USA

F. Tamimi
College of Dental Medicine, Qatar University, Doha, Qatar
e-mail: fmarino@qu.edu.qa

P. Blinvignac · R. Richert
Faculty of Dentistry, Claude Bernard Lyon 1 University, University of Lyon, Lyon, France

Dentistry Department, Hospices Civils de Lyon, Lyon, France
e-mail: raphael.richert@univ-lyon1.fr

M. Ducret (✉)
Faculty of Dentistry, Claude Bernard Lyon 1 University, University of Lyon, Lyon, France

Dentistry Department, Hospices Civils de Lyon, Lyon, France

Faculté d'Odontologie Université Claude Bernard Lyon 1, Université de Lyon, Lyon, France
e-mail: maxime.ducret@univ-lyon1.fr

Artificial intelligence (AI) refers to the simulation of human intelligence in machines that are programmed to think like humans and mimic their actions. These systems can learn from data, identify patterns, and make decisions with minimal human intervention. In the context of digital dentistry, practitioners who anticipated the shift toward digital technologies may find the integration of AI more intuitive. AI solutions are increasingly being offered for various applications, including treatment planning, digitizing patient information, and aiding in the design and manufacturing of dental prostheses [2–4] (Fig. 5.1).

This chapter provides a comprehensive overview of AI applications in the field of prosthetic and implant dentistry. The literature reported consists of pilot studies, case reports, and preclinical studies. As such, the content of this chapter should be critically assessed, recognizing that it represents an initial snapshot of the first medical devices available. It is expected that more sophisticated and robust solutions will be developed in the near future [5].

AI solutions (AIS) in prosthetic and implant dentistry are vast, encompassing applications for identification, communication prediction, and the design and manufacturing of prosthetics and implants. Also, this chapter will explore future possibilities in prosthetic dentistry brought about by the advancement of AIS, including robotics, augmented reality, and patient-specific modeling [6–9].

F. Schwendicke et al. (eds.), *Artificial Intelligence for Oral Health Care*,
https://doi.org/10.1007/978-3-031-84047-0_5

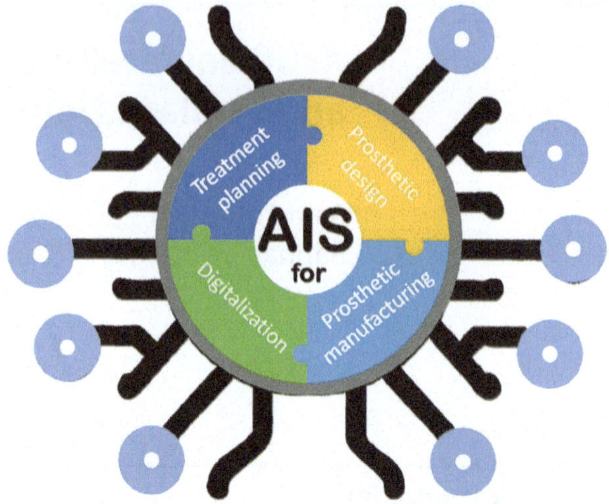

Fig. 5.1 Overview of AI solutions (AIS) in prosthetic and implant dentistry for treatment planning, digitalization of patients, design, and prosthesis manufacturing

5.1.1 Identification of Structures, Assisting Treatment Planning, and Communication

A common problem in implant and prosthetic dentistry is determining the implant type according to patient's dental radiographs. A pretrained deep convolutional neural network (CNN), specifically the GoogLeNet Inception-v3 model, which was trained on a substantial dataset of panoramic and periapical radiographs, demonstrated superior performance compared to a board-certified periodontist in identifying implant types. The CNN achieved an area under the curve (AUC) of 0.971, with a 95% confidence interval of 0.963–0.978, surpassing the periodontist's AUC of 0.925 (95% CI, 0.913–0.935) [10]. Also, based on Hsaio et al., with an average accuracy rate of over 95%, three different implant manufacturers and their respective subtypes were identified [11].

For treatment planning, various AI tools are currently available that identify dental structures and aid clinicians in the planning process marketed (Fig. 5.2). For instance, Chen et al. developed a decision-support model to help less experienced dentists select suitable removable prosthetic options [12]. Likewise, Takahashi et al. achieved outstanding results in classifying four types of dental arches using a CNN, with diagnostic accuracies of 99.5% for maxillary arches and 99.7% for mandibular arches [13].

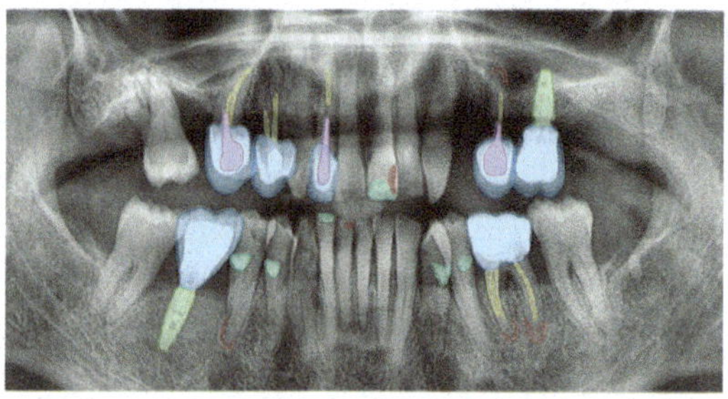

Fig. 5.2 Illustration of AIS that identifies various structures on panoramic radiographs and assist clinicians during treatment planning or to improve communication. (Software from Allisone company)

The performance remained consistently high, with over 95% accuracy when classifying new images, indicating that CNNs could play a significant role in the future of dental arch classification and removable partial denture design [13]. Moreover, AI has been applied in smile design software, which aids clinicians in treatment planning and enhances communication with patients [14].

5.1.2 Static and Dynamic Occlusion Analysis

A recent review examined various jaw-tracking systems, including those using ultrasonic and photometric technologies, some of which incorporate AI algorithms [15]. These systems have been evaluated for their ability to analyze occlusal contacts and the distribution of pressure across occlusal surfaces. The review concluded that while digital technologies provide valuable diagnostic and design tools for prosthodontic treatment, further research is necessary to determine their precision in recording and analyzing both static and dynamic aspects of the occlusion [15]. However, another systematic review highlighted many concerns regarding the use of machine learning to diagnose functional and parafunctional occlusal parameters; the absence of established baselines for model evaluation led to subjective validation by clinicians and introduced potential bias based on professional experience [16]. Furthermore, a recent study also reported that the scanner and the type of AI model influenced the maxillomandibular relationship. Indeed, better occlusal trueness was obtained when adjusted by the AIS included in the intraoral scanner compared with CAD software [17].

5.1.3 AIS for Shade Selection or Guide Fitting

AIS models used for tooth shade selection were reported to have shown promise in the realm of tooth shade selection, where they have achieved better matches than traditional visual methods [18]. Additionally, AIS has been proposed for aligning intraoral scans with CAD files to evaluate the fit of dental guides and prostheses [19].

5.1.4 Prediction of the Performance of Dental Prosthesis and Implant

AIS was used to predict the outcome of dental prostheses. Deep learning models were trained to predict the deboning probability of a CAD-CAM fabricated crowns and achieved a final accuracy of 98.5% and a precision of 97.0% [20]. Furthermore. AI models have provided prediction of wear resistance for nanohybrid composite, polymethyl methacrylate with microfillers, CAD-milled, and 3D-printed teeth materials [21].

In predicting the performance of dental prostheses, deep learning models have been trained with high success. One such model forecasted the debonding probability of CAD-CAM fabricated crowns with an impressive accuracy of 98.5% and precision of 97%. AI models have also been effective in predicting the wear of denture teeth [22]. A random forest model trained on data from 942 implants from 398 patients achieved an AUC of 0.872 to predict dental implant failures and 0.840 to predict peri-implantitis [23]. Another deep learning model trained on the preoperative CBCT of 603 patients could predict implant fate within 5 years with an AUC of 0.87 [24]. Moreover, an AI model predicted implant osseointegration using plain radiography and achieved mean AUROC values ranging from 0.890 to 0.922 [25]. In addition, a Faster region-based convolutional neural network (R-CNN) trained on 1670 periapical radiographs achieved a performance equal to that of resident dentists to detect marginal bone loss around dental implants [26].

5.1.5 Recognition of Dental Structures and Margin Line

CNN algorithms can recognize dental structures accurately; for instance, in a study by Raith et al., cusps were recognized at 93.5% accuracy [27], and a CNN based on sparse octree (S-Octree) structure achieved an accuracy of 97.43% to automatically detect the margin line of a tooth preparation [28]. Moreover, another study on implant-supported monolithic zirconia crowns (MZCs) cemented on customized hybrid abutments found that an AIS can effectively automate the process of tracing the margin line of the implant abutment, even when it extends subgingivally with a cumulative survival rate of 99.0% and a success rate of 91.3% [9].

5.1.6 Designing Dental Prosthesis

The application of AIS to prosthodontics mainly lies in restoration design, which is already in several marketed products. However, it should be mentioned that human expertise still plays a crucial role in this process. While AI can generate proposals quickly, dental professionals bring invaluable expertise that includes consideration of aesthetic and functional aspects that may not be fully captured by AI algorithms. For instance, a dentist's experience and understanding of a patient's unique occlusion, tooth morphology, and aesthetics can guide adjustments to the CAD design that better suit the individual patient. Moreover, the current state of AI in dental CAD systems might be more accurately described as assisted design rather than fully autonomous creation. Dentists and dental technicians often use AI-generated designs as a starting point and then make manual adjustments to tailor the restoration specifically to the patient's needs I [29].

In the study reported by Ding et al., 3D-DCGAN was used to design dental crowns to mimic both the morphology and biomechanics of natural teeth; the authors compared lithium disilicate crowns designed with 3D-DCGAN to those designed using CEREC Bioengineering and found that the former had the better match regarding the stress distribution and morphology [30]. Using another approach, Hwang et al. [31] and Tian et al. [32] trained 2D-GAN models to generate a crown by learning from technicians' designs.

ML algorithms are increasingly becoming integrated into various aspects of dental prosthesis design and manufacturing, including the creation of removable dentures. While expert systems have been established in the field, the introduction of ML algorithms for designing removable dentures represents an innovative step forward [33–35]. Recently, a study reported using a patient-specific approach of removable partial dentures with a clasp design adapted to the morphology of the crown. However, further studies are required before applying this type of software to clinical practice [36]. Finally, a recent study showed that two AIS could replicate the performance of a laboratory technician in creating occlusal devices, which is particularly encouraging. AIS developed for occlusal devices could mimic the performance of a laboratory technician [37]. This suggests that AIS can be trained to perform complex tasks that traditionally require the skill and expertise of experienced technicians.

5.1.7 Computer-Aided Manufacturing (CAM)

The production of dental prostheses through digital milling and printing is significantly enhanced by the use of AI models [38, 39]. These systems optimize manufacturing efficiency, reduce material wastage, and ensure high precision and reliability in the final product. A prime example of such technological integration is found in dental 3D printers that incorporate AIS, enabling the precise and optimal arrangement of components, which in turn saves time for the user [40] (Fig. 5.3).

Manufacturing techniques in dentistry face certain challenges, which AI is poised to address by optimizing operational parameters [41]. These enhancements aim to reduce tool wear, prevent overheating of components, and minimize material waste, all of which contribute to poor milling quality and potentially unusable outcomes. As CAM in dentistry benefits from the implementation of AI solutions, further research is anticipated to thoroughly explore the potential for cost reduction, improved manufacturing quality, and enhanced productivity.

5.1.8 Robot-Assisted Implant Placement

AIS has recently been used to assist clinicians during the placement of dental implants using robotic devices [42–44]. Additionally, emerging technologies are providing dynamic surgical guidance through visual and haptic feedback,

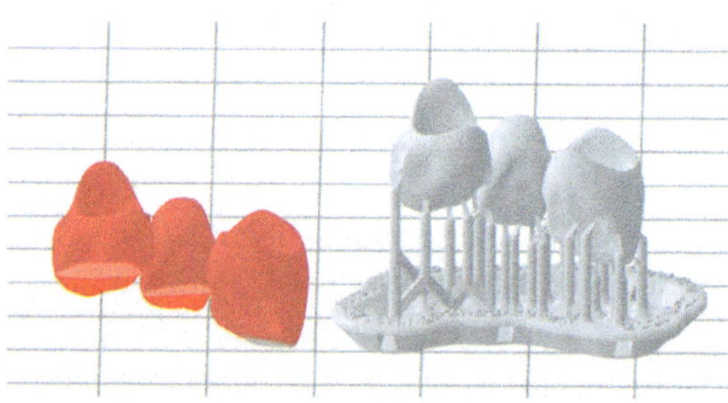

Fig. 5.3 AIS in 3D printers to optimize the manufacturing process. Here, using the "One-Click Print" optimizes the printing strategy for each device. Left is before and right after using this button

aiding osteotomy preparation and implant placement. Case reports have shown promising results, particularly in the accuracy of prosthetically driven planning and the immediate placement of single-tooth dental implants using such advanced systems [45]. Robotic assistance can also help guide the placement of zygomatic implants based on preoperative computed tomography scans. Four zygomatic implants were placed in the case patient according to the flapless protocol, with a mean vector error of 1.78 mm (range 0.52–4.70 mm). This approach guarantees a very high degree of precision and minimal inaccuracies in the placement of zygomatic implants through a safe flapless surgery technique [46].

5.1.9 Augmented Reality

Augmented reality (AR) represents a technological concept, wherein the physical environment is enriched by overlaying computer-generated virtual content onto real-world structures [47, 48]. While AR tools have traditionally been associated with video games and animations, the medical field is actively exploring their integration for applications in diagnosis, surgery, education, and patient communication [49]. Within dentistry, AR initially found use in education, serving as a tool for objectively assessing students and providing immediate feedback [49]. Recently, AR was also used to assist clinicians and patients during communication regarding smile design [50, 51]. However, these devices are relatively new, and only a limited number of studies were identified, suggesting caution before use in the clinic.

5.1.10 Patient-Specific Modeling

Precision medicine is leveraging imaging and electronic health records to train various AIS for the creation and utilization of patient-specific digital twins [52] (Fig. 5.4).

This digital twin concept offers the development of patient-specific modeling (PSM) for medical devices. This approach starts by recording patient data, such as teeth and bone, and importing them into specialized platforms for finite element (FE) analysis such as Amira or Mimics. Subsequently, the segmented objects are meshed to facilitate biomechanical calculations. PSM allows clinicians and researchers to digitally evaluate the influence of various biological and biomechanical parameters, aiding clinical decision-making [53–57]. This approach aims to find optimal mathematical solutions and propose the most conservative treatment options, considering minimal stress constraints, to increase the durability of devices for each patient [58] (Fig. 5.5).

This innovative approach has sparked discussions on refining prosthesis sizing, and finite element (FE) models and analyses have become critical tools for investigating and enhancing the design of clasps and crowns, particularly regarding the distribution of stresses they can support [35, 53, 59]. The potential of PSM lies in proposing the most biomechanically adapted prosthetic treatment option for each patient. This could be particularly valuable in intricate clinical scenarios, such as removable prostheses, where multiple prosthetic components interact.

Regarding implant dentistry, several PSM parameters, including bone quality and quantity, were reported to significantly influence mechanical failure in dental implants or bone analogs [60]. These parameters can now be accurately replicated in PSMs derived from CBCT scans, facilitating the development and evaluation of customized prosthetic solutions through FE analysis and modeling [61–64]. Personalized implant-based prosthetic rehabilitations were reported as having more favorable stress distributions than traditional prosthetics [62]. Customized bone analogs have also shown to have lower bone stresses and higher success rates after 1 year compared to conventional methods [63]. These positive results strongly encourage simulating approaches, and software were developed to mathematically optimize the design of plates and bone analogues to minimize bone stresses, thus favoring osteointegration [61, 64].

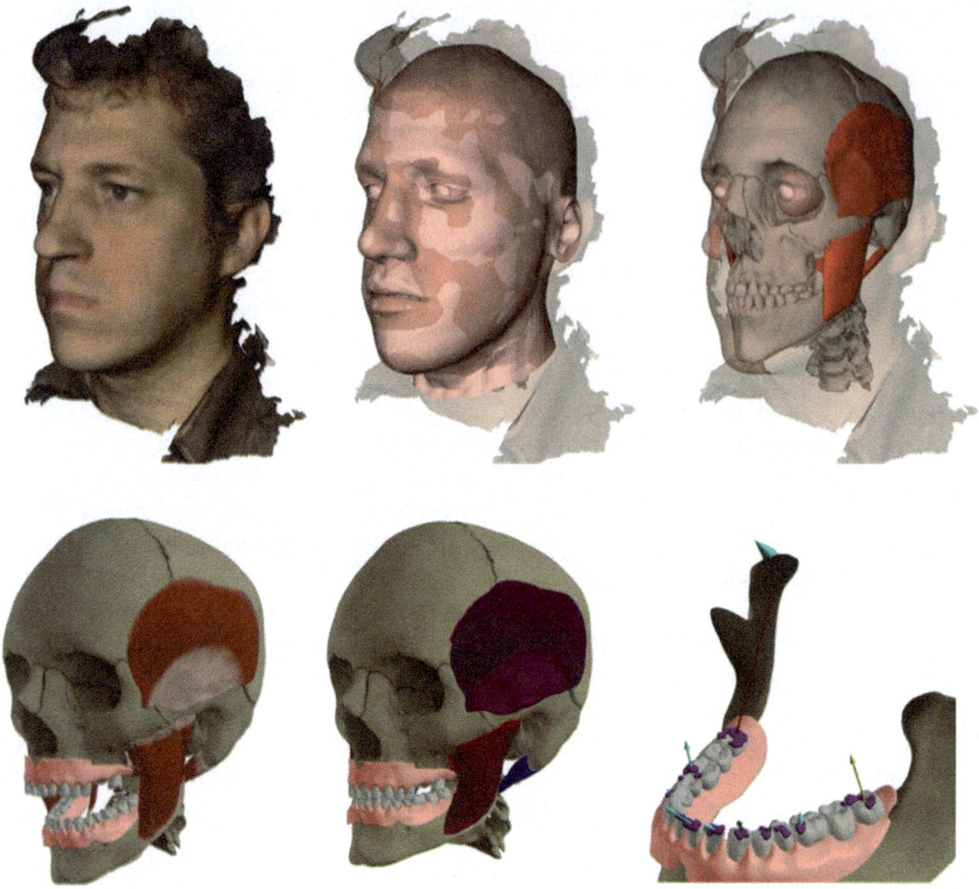

Fig. 5.4 Semi-personalized digital twin using patient data (face and intraoral scans) and an AIS that can match these data with a universal model. The scan could secondly be animated according to muscular activation to mimic patient occlusion and use it for CAD of prothesis. (Software from Circle Company)

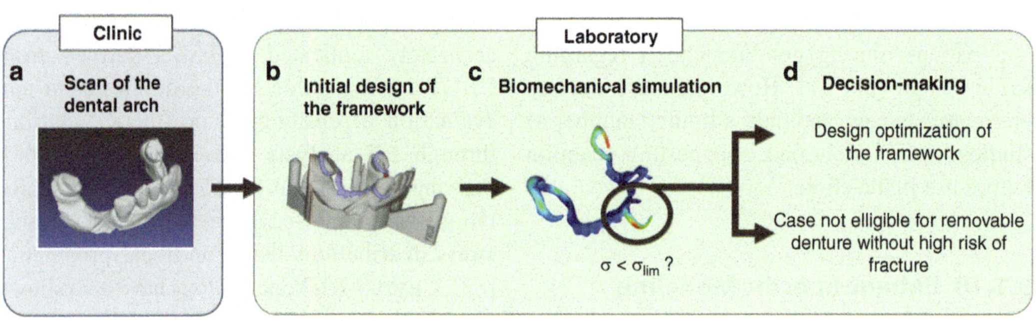

Fig. 5.5 Digital workflow following patient-specific modeling

PSM, using various AIS tools, could now bring dental practitioners into a new more predictive era of medicine, but such evolutions raise technical, ethical, and economic questions among the different stakeholders, and further investigations are required before to integrate all these AIS in everyday practice.

5.2 Conclusion

While the application of AIS in prosthetic and implant dentistry is promising, it should be noted that these technologies are still in their nascent stages, with a limited body of published studies. The questions and challenges they present require thorough scrutiny. This discussion highlights the need for caution in the integration of AIS into everyday clinical practices. Further advancements are crucial to improve the maturity and validation of these technologies, especially regarding user interfaces that can enable more effective human oversight of AIS.

Referenes

1. Richert R, Goujat A, Venet L, Viguie G, Viennot S, Robinson P, Farges J-C, Fages M, Ducret M. Intraoral scanner technologies: a review to make a successful impression. J Healthc Eng. 2017;2017:8427595. https://doi.org/10.1155/2017/8427595.
2. Mörch CM, Atsu S, Cai W, Li X, Madathil SA, Liu X, Mai V, Tamimi F, Dilhac MA, Ducret M. Artificial intelligence and ethics in dentistry: a scoping review. J Dent Res. 2021;100:1452–60. https://doi.org/10.1177/00220345211013808.
3. Singi SR, Sathe S, Reche AR, Sibal A, Mantri N. Extended arm of precision in prosthodontics: artificial intelligence. Cureus. 2022;14:1–9. https://doi.org/10.7759/cureus.30962.
4. Ding H, Wu J, Zhao W, Matinlinna JP, Burrow MF, Tsoi JKH. Artificial intelligence in dentistry—a review. Front Dent Med. 2023;4:1–13. https://doi.org/10.3389/fdmed.2023.1085251.
5. Bernauer SA, Zitzmann NU, Joda T, Bernauer SA, Zitzmann NU, Joda T. The use and performance of artificial intelligence in prosthodontics: a systematic review. Sensors. 2021;21(19):6628.
6. Revilla-León M, Gómez-Polo M, Vyas S, Barmak AB, Gallucci GO, Att W, Özcan M, Krishnamurthy VR. Artificial intelligence models for tooth-supported fixed and removable prosthodontics: a systematic review. J Prosthet Dent. 2023;129:276–92. https://doi.org/10.1016/j.prosdent.2021.06.001.
7. Alshadidi AAF, Alshahrani AA, Aldosari LIN, Chaturvedi S, Saini RS, Awod S, Hassan B, Cicci M, Minervini G. Investigation on the application of artificial intelligence in prosthodontics. Appl Sci. 2023;13(8):5004. https://doi.org/10.3390/app13085004.
8. Revilla-León M, Gómez-Polo M, Vyas S, Barmak BA, Galluci GO, Att W, Krishnamurthy VR. Artificial intelligence applications in implant dentistry: a systematic review. J Prosthet Dent. 2023;129:293–300. https://doi.org/10.1016/j.prosdent.2021.05.008.
9. Lerner H, Mouhyi J, Admakin O, Mangano F. Artificial intelligence in fixed implant prosthodontics: a retrospective study of 106 implant-supported monolithic zirconia crowns inserted in the posterior jaws of 90 patients. BMC Oral Health. 2020;20:1–17. https://doi.org/10.1186/s12903-020-1062-4.
10. Lee J-H, Jeong S-N. Efficacy of deep convolutional neural network algorithm for the identification and classification of dental implant systems, using panoramic and periapical radiographs. Medicine (Baltimore). 2020;99:e20787. https://doi.org/10.1097/MD.0000000000020787.
11. Hsiao CY, Bai H, Ling H, Yang J. Artificial intelligence in identifying dental implant systems on radiographs. Int J Periodontics Restorative Dent. 2023;43:363–8. https://doi.org/10.11607/prd.5781.
12. Chen Q, Wu J, Li S, Lyu P, Wang Y, Li M. An ontology-driven, case-based clinical decision support model for removable partial denture design. Sci Rep. 2016;6:27855. https://doi.org/10.1038/srep27855.
13. Takahashi T, Nozaki K, Gonda T, Ikebe K. A system for designing removable partial dentures using artificial intelligence. Part 1. Classification of partially edentulous arches using a convolutional neural network. J Prosthodont Res. 2021;65:115–8. https://doi.org/10.2186/jpr.JPOR_2019_354.
14. Gurel G. The artificial intelligence-based 3D smile design: REBEL. In: Esthetic Oral rehabilitation with veneers. Cham: Springer International Publishing; 2020. p. 235–63. https://doi.org/10.1007/978-3-030-41091-9_9.
15. Revilla-León M, Kois DE, Zeitler JM, Att W, Kois JC. An overview of the digital occlusion technologies: intraoral scanners, jaw tracking systems, and computerized occlusal analysis devices. J Esthet Restor Dent. 2023;35:735–44. https://doi.org/10.1111/jerd.13044.
16. Farook TH, Rashid F, Ahmed S, Dudley J. Clinical machine learning in parafunctional and altered functional occlusion: a systematic review. J Prosthet Dent. 2025;133(1):124–8. https://doi.org/10.1016/j.prosdent.2023.01.013.
17. Revilla-León M, Gómez-Polo M, Barmak AB, Kois JC, Yilmaz B, Alonso Pérez-Barquero J. Influence of occlusal collision corrections completed by two intraoral scanners or a dental design program on the accuracy of the maxillomandibular relationship. J Prosthet Dent. 2024;132(1):191–203. https://doi.org/10.1016/j.prosdent.2023.05.015.
18. Wei J, Peng M, Li Q, Wang Y. Evaluation of a novel computer color matching system based on the improved back-propagation neural network model. J Prosthodont. 2018;27:775–83. https://doi.org/10.1111/jopr.12561.
19. Bittar E, Binvignat P, Villat C, Maurin J-C, Ducret M, Richert R. Assessment of guide fitting using an intra-oral scanner: an in vitro study. J Dent. 2023;135:104590. https://doi.org/10.1016/j.jdent.2023.104590.

20. Yamaguchi S, Lee C, Karaer O, Ban S, Mine A, Imazato S. Predicting the debonding of CAD/CAM composite resin crowns with AI. J Dent Res. 2019;98:1234–8. https://doi.org/10.1177/0022034519867641.
21. Grymak A, Tieh MT, Yang AHX, Choi JJE. Development of predictive algorithms for the wear resistance of denture teeth materials. J Mech Behav Biomed Mater. 2023;144:105984. https://doi.org/10.1016/j.jmbbm.2023.105984.
22. Alarifi A, AlZubi AA. Memetic search optimization along with genetic scale recurrent neural network for predictive rate of implant treatment. J Med Syst. 2018;42:202. https://doi.org/10.1007/s10916-018-1051-1.
23. Rekawek P, Herbst EA, Suri A, Ford BP, Rajapakse CS, Panchal N. Machine learning and artificial intelligence: a web-based implant failure and peri-implantitis prediction model for clinicians. Int J Oral Maxillofac Implants. 2023;38:576–582b. https://doi.org/10.11607/jomi.9852.
24. Huang N, Liu P, Yan Y, Xu L, Huang Y, Fu G, Lan Y, Yang S, Song J, Li Y. Predicting the risk of dental implant loss using deep learning. J Clin Periodontol. 2022;49:872–83. https://doi.org/10.1111/jcpe.13689.
25. Oh S, Kim YJ, Kim J, Jung JH, Lim HJ, Kim BC, Kim KG. Deep learning-based prediction of osseointegration for dental implant using plain radiography. BMC Oral Health. 2023;23:208. https://doi.org/10.1186/s12903-023-02921-3.
26. Liu M, Wang S, Chen H, Liu Y. A pilot study of a deep learning approach to detect marginal bone loss around implants. BMC Oral Health. 2022;22:11. https://doi.org/10.1186/s12903-021-02035-8.
27. Raith S, Vogel EP, Anees N, Keul C, Güth J-F, Edelhoff D, Fischer H. Artificial neural networks as a powerful numerical tool to classify specific features of a tooth based on 3D scan data. Comput Biol Med. 2017;80:65–76. https://doi.org/10.1016/j.compbiomed.2016.11.013.
28. Zhang B, Dai N, Tian S, Yuan F, Yu Q. The extraction method of tooth preparation margin line based on S-Octree CNN. Int J Numer Method Biomed Eng. 2019;35(10):e3241. https://doi.org/10.1002/cnm.3241.
29. Chen Y, Lee JKY, Kwong G, Pow EHN, Tsoi JKH. Morphology and fracture behavior of lithium disilicate dental crowns designed by human and knowledge-based AI. J Mech Behav Biomed Mater. 2022;131:105256. https://doi.org/10.1016/j.jmbbm.2022.105256.
30. Ding H, Cui Z, Maghami E, Chen Y, Matinlinna JP, Pow EHN, Fok ASL, Burrow MF, Wang W, Tsoi JKH. Morphology and mechanical performance of dental crown designed by 3D-DCGAN. Dent Mater. 2023;39:320–32. https://doi.org/10.1016/j.dental.2023.02.001.
31. Hwang JJ, Azernikov S, Efros AA, Yu SX. Learning beyond human expertise with generative models for dental restorations. arXiv:1804.00064. 2018. https://doi.org/10.48550/arXiv.1804.00064.
32. Tian S, Wang M, Dai N, Ma H, Li L, Fiorenza L, Sun Y, Li Y. DCPR-GAN: dental crown prosthesis restoration using two-stage generative adversarial networks. IEEE J Biomed Heal Informatics. 2022;26:151–60. https://doi.org/10.1109/JBHI.2021.3119394.
33. Chen Q, Lin S, Wu J, Lyu P, Zhou Y. Automatic drawing of customized removable partial denture diagrams based on textual design for the clinical decision support system. J Oral Sci. 2020;62:236–8. https://doi.org/10.2334/josnusd.19-0138.
34. Zhang J, Xia JJ, Li J, Zhou X. Reconstruction-based digital dental occlusion of the partially edentulous dentition. IEEE J Biomed Heal Informatics. 2017;21:201–10. https://doi.org/10.1109/JBHI.2015.2500191.
35. Sporring J, Hommelhoff Jensen K. Bayes reconstruction of missing teeth. J Math Imaging Vis. 2008;31:245–54. https://doi.org/10.1007/s10851-008-0081-6.
36. Richert R, Alsheghri AA, Alageel O, Caron E, Song J, Ducret M, Tamimi F. Analytical model of I-bar clasps for removable partial dentures. Dent Mater. 2021;37:1066–72. https://doi.org/10.1016/j.dental.2021.03.018.
37. Kois JC, Zeitler JM, Barmak AB, Yilmaz B, Gómez-Polo M, Revilla-León M. Discrepancies in the occlusal devices designed by an experienced dental laboratory technician and by 2 artificial intelligence-based automatic programs. J Prosthet Dent. 2023:S0022-3913(23)00551-6. https://doi.org/10.1016/j.prosdent.2023.08.015.
38. Dawood A, Marti BM, Sauret-Jackson V, Darwood A. 3D printing in dentistry. Br Dent J. 2015;219:521–9. https://doi.org/10.1038/sj.bdj.2015.914.
39. Grischke J, Johannsmeier L, Eich L, Griga L, Haddadin S. Dentronics: towards robotics and artificial intelligence in dentistry. Dent Mater. 2020;36:765–78. https://doi.org/10.1016/j.dental.2020.03.021.
40. Regassa Hunde B, Debebe Woldeyohannes A. Future prospects of computer-aided design (CAD)—a review from the perspective of artificial intelligence (AI), extended reality, and 3D printing. Results Eng. 2022;14:100478. https://doi.org/10.1016/j.rineng.2022.100478.
41. Hashmi AW, Mali HS, Meena A, Khilji IA, Hashmi MF, Mohd Saffe SN. Artificial intelligence techniques for implementation of intelligent machining. Mater Today Proc. 2022;56:1947–55. https://doi.org/10.1016/j.matpr.2021.11.277.
42. Shan T, Tay FR, Gu L. Application of artificial intelligence in dentistry. J Dent Res. 2021;100:232–44. https://doi.org/10.1177/0022034520969115.
43. van Riet TCT, Chin Jen Sem KTH, Ho JTF, Spijker R, Kober J, de Lange J. Robot technology in dentistry, part two of a systematic review: an overview of initiatives. Dent Mater. 2021;37(8):1227–36. https://doi.org/10.1016/j.dental.2021.06.002.
44. Westgarth D. Artificial intelligence vs assisted intelligence in dentistry. BDJ In Practice. 2023;36(6):14–8. https://doi.org/10.1038/s41404-023-2039-1.

45. Rawal S. Guided innovations: robot-assisted dental implant surgery. J Prosthet Dent. 2022;127:673–4. https://doi.org/10.1016/j.prosdent.2022.03.029.
46. Olivetto M, Bettoni J, Testelin S, Lefranc M. Zygomatic implant placement using a robot-assisted flapless protocol: proof of concept. Int J Oral Maxillofac Surg. 2023;52:710–5. https://doi.org/10.1016/j.ijom.2022.12.002.
47. Kwon H-B, Park Y-S, Han J-S. Augmented reality in dentistry: a current perspective. Acta Odontol Scand. 2018;76:497–503. https://doi.org/10.1080/00016357.2018.1441437.
48. Farronato M, Maspero C, Lanteri V, Fama A, Ferrati F, Pettenuzzo A, Farronato D. Current state of the art in the use of augmented reality in dentistry: a systematic review of the literature. BMC Oral Health. 2019;19:135. https://doi.org/10.1186/s12903-019-0808-3.
49. Huang T, Yang C, Hsieh Y, Wang J, Hung C. Augmented reality (AR) and virtual reality (VR) applied in dentistry. Kaohsiung J Med Sci. 2018;34:243–8. https://doi.org/10.1016/j.kjms.2018.01.009.
50. Touati R, Richert R, Millet C, Farges J-C, Sailer I, Ducret M. Comparison of two innovative strategies using augmented reality for communication in aesthetic dentistry: a pilot study. J. Healthc. Eng. 2019;2019:1–6. https://doi.org/10.1155/2019/7019046.
51. Marchand L, Touati R, Fehmer V, Ducret M, Sailer I. Latest advances in augmented reality technology and its integration into the digital workflow. Int J Comput Dent. 2020;23:397–408. http://www.ncbi.nlm.nih.gov/pubmed/33491935
52. Lahoud P, Jacobs R, Boisse P, EzEldeen M, Ducret M, Richert R. Precision medicine using patient-specific modelling: state of the art and perspectives in dental practice. Clin Oral Investig. 2022;26(8):5117–28. https://doi.org/10.1007/s00784-022-04572-0.
53. Rodrigues MP, Soares PBF, Valdivia ADCM, Pessoa RS, Veríssimo C, Versluis A, Soares CJ. Patient-specific finite element analysis of Fiber post and ferrule design. J Endod. 2017;43(9):1539–44. https://doi.org/10.1016/j.joen.2017.04.024.
54. Richert R, Farges JC, Villat C, Valette S, Boisse P, Ducret M. Decision support for removing fractured endodontic instruments: a patient-specific approach. Appl Sci. 2021;11:2602. https://doi.org/10.3390/app11062602.
55. Knoops PGM, Papaioannou A, Borghi A, Breakey RWF, Wilson AT, Jeelani O, Zafeiriou S, Steinbacher D, Padwa BL, Dunaway DJ, Schievano S. A machine learning framework for automated diagnosis and computer-assisted planning in plastic and reconstructive surgery. Sci Rep. 2019;9:1–12. https://doi.org/10.1038/s41598-019-49506-1.
56. Barone S, Paoli A, Razionale AV, Savignano R. Computational design and engineering of polymeric orthodontic aligners. Int J Numer Method Biomed Eng. 2017;33:1–15. https://doi.org/10.1002/cnm.2839.
57. Juloski J, Apicella D, Ferrari M. The effect of ferrule height on stress distribution within a tooth restored with fibre posts and ceramic crown: a finite element analysis. Dent Mater. 2014;30:1304–15. https://doi.org/10.1016/j.dental.2014.09.004.
58. Sigmund O. A 99 line topology optimization code written in matlab. Struct Multidiscip Optim. 2001;21:120–7. https://doi.org/10.1007/s001580050176.
59. Alageel O, Alsheghri AA, Algezani S, Caron E, Tamimi F. Determining the retention of removable partial dentures. J Prosthet Dent. 2019;122:55–62.e3. https://doi.org/10.1016/j.prosdent.2018.06.015.
60. Kuroshima S, Kaku M, Ishimoto T, Sasaki M, Nakano T, Sawase T. A paradigm shift for bone quality in dentistry: a literature review. J Prosthodont Res. 2017;61:353–62. https://doi.org/10.1016/j.jpor.2017.05.006.
61. Roy S, Dey S, Khutia N, Roy A, Datta S. Design of patient specific dental implant using FE analysis and computational intelligence techniques. Appl Soft Comput J. 2018;65:272–9. https://doi.org/10.1016/j.asoc.2018.01.025.
62. Parthasarathy J. 3D modeling, custom implants and its future perspectives in craniofacial surgery. Ann Maxillofac Surg. 2014;4:9. https://doi.org/10.4103/2231-0746.133065.
63. Tamura N, Takaki T, Takano N, Shibahara T. Three-dimensional finite element analysis of bone fixation in bilateral sagittal split ramus osteotomy using individual models. Bull Tokyo Dent Coll. 2018;59:67–78. https://doi.org/10.2209/tdcpublication.2013-3000.
64. Cheng K, Liu Y, Wang R, Zhang J, Jiang X. Topological optimization of 3D printed bone analog with PEKK for surgical mandibular reconstruction. J Mech Behav Biomed Mater. 2020;107:103758. https://doi.org/10.1016/j.jmbbm.2020.103758.

6 Artificial Intelligence Applications in Orthodontics

Yashodhan M. Bichu, Bingshuang Zou, Prabhat Kumar Chaudhari, Samar M. Adel, and Nikhillesh Vaiid

6.1 Simplifying the AI Jargon

Terms, such as artificial intelligence (AI), machine learning (ML), neural networks (NN), and deep learning (DL), slowly crept into our lives over the last few decades and have now become deeply entwined in our day-to-day lives rapidly over the last few years with the result that we have become accustomed to them, perhaps without properly comprehending their true connotations. These terms often tend to be used interchangeably in conversations, and although these technologies are inter-related, they do exhibit innate differences [1].

Perhaps the easiest way to think about them is like a Venn diagram, where each next entity is essentially a subset of the prior term, when arranged as AI, ML, and DL. AI, the broadest term, is used to classify machines that mimic human intelligence and can be used to predict, automate, and optimize tasks that humans have historically performed, such as speech and facial recognition, decision-making, and translation. Artificial narrow intelligence (ANI), artificial general intelligence (AGI), and artificial super intelligence (ASI) are the three main categories of AI, with ANI considered as "weak" AI and the other two types classified as "strong" AI [1].

Machine learning is a subset of artificial intelligence that allows for optimization. Classical or "non-deep" machine learning is more dependent on human intervention to learn, where human experts determine the hierarchy of features to understand the differences between data inputs, usually requiring more structured data to learn. "Deep" machine learning or simply deep learning, a subdomain of ML, can leverage labeled datasets, also known as supervised learning, to inform its algorithm, but it doesn't necessarily require a labeled dataset. It can ingest unstructured data in its raw form, such as text and/or images, and it can automatically determine the set of features, which distinguish different entities from one another.

Y. M. Bichu
Graduate Orthodontics, Faculty of Dentistry, University of British Columbia, Vancouver, BC, Canada

B. Zou
Oral Health Sciences, Faculty of Dentistry, University of British Columbia, Vancouver, BC, Canada
e-mail: drzou@dentistry.ubc.ca

P. K. Chaudhari
Division of Orthodontics and Dentofacial Deformities, Centre for Dental Education Research (CDER), All India Institute of Medical Sciences, New Delhi, New Delhi, India
e-mail: dr.prabhatkc@aiims.edu

S. M. Adel
Department of Orthodontics, Faculty of Dentistry, Alexandria University, Alexandria, Egypt

N. Vaiid (✉)
National University of Singapore, Singapore, Singapore

Saveetha Dental College, Chennai, Tamil Nadu, India

F. Schwendicke et al. (eds.), *Artificial Intelligence for Oral Health Care*,
https://doi.org/10.1007/978-3-031-84047-0_6

DL's precursor is an artificial neural network (ANN), which mimics the human brain through a set of algorithms. At a basic level, a neural network is comprised of four main components: inputs, weights, a bias or threshold, and an output. The "deep" in deep learning refers to the depth of layers in a neural network. A neural network that typically consists of more than three layers, inclusive of the inputs and the output, can be considered a form of deep learning algorithm. Figure 6.1 provides a simplistic classification of common AI terminologies and popular ML algorithms.

Liu et al. [2] have mentioned that classification, regression, detection, and segmentation can be considered to be the four major AI-driven tasks in dentistry (Fig. 6.2). Specific to orthodontics, classification can be applied to skeletal patterns or assessment of growth and development. Regression could be applied for clinical decision-making, such as to determine the extraction decision. Detection could include automatic identification of landmarks and acquisition of tooth segmentation can be categorized under segmentation tasks. ANN and its variants, along with DT and RF, constitute bulk of the ML algorithms utilized for diverse orthodontic applications. Table 6.1 depicts commonly utilized ML algorithms with their description and specific orthodontic applications pertaining to these tasks.

Classification is the most well-known of these tasks and refers to assigning objects or features to prespecified categories. The common classification algorithms include Naïve Bayes (NB), support vector machine (SVM), logistic regression (LR), decision trees (DT) and Forests (RF), and artificial neural network (ANN). In orthodontics, classification algorithms have been utilized for various clinical applications, such as automatic detection of cephalometric landmarks, prediction of need for orthodontic treatment, determination of cervical vertebrae maturation, determination of facial attractiveness from orthodontic photographs, and for classification of skeletal patterns.

Regression analysis can be applied to investigate the relationships between multiple variables and predict dependent variables based on independent variables. Regression methods could be linear or logistic and can also be integrated into ML models based on DT and RF. Some of the hitherto published orthodontic applications of LR models include determination of cervical vertebrae maturation and genetic risk assessment of infants with non-syndromic orofacial clefts.

Segmentation in AI refers to defining the contours of an object, whereas detection looks to define the position of objects. CNN algorithms have been utilized in orthodontics for automatic individual teeth segmentation from digital dental casts and RNN programs have been used for automatic tooth root segmentation of CBCT images. One of the most advanced object detection algorithms currently available is the you only look once (YOLO), which has been utilized in orthodontics for automated cephalometric landmark detection as well as automatic detection of facial landmarks on 2D facial images [2].

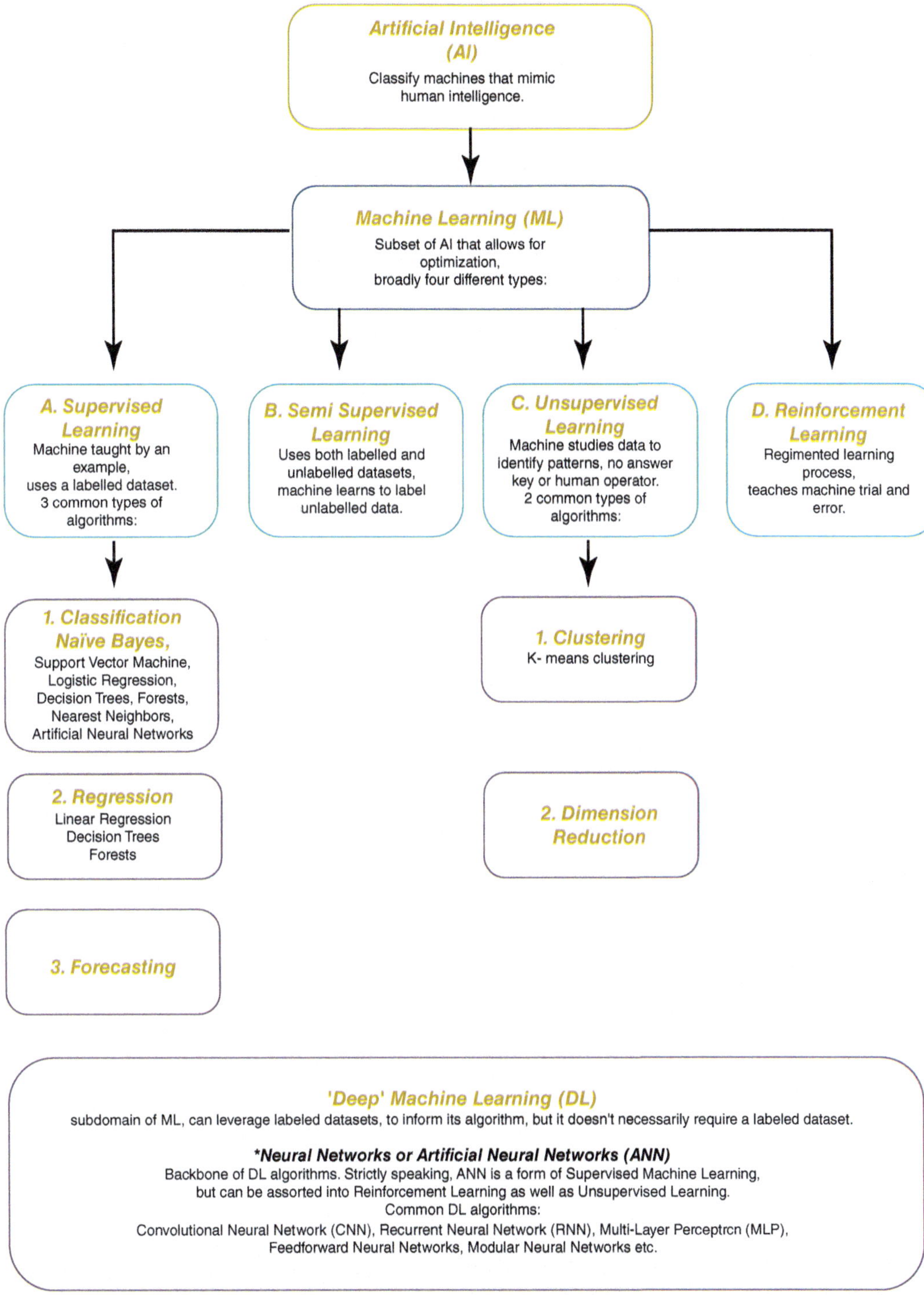

Fig. 6.1 Simplistic classification of common AI terminologies and popular ML algorithms

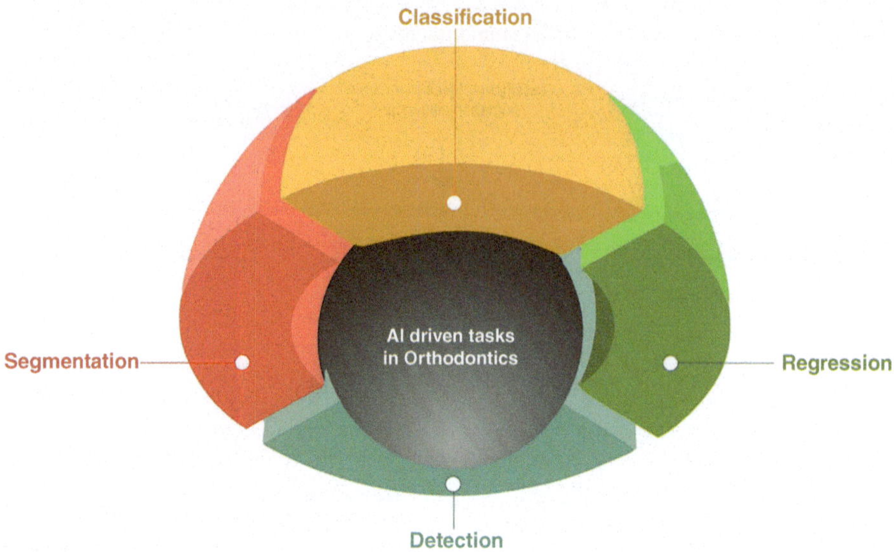

Fig. 6.2 Four major AI-driven task groups in orthodontics

Table 6.1 Commonly utilized ML algorithms with their description and previously studied orthodontic applications

Sr. no.	Name of ML algorithm	Algorithm type	Algorithm description	Orthodontic applications investigated previously utilizing this algorithm
1.	Naïve Bayes (NB)	Supervised learning: classification type	• Classifies every value as independent of other values • Predicts category based on given set of features utilizing probability	• Automatic detection of cephalometric landmarks • Prediction of need for orthodontic treatment • Determination of cervical vertebrae maturation
2.	Support vector machine (SVM)	Supervised learning: classification type	• Filters data into categories, by providing set of training examples • Marks each set as belonging to one or the other category • Builds a model that assigns new values to either category	• Determination of cervical vertebrae maturation • Genetic risk assessment of infants with non-syndromic orofacial clefts • Design treatment plan based on freeform documents written by dentists • Determination of facial attractiveness from orthodontic photographs • Classification of skeletal patterns
3.	Logistic regression (LR)	Supervised learning: classification type	• Estimates probability of an event occurring based on previous data provided • Covers a binary dependent variable, where only 2 values, 0 and 1, represent outcomes	• Determination of cervical vertebrae maturation • Genetic risk assessment of infants with non-syndromic orofacial clefts
4.	Decision trees (DT)	Supervised learning: classification/ regression type	• Flowchart like tree structure that uses a balancing method to illustrate every possible outcome of a decision • Each node within a tree represents a test on a specific variable • Each branch is the outcome of that test	• Determination of cervical vertebrae maturation • Detection of craniofacial morphology patterns • Automatic detection of cephalometric landmarks • Evaluation of orthodontic treatment progression
5.	Forests (RF)	Supervised learning: classification/ regression	• Random decision forest is an ensemble learning method, combining multiple algorithms to generate better results for classification, regression, and other tasks • Starts with a decision tree with input entered at the top that then travels down the tree with data segmented into progressively smaller sets, based on specific variables	• Assessment of maxillary structure variation in unilateral canine impaction • Determination of cervical vertebrae maturation • Automatic detection of cephalometric landmarks • Determination of tooth extraction decision • Prediction of cessation of orthodontic treatment • Prediction of blood loss prior to orthognathic surgery • Prediction of features in success of pre-orthodontic treatment in cleft lip and palate patients
6.	Nearest neighbors (KNN)	Supervised learning	• K-nearest neighbor estimates how likely a datapoint is to being a member of one group or another • Looks at datapoints around a single data point to determine what group it actually is in	• Determination of cervical vertebrae maturation

(continued)

Table 6.1 (continued)

Sr. no.	Name of ML algorithm	Algorithm type	Algorithm description	Orthodontic applications investigated previously utilizing this algorithm
7.	K-means clustering	Unsupervised learning clustering	• Categorizes unlabeled data or data without defined categories or groups • Works by finding groups within data, number of groups represented by variable K • Works iteratively to assign each data point to one of K groups based on features provided	• Detection of craniofacial morphology patterns
8.	Artificial neural networks (ANN) Backbone of DL. Common algorithms: Convolutional neural network (CNN), recurrent neural network (RNN), multilayer perceptron (MLP), etc.	Strictly speaking, ANN form of supervised learning But can be assorted into reinforcement as well as unsupervised learning	• Large number of interconnected processing elements, working in unison to solve specific problems • Learn by examples as well as experience • Extremely useful for modeling nonlinear relationships in high-dimensional data or where relationship among input variables is difficult to understand	• Determination of extraction decision, prediction of extraction patterns, and anchorage planning • Determination of cervical vertebrae maturation (ANN) • Automatic determination of archform shape (ANN) • Automatic detection of cephalometric landmarks (CNN most commonly used) • Estimation of human age based on OPG samples (CNN) • Automatic orthodontic diagnostic imaging system (CNN) • Automatic individual teeth segmentation from digital dental casts (CNN) • Quantification of 3D asymmetry of maxilla in patients with unilateral cleft lip and palate (CNN) • Automatic tooth root segmentation of CBCT images (RNN) • Prediction of need and type of orthognathic surgery in skeletal malocclusions (ANN, RNN) • Diagnosis of facial distortions (CNN, RNN)

6.2 Mapping Contemporary Evidence

Literature on the applications of AI and ML across various healthcare fields has grown exponentially over the last two decades [3–6]. Orthodontics, although a slow starter on this terrain, has now been enriched with a considerable number of systematic and scoping reviews on these applications, especially over the last 5 years.

Bichu et al. [1] conducted one of the first scoping reviews mapping the diverse applications of AI and ML in the field of orthodontics in 2021. The authors mentioned that one of the earliest studies to document the utilization of AI in the field of orthodontics was published in a non-orthodontic journal back in 1986. Their scoping review, which included 62 original studies, outlined the fact that there was a progressive increase in publications related to the applications of AI and ML in orthodontics from 7 in 1991–2000 to 12 in 2001–2010 to 43 in 2011–2020, with majority of studies originating from the USA, South Korea, Japan, and China and also the fact that studies on this topic tended to be published more commonly in non-orthodontic journals rather than orthodontic specialty journals. This scoping review also revealed that artificial neural networks (ANN), convolutional neural networks (CNN), and support vector machine (SVM) were some of the commonly utilized AL/ML algorithms. Furthermore, orthodontic diagnosis and treatment planning, automated anatomic landmark detection, and assessment of growth and development were the most commonly studied domains in orthodontics.

A similar scoping review by Monill-Gonzalez and coauthors [7], searched electronic literature from January 2010 till March 2021 and included 17 eligible publications that evaluated various applications of AI and ML in orthodontics. This scoping review demonstrated that CNN was the most commonly utilized ML algorithm and that automated detection of cephalometric landmarks, determination of extractions for orthodontic treatment, evaluation of cervical vertebral maturation for assessment of growth, and automated tooth segmentation were the commonly assessed AI applications. The authors concluded that AI could improve orthodontic diagnostic accuracy and help the orthodontist work more efficiently and accurately.

Another scoping review in 2021, by Mohammad-Rahimi and coworkers [8], included 49 papers published between January 2010 and July 2020. These authors reaffirmed that AI technology had achieved state-of-the-art results in various orthodontic applications, such as automated landmark detection on lateral cephalograms and photography images, cervical vertebra maturation degree determination, skeletal classifications, orthodontic tooth extraction decisions, prediction of the need for orthodontic treatment or orthognathic surgery, and determination of facial attractiveness. This scoping review found that majority of the AI models used in these applications were based on ANN.

In addition to the aforementioned studies, evidence gleaned from contemporary studies and recent systematic reviews specific to major clinical applications of AI and ML in orthodontics has been outlined in the ensuing section of this chapter.

6.3 Applications of AI and ML in Orthodontics: Key Domains

Although previously mentioned scoping reviews and other published studies document numerous applications of AI and ML algorithms in the field of orthodontics, majority of these applications can typically be organized into four major domains as succinctly summarized by Orhan and Amasya [9] and have been illustrated in Fig. 6.3.

1. Diagnosis and treatment planning: either broad-based or for specific condition(s)
2. Prediction analysis and/or evaluation of treatment outcomes
3. Appliance and/or treatment monitoring
4. Patient engagement

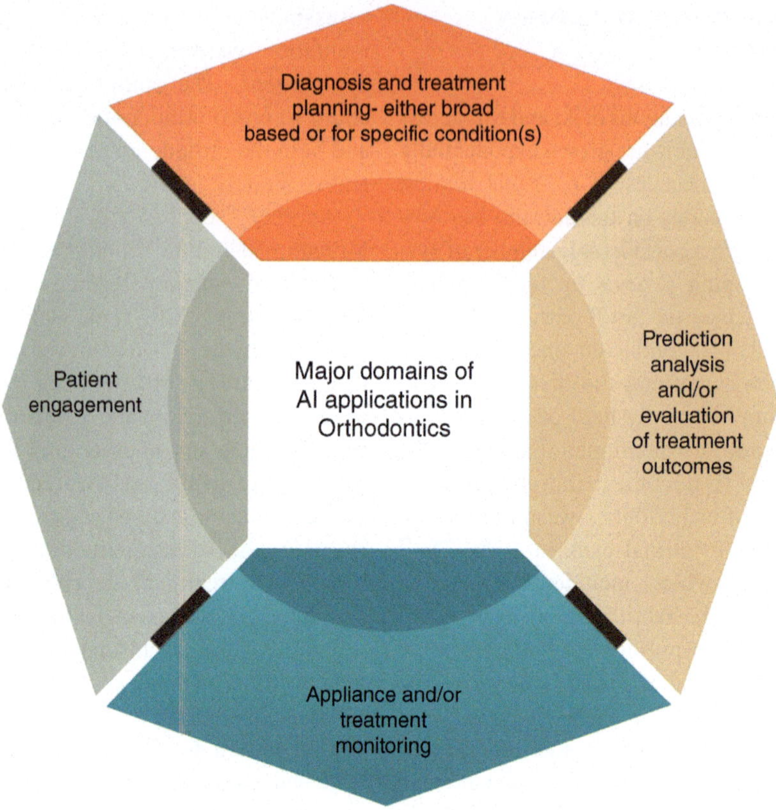

Fig. 6.3 Major domains of AI applications in orthodontics

6.3.1 Diagnosis and Treatment Planning: Either Broad-Based or for Specific Condition(S)

Diagnosis remains the cornerstone of successful orthodontic treatment, and, unsurprisingly, the major clinical domain, where varied AI and ML algorithms find majority of their application in orthodontics, is for diagnosis and treatment planning. AI and ML algorithms are based on the availability of digital patient data. Digital data in orthodontics could be radiographic, as obtained from two-dimensional imaging techniques, such as lateral cephalograms, frontal cephalograms, or panoramic radiographs, or as obtained from three-dimensional imaging techniques, such as cone-beam computed tomography (CBCT). Further, intraoral and extraoral volumetric optical scanners now provide detailed information related to intraoral and extraoral surfaces respectively. Data from the above sources can be combined together to constitute a patient-specific data input set, which can then be analyzed by various ML algorithms to create a partial or fully automated digital workflow system that may help improve diagnostic accuracy and treatment planning efficiency [9].

Literature shows that a large number of publications have focused on automated anatomic landmark detection and/or analyses, chiefly from lateral cephalograms initially and increasingly from CBCT images recently, to improve the accuracy of landmark detection and analyses and to reduce human time and effort spent in these applications.

Liu et al. [2] have previously highlighted some of the commercially available applications based on ML algorithms for orthodontic purposes. These have been presented in Table 6.2.

Schwendicke and coauthors [10] in 2021 performed a systematic review (SR) and meta-analysis to assess the accuracy and underlying

Table 6.2 Commercial applications based on ML algorithms for orthodontic purposes

Commercial manufacturer	Country of origin	Application name	Website	Application purpose
ORCA dental AI	Las Vegas, USA	Cephx	https://www.orca-ai.com/	Cephalometric analysis, teeth segmentation, and airway analysis
CellmatiQ GmbH	Hamburg, Germany	DentaliQ ortho DentaliQ opg	https://cellmatiq.com/	Cephalometric analysis, detection of dental disease
Uceph	Chengdu, China	Uceph	http://www.uceph.com/	Cephalometric analysis
Zhibeicloud	Chengdu, China	Zhibeicloud	https://www.aortho360.com/	Cephalometric analysis, analysis of bone age, and analysis facial esthetics

evidence for DL for cephalometric landmark detection on 2D and 3D radiographs. This paper included 19 eligible studies published between 2017 and 2020, all utilizing CNN algorithms. The authors found that applicability concerns were detected for most studies, chiefly with regard to selection of data and conduct of reference test. This SR concluded that DL showed relatively high accuracy for detecting landmarks on cephalometric imagery and that, although the overall body of evidence was consistent, it suffered from high risk of bias. Furthermore, majority of studies focused on 2D imaging and data on 3D imagery although sparse, looked promising. The authors suggested that future studies could focus on improving generalizability, robustness, and clinical usefulness of DL for this specific application.

"To extract or not to extract" has been the question in orthodontics since time immemorial, with substantial variability noted between extraction decision planning of different orthodontists. The second major diagnostic and treatment planning application of ML algorithms is the development of decision support systems that minimize the relative subjectivity associated with orthodontic extraction decision-making. Li et al. [11] in 2019 demonstrated that ANNs were successful in prediction of extraction decision, determination of extraction pattern, as well determination of the anchorage pattern. Choi et al. [12] in 2019 further expanded their use for the diagnosis of orthognathic surgery decision and the type of surgery selection in addition to the extraction decision. Evangelista and coworkers [13] outlined the accuracy of artificial intelligence algorithms to determine the decision of tooth extraction in orthodontics through a systematic review and meta-analysis in 2022. This paper included six studies and showed an unclear risk of bias of patient selection. Data were pooled in a random model and yielded an accuracy value of 0.87 (95% CI = 0.75–0.96) for all studies, 0.89 (95% CI = 0.70–1.00) for multilayer perceptron, and 0.88 (95% CI = 0.73–0.98) for back propagation models. Sensitivity, specificity, and area under the curve of the multilayer perceptron model yielded 0.84 (95% CI = 0.58–1.00), 0.89 (95% CI = 0.74–0.98), and 0.92 (95% CI = 0.72–1.00) scores, respectively. Sagittal discrepancy, upper crowding, and protrusion showed the highest ranks weighted in the models. This paper concluded that orthodontic tooth extraction decision-making using AI presented promising accuracy but should be considered with caution due to the very low certainty of evidence.

Apart from automatic anatomic landmark detection and extraction decision planning, the third common application of ML algorithms in orthodontic diagnosis and treatment planning has been found to be the evaluation of cervical vertebral maturation for the assessment of growth and development of the orthodontic patient. Mathew et al. [14] in 2022 conducted a systematic review to assess the accuracy of identification and/or classification of the stage of cervical vertebrae maturity on lateral cephalograms by neural networks and compare it to that determined by human observers. This SR included eight eligible publications and found that the accuracy of the models on the test data ranged from 50% to more than 90%. All the studies were found to exhibit concerns regarding the risk of bias in the index test and the reference standards. The authors concluded that although neural networks could detect and classify cervical vertebrae maturation stages on lateral cephalograms, future studies should be conducted to develop robust models using appropriate reference standards.

Apart from the aforementioned three major applications, ML algorithms have been utilized to investigate a multitude of other diagnostic clinical applications in orthodontics including but not limited to the detection of temporomandibular joint osteoarthritis (TMJ-OA), assessment of maxillary constriction and/or impaction of maxillary canines, screening of osteoporosis from panoramic radiographs, classification of skeletal patterns, assessment of airflow dynamics and prediction of obstructive sleep apnea (OSA), genetic risk assessment of non-syndromic orofacial clefts, and selection of orthodontic appliances, including headgears, fixed appliances and removable appliances, and devise models to create referral application to optimize orthodontic referrals in a public oral healthcare system and to examine postoperative infections following orthognathic surgeries [1, 7, 8, 15, 16].

6.3.2 Prediction Analysis and/or Evaluation of Treatment Outcomes

ML tools have been utilized for predictive analytics, such as assessing the need for orthodontic treatment, predicting the outcome of planned orthodontic treatment for specific types of malocclusions, as well evaluating the outcome of orthodontic and/or combined ortho-surgical treatment.

Wang et al. [17] in 2016 investigated an eye-tracking method to predict orthodontic treatment need and treatment outcome from the lay perspective in an objective way and compared it to traditional methods. The study utilized support vector machine techniques and concluded that the eye-tracking device was able to objectively quantify the effect of malocclusion on facial perception and the impact of orthodontic treatment on malocclusion from a lay perspective. Thanathornwong [18] utilized the Bayesian network for an assessment of the need for orthodontic treatment and concluded that the results obtained by the decision support system were comparable with those suggested by expert orthodontists.

In addition to the assessment of need for orthodontic treatment, predictions of orthodontic treatment outcomes in patients with class II malocclusions utilizing ML algorithms have also been reported [19]. Kim et al. [20], as early as in 2009, evaluated a feature wrapping method for the prediction of prognosis for class III malocclusions. Auconi et al. [21] then developed a system to predict treatment outcomes in patients with untreated class III malocclusions through orthodontic data mining. Unsupervised learning was utilized to cluster patients as hypermandibular, hyperdivergent, or balanced based on their cephalometric variables. The system was then applied to a treated sample, where it showed that all of the unsuccessful cases belonged to either the hypermandibular or the hyperdivergent cluster. Auconi et al. [22] had previously also attempted to identify critical peculiarities of class II and class III malocclusions and demonstrated that class II subjects exhibited few highly connected orthodontic features, while class III patients showed more compact network structure characterized by strong co-occurrence of normal and abnormal clinical functional and radiological features. The authors concluded that network analysis could allow orthodontists to visually evaluate and anticipate the co-occurrence of auxological anomalies during individual craniofacial growth and possibly localize reactive sites for a therapeutic approach to a malocclusion.

The third area of applicability of AI algorithms within the predictive analytics domain is the evaluation of treatment outcomes and the effect of orthognathic surgery on facial appearance and age perception as evidenced by two studies of Patcas et al. [23, 24] Algorithms employed in these studies concluded that the appearance of majority of patients appearance improved with treatment (66.4%), resulting in a younger appearance of nearly 1 year, especially after a profile altering surgery. Similar improvement was noted on facial attractiveness in 74.7% of patients, especially after lower jaw surge, and the authors concluded that AI might be considered to score facial attractiveness and apparent age in orthognathic patients.

AI tools can pool past treatment data, combine it with patient specific characteristics including malocclusion complexity and patient compliance, and incorporate multiple treatment plans to make precise predictions of expected treatment outcome. This may help estimate treatment duration, predict treatment success, evaluate long-term treatment stability, and thus guide customized treatment planning. Incorporation of these tools in routine clinical practice may help the patient better understand the nuances involved in orthodontic treatment and offer the opportunity to make shared decisions for more predictable results. As every individual's growth and development varies, each patient's response to treatment differs as well, and individualized predictive analytics could help attain results closer to patient expectations. However, it is essential to impress upon the patient that the AI/ML simulations are merely estimates and may not accurately reflect the definitive final treatment outcomes, especially in the early stages of development of these algorithms [9].

6.3.3 Appliance and/or Treatment Monitoring

Orthodontics traditionally relies upon patient compliance and regular follow up examinations to monitor treatment progress and clinicians plan chairside appointment schedules that can be optimally coordinated with patient's biological response to the forces applied. Typical schedules can range from weekly changes for aligner patients to 4-to-8-week intervals for traditional orthodontic patients. The advent of teleorthodontics has now enabled remote and proactive monitoring of patient's orthodontic treatment, thereby allowing customization of appointment frequency on the basis of an actual requirement for in-office visits, rather than conventional scheduling [25].

Artificial Intelligence Driven Remote Monitoring (AIDRM) technology has now made it possible for patients to capture pictures or videos of their mouths at home, which are then analyzed by AI-powered image analysis software trained to recognize specific features. By using DL, the neural network of the software improves its ability to detect these attributes. Dental monitoring (DM; Paris, France) utilizes smartphone technology to facilitate orthodontist-patient interaction and remotely monitor treatment progress. DM relies on patients recording images of their dentition (DM scans) using their smartphones and a standardized check retractor, on regular intervals prescribed by the clinician, and then uploading them to the DM application on their smartphone. DM software then uses AI to detect occlusal changes during orthodontic treatment, tooth movement tracking, aligner unseating, missing brackets, and patient compliance. The DM software then sends specific notifications to the patient and real-time data to the clinician on the basis of the conditions detected by the AI algorithm [26].

Proponents of DM mention a reduction in tooth movement tracking problems, a reduction in the number of additional or refinement clear aligners, and an overall treatment duration, in addition to a reduction in the number of clinic visits and enhanced patient convenience. Hansa et al. [25] showed that the use of DM with Invisalign clear aligner therapy resulted in a reduced number of appointments by 3.5 visits (33.1%). The DM group also achieved a clinically similar accuracy in obtaining predicted tooth movements compared with the control group in 1.7 fewer months, indicating improved aligner tracking in the DM group. Homsi et al. [26] demonstrated that DM AI algorithm can track tooth movement and reconstruct 3D digital models to a clinically acceptable degree for orthodontic application. Although remote monitoring systems cannot completely substitute detailed clinical examination, they can help identify problems during treatment issues early on, allowing orthodontists to initiate suitable intervention and alter the treatment plan as needed.

6.3.4 Patient Engagement

The advent of smartphones and wearable smart devices, ubiquitous Internet connectivity, and highly evolved DL algorithms have now resulted in significantly greater patient engagement in their orthodontic treatment as compared to couple of decades earlier. Virtual orthodontic consultations, retainer follow-up monitoring, tracking progress of clear aligner therapy, detection and monitoring of oral hygiene during orthodontic treatment, detection and monitoring of sleep disturbances and parafunctional oral habits, gaming, and app-based rewards related to compliance during orthodontic treatment are just some of the ways in which patient experience and engagement are undergoing a paradigm shift.

Communication systems, especially in the aftermath of COVID-19 pandemic, were specifically focused on virtual rather than in-person consultations and continue to be an increasing trend, providing benefits of reduction of chairside time for the clinician as well as time and finance benefits for both the patient and the clinician. AI integrated tools and technologies endeavor to provide user-friendly and secure remote communication between the patient and the orthodontist, allowing orthodontists and patients to collaborate effectively by enabling real-time videoconferencing and data sharing. Remote monitoring of clear aligners and retainers combined with virtual consultations can be used to make personalized recommendations. AI algorithms can also help maintain patient information private and secure during the virtual consultations, by protecting sensitive data by encryption and authentication systems as well as by discovering and stopping unwanted access or data breaches [9].

In addition to virtual consultations, wearable devices, and technologies specific to the orofacial region and important from an orthodontic perspective, for continuous, unobtrusive, and objective monitoring of appliance compliance, sleep disorders and obstructive sleep apnea, jaw function, and parafunction have been slowly gaining traction since the 1990s. Over the years, microelectronic sensors for monitoring compliance have been successfully embedded in functional appliances, appliances for sleep disorders, facemasks, headgears, removable appliances, and retainers. Long-term removable retainer wear is recommended post-orthodontic treatment, and microsensor-embedded retainers have been used to overcome the practical challenges associated with monitoring compliance. The majority of the sensors used intraorally are temperature-sensitive microsensors that detect and measure intraoral temperature when the appliances are in the mouth and translate the information into wear time. Dedicated software (Braebon Medical Corporation, Ottawa, ON, Canada) is used to convert data recorded by the sensor into wear time. Data from intra-oral microelectronic sensors are read using dedicated stations or may be transferred to a smartphone via Bluetooth in real-time [27].

Vaid et al. [28, 29] evaluated the scope and extent of the published literature on mobile apps in orthodontics and found that the domain outcome with the greatest representation in the literature was apps used in reminder therapy (41%). Patient reminders have been shown to improve compliance, reduce the number of missed appointments, improve oral hygiene, reduce white spot lesions, and reduce treatment times and bracket failure. The advantages of using these apps for reminder therapy are their low costs and simple implementation.

Smartphone apps are now available that allow users to perform an audio recording while they sleep to detect sounds related to teeth clenching and/or grinding as well as snoring and/or apnea-hypopnea episodes (Do I snore or grind, SleepScore Labs). ML algorithms then analyze these sounds to caution the patient about the possibility of parafunctional oral habits and snoring or sleep disorders, respectively, and seek appropriate dental and medical attention. The algorithms typically incorporate reinforcement learning in which increased data from multiple recordings from a greater number of patients further improves the capacity of the ML algorithms to detect abnormal patterns.

Virtual reality (VR) and augmented reality (AR) technologies can be utilized for educational purposes as well as providing patient care.

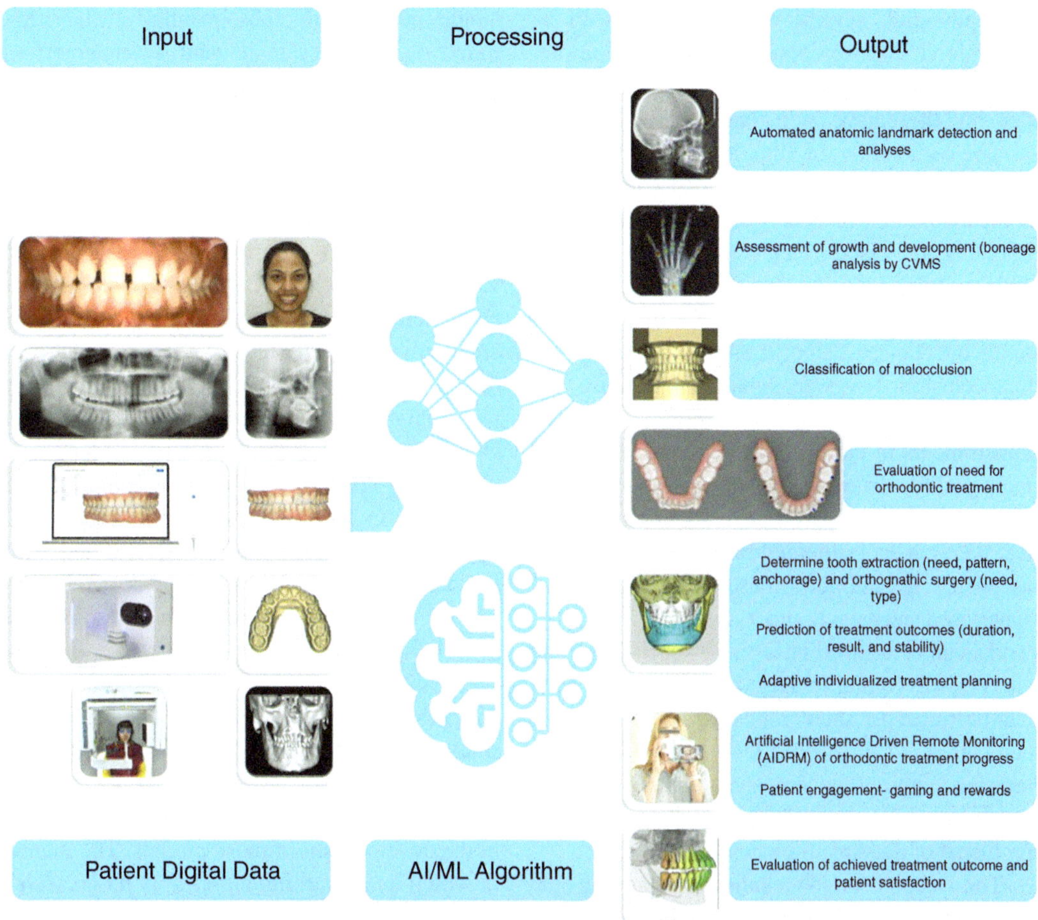

Fig. 6.4 Schematic illustration encapsulating the diverse applications of AI in orthodontics

Patients can experience 3D virtual simulations and visualize predictions about changes to their teeth alignment and dentofacial esthetics with orthodontic treatment over time. Expected treatment scenarios may be virtually demonstrated to the patient along with possible simulations of unexpected outcomes based on real patient data; this may help patients better comprehend the nature and course of their treatment, as well as help in pain and anxiety management [30]. Finally, gamification techniques, such as rewards or challenges, from smartphone-based apps can help increase patient compliance and motivation. Patients may earn points or badges for following prescribed treatment guidelines, practicing good oral hygiene, or attending appointments, which foster motivation and engagement throughout their orthodontic treatment journey [9]. Figure 6.4 provides a schematic illustration encapsulating the diverse applications of AI in orthodontics.

6.4 Translating Algorithms to Clinical Fruition: Possibilities and Challenges

AI and ML could potentially help provide high-quality diagnosis as well as assist optimal decision-making and in clinical orthodontics. DL algorithms can simplify protocols, save time, and provide objective predictable outcomes, especially in comparison to traditional procedures. Liu et al. [2] and Lee et al. [31] recently have aptly summarized how, despite their significant potential, several challenges need to be understood and overcome before AI can be successfully implemented into routine clinical practice, and these have been elucidated below.

The availability of high-quality datasets for orthodontic research is quite limited, especially in comparison to several other medical fields. Furthermore, discrepancies in training datasets make comparison between various AI-based models questionable. Supervised learning is currently the choice of algorithm for the diagnosis of malocclusion; however, significant expense and manpower associated with labeling are major impediments in the creation of standardized and high-quality datasets for orthodontic studies. When training data are repeatedly applied in the test stages, a data snooping bias is bound to occur as well. To mitigate these problems, semi-supervised and weakly supervised learning frameworks can be utilized in instances such as for the analysis of original images, and these have been demonstrated to show robustness and accuracy comparable to supervised learning. Additionally, transfer learning and few-shot learning methodologies could present alternatives to address the problems of data insufficiency [2].

The second major challenge plaguing the seamless clinical transition of AI algorithms into clinical applications is the reproducibility crisis, indicating that many of previously obtained research results cannot be successfully replicated when an identical investigation is conducted by another research team. Furthermore, researchers may inadvertently neglect the sensitivity of results to hyper-parameters, including but not limited to study rates, iteration times and initialization strategies. To address these issues, appropriate sensitivity tests should be performed to determine performance of the algorithm. Data cleaning technique could present itself as a viable alternative to minimize manual errors during data labeling and measurement that could improve the reproducibility of ML models [2].

Majority of the engineering models are saddled with "overfitting" issues, indicating the poor performance of these models in predicting unknown samples. AI-related studies tend to focus on homogenous samples sourced from a single center, and subsequentially, algorithms based on such a sample tend to underperform when applied to a larger and a more heterogenous population. Algorithm developers as well as healthcare providers should be aware of the pitfalls of applying AI tools to populations on which the algorithms were not developed or meant to represent [31]. Overfitting could be addressed in various ways, such as by a betterment in the external generalization abilities of ML models and by creation of diverse clinical scenarios for the validation of the model. Selecting the appropriate representative datasets is another means to address overfitting. Finally, various algorithms have been devised to specifically avoid overfitting issues, and these include early stopping, dropout, and regularization penalty. Multimodal learning methods can help integrate different types of data, such as images, and help attain superior results when processing imbalanced data [2].

Finally, integration of AI systems into contemporary orthodontic practice extends beyond solely clinical concerns. Deep learning typically relies on a black box method for the development of algorithms, with minimal human intervention in the development of these models. The manner in which deep learning algorithms progressively train and learn from hidden sequential layers of data is not very well understood. It can be surmised that neither the healthcare provider nor the algorithm developer of deep learning models can be fully cognizant as to why a particular decision was arrived at from the provided inputs. This could have far-reaching ethical and patient safety implications [31]. Possible risks related to the use of AI algorithms, especially in the aftermath of a medical or dental error, need to be clearly outlined to the patient, treating orthodontist and professional organizations, with legislations in place to protect orthodontists relying on these algorithms. AI algorithms could be utilized merely as support systems to assist healthcare professionals, or they may represent a fully functioning, independent, automated decision-making entity, in which the AI systems may be held accountable. Policymakers must work closely with the AI developers and healthcare providers, patients, and payers to ensure legal accountability [31].

6.5 Crystal Ball Gazing? Overcoming the Challenges!

AI-based systems are likely to profoundly influence and alter the fundamental manner in which clinicians practice, necessitating clinicians to continually adapt and evolve with emerging technologies to stay relevant in contemporary healthcare milieu. Successful incorporation of AI technologies in healthcare systems mandates keen interest and firm commitment from stakeholders within the healthcare systems, continuous technical support from ML algorithm developers, and relevant modifications within legal frameworks to protect all stakeholders [31].

The ethical problems in implementing ML in routine orthodontic procedures will need to be addressed. The "black-box" nature of ML algorithms necessitates the visualization and establishment of trust of both the patients and doctors, before clinical application can be considered. It is the inherent right of patients to completely understand about the basis, utility, and limitations of AI algorithms and ML models. Secondly, health data privacy may need to be expanded appropriately and redefined due to the increasing usage of electronic medical records. Finally, the legal liability distribution between treating orthodontists and ML models will need to be defined and continually improved [2].

Although interpretability of ML poses a daunting task, standardized clinical trials will need to be conducted regularly to serve as strong medical evidence for guidance, incorporating robust methods to control various biases during the trial design. For instance, it is essential to perform a calibration of the inter-rater reliability by consistency validation; additionally, reviewers should be blinded to the allocation schemes to prevent subjective bias. Finally, providing context-specific empirical validation could also make it easier to audit bias and enhance trust of practitioners [2].

Over the next few years, AI-based orthodontic systems could potentially serve as auxiliary tools for diverse clinical procedures. However, the outcomes derived from various ML models should be interpreted with caution and used as a reference, rather than absolute norms, at least during the nascent stages of AI influenced clinical practice. AI-based models may serve to simulate nonconventional ways of thinking for experts and provide important initial support for young orthodontists, who may benefit by easier and faster acquisition of theories and practice experiences through ML models [2].

The myriad of possibilities resulting from the diverse applications of AI and ML can be astounding and at the same time misleading, especially for patients. Diverse tools offered by these systems may cause dependence and overconfidence in these systems, heightened patient expectations regarding the predictability of treatment results, and possibly disappointment on the process completion. Patients need to be adequately educated that predictions and simulations designed by AI-based systems are merely an estimate and the actual treatment experience may significantly differ based on individual biological response as well as factors beyond the clinician's control. Likewise, orthodontists should not be hesitant to question clinical decisions generated by decision systems and/or intervene in case these decisions are in conflict with overall patient benefit [9].

The advancement of AI/ML algorithms and their subsequent incorporation into day-to-day clinical orthodontics should ideally help encourage data-driven diagnosis and adaptive treatment planning, enhance clinician-patient communication, and, consequentially, continually enhance orthodontic treatment standards in the near future. Clinicians could well benefit by viewing AI as a support system, rather than a threat.

References

1. Bichu YM, Hansa I, Bichu AY, Premjani P, Flores-Mir C, Vaid NR. Applications of artificial intelligence and machine learning in orthodontics: a scoping review. Prog Orthod. 2021;22(1):18. https://doi.org/10.1186/s40510-021-00361-9.
2. Liu J, Chen Y, Li S, Zhao Z, Wu Z. Machine learning in orthodontics: challenges and perspectives. Adv Clin Exp Med. 2021;30(10):1065–74. https://doi.org/10.17219/acem/138702.

3. Vaid NR. Artificial intelligence (AI) driven orthodontic care: a quest toward utopia? Semin Orthod. 2021;27(2):57–61.
4. Gandedkar NH, Vaid NR, Darendeliler MA, Premjani P, Ferguson DJ. The last decade in orthodontics: a scoping review of the hits, misses and the near misses! Semin Orthod. 2019;25(4):339–55.
5. Vaid N, Doshi V, Vandekar M. What's "trend" ing in orthodontic literature? APOS Trends Orthod. 2016;6(1):1–4.
6. Vaid NR. Digital technologies in orthodontics–an update. Semin Orthod. 2018;24(4):373–5.
7. Monill-González A, Rovira-Calatayud L, d'Oliveira NG, Ustrell-Torrent JM. Artificial intelligence in orthodontics: where are we now? A scoping review. Orthod Craniofac Res. 2021;24(Suppl 2):6–15. https://doi.org/10.1111/ocr.12517.
8. Mohammad-Rahimi H, Nadimi M, Rohban MH, Shamsoddin E, Lee VY, Motamedian SR. Machine learning and orthodontics, current trends and the future opportunities: a scoping review. Am J Orthod Dentofacial Orthop. 2021;160(2):170–192.e4. https://doi.org/10.1016/j.ajodo.2021.02.013.
9. Orhan K, Amasya H. AI in orthodontics. In: Orhan K, Jagtap R, editors. Artificial intelligence in dentistry. Cham: Springer Nature. p. 131–41. https://doi.org/10.1007/978-3-031-43827-1_8.
10. Schwendicke F, Chaurasia A, Arsiwala L, Lee JH, Elhennawy K, Jost-Brinkmann PG, Demarco F, Krois J. Deep learning for cephalometric landmark detection: systematic review and meta-analysis. Clin Oral Investig. 2021;25(7):4299–309. https://doi.org/10.1007/s00784-021-03990-w.
11. Li P, Kong D, Tang T, et al. Orthodontic treatment planning based on artificial neural networks. Sci Rep. 2019;9:2037. https://doi.org/10.1038/s41598-018-38439-w.
12. Choi HI, Jung SK, Baek SH, Lim WH, Ahn SJ, Yang IH, Kim TW. Artificial intelligent model with neural network machine learning for the diagnosis of orthognathic surgery. J Craniofac Surg. 2019;30(7):1986–9. https://doi.org/10.1097/SCS.0000000000005650.
13. Evangelista K, de Freitas Silva BS, Yamamoto-Silva FP, Valladares-Neto J, Silva MAG, Cevidanes LHS, de Luca CG, Massignan C. Accuracy of artificial intelligence for tooth extraction decision-making in orthodontics: a systematic review and meta-analysis. Clin Oral Investig. 2022;26(12):6893–905. https://doi.org/10.1007/s00784-022-04742-0.
14. Mathew R, Palatinus S, Padala S, Alshehri A, Awadh W, Bhandi S, Thomas J, Patil S. Neural networks for classification of cervical vertebrae maturation: a systematic review. Angle Orthod. 2022;92(6):796–804. https://doi.org/10.2319/031022-210.1.
15. Mohamed M, Ferguson DJ, Venugopal A, Alam MK, Makki L, Vaid NR. An artificial intelligence based referral application to optimize orthodontic referrals in a public oral healthcare system. Semin Orthod. 2021;27(2):157–63.
16. Allareddy V, Lee MK, Vaid NR, Yadav S. Use of neural network model to examine post-operative infections following orthognathic surgeries in the United States. Semin Orthod. 2021;27(2):130–7.
17. Wang X, Cai B, Cao Y, Zhou C, Yang L, Liu R, Long X, Wang W, Gao D, Bao B. Objective method for evaluating orthodontic treatment from the lay perspective: an eye-tracking study. Am J Orthod Dentofacial Orthop. 2016;150(4):601–10. https://doi.org/10.1016/j.ajodo.2016.03.028.
18. Thanathornwong B. Bayesian-based decision support system for assessing the needs for orthodontic treatment. Healthc Inform Res. 2018;24(1):22–8. https://doi.org/10.4258/hir.2018.24.1.22.
19. Park JH, Kim YJ, Kim J, Kim J, Kim IH, Kim N, Vaid NR, Kook YA. Use of artificial intelligence to predict outcomes of nonextraction treatment of class II malocclusions. Semin Orthod. 2021;27(2):87–95.
20. Kim BM, Kang BY, Kim HG, Baek SH. Prognosis prediction for class III malocclusion treatment by feature wrapping method. Angle Orthod. 2009;79(4):683–91. https://doi.org/10.2319/071508-371.1.
21. Auconi P, Scazzocchio M, Cozza P, McNamara JA Jr, Franchi L. Prediction of class III treatment outcomes through orthodontic data mining. Eur J Orthod. 2015;37(3):257–67. https://doi.org/10.1093/ejo/cju038.
22. Auconi P, Caldarelli G, Scala A, Ierardo G, Polimeni A. A network approach to orthodontic diagnosis. Orthod Craniofac Res. 2011;14(4):189–97. https://doi.org/10.1111/j.1601-6343.2011.01523.x.
23. Patcas R, Timofte R, Volokitin A, Agustsson E, Eliades T, Eichenberger M, et al. Facial attractiveness of cleft patients: a direct comparison between artificial-intelligence-based scoring and conventional rater groups. Eur J Orthod. 2019;41(4):428–33. https://doi.org/10.1093/ejo/cjz007.
24. Patcas R, Bernini DAJ, Volokitin A, Agustsson E, Rothe R, Timofte R. Applying artificial intelligence to assess the impact of orthognathic treatment on facial attractiveness and estimated age. Int J Oral Maxillofac Surg. 2019;48(1):77–83. https://doi.org/10.1016/j.ijom.2018.07.010. Epub 2018 Aug 4
25. Hansa I, Katyal V, Semaan SJ, Coyne R, Vaid NR. Artificial intelligence driven remote monitoring of orthodontic patients: clinical applicability and rationale. Semin Orthod. 2021;27(2):138–56., ISSN 1073-8746. https://doi.org/10.1053/j.sodo.2021.05.010.
26. Homsi K, Snider V, Kusnoto B, Atsawasuwan P, Viana G, Allareddy V, Gajendrareddy P, Elnagar MH. In-vivo evaluation of artificial intelligence driven remote monitoring technology for tracking tooth movement and reconstruction of 3-dimensional digital models during orthodontic treatment. Am J Orthod Dentofacial Orthop. 2023;164(5):690–9. https://doi.org/10.1016/j.ajodo.2023.04.019.
27. Prasad S, Arunachalam S, Boillat T, Ghoneima A, Gandedkar N, Diar-Bakirly S. Wearable orofacial technology and orthodontics. Dent J (Basel). 2023;11(1):24. https://doi.org/10.3390/dj11010024.

28. Vaid NR, Hansa I, Bichu Y. Smartphone applications used in orthodontics: a scoping review of scholarly literature. J World Fed Orthod. 2020;9(3S):S67–73. https://doi.org/10.1016/j.ejwf.2020.08.007.
29. Gupta G, Vaid N. The world of orthodontic apps. APOS Trends Orthod. 2017;7(2):79–3.
30. Gandedkar NH, Wong MT, Darendeliler MA. Role of virtual reality (VR), augmented reality (AR) and artificial intelligence (AI) in tertiary education and research of orthodontics: an insight. Semin Orthod. 2021;27(2):69–77.
31. Lee MK, Allareddy V, Rampa S, Elnagar MH, Oubaidin M, Yadav S, Venugopalan SR. Applications and challenges of implementing artificial intelligence in orthodontics: a primer for orthodontists. Semin Orthod. 2024;30(1):72–6., ISSN 1073-8746. https://doi.org/10.1053/j.sodo.2024.01.005.

Artificial Intelligence in Cariology 7

Falk Schwendicke and Sergio E. Uribe

7.1 Artificial Intelligence and Data Dentistry

Artificial intelligence (AI) is on everyone's lips—from self-driving cars to security technology and medicine: AI has become an everyday phenomenon. In this book, numerous definitions can be found. In principle, AI is understood as the ability of a machine to imitate active cognitive processes of humans (e.g., thinking, reacting, or acting). A central component of AI technologies is machine learning. This method is particularly suitable when classical rule-based programming approaches reach their limits. This is the case, for example, when analyzing complex data such as images, language, or large numerical data (such as claims data). In machine learning, it is not human programmers who provide the machine with certain rules according to which it performs defined tasks. Rather, the machine itself learns to understand the structure of the data and statistical patterns in it and derives rules based on this. For complex data such as images or language, deep learning has been used for about a decade. Complex algorithms and powerful mathematical models, especially neural networks, are used.

The reported successes of AI across diverse application fields, including dentistry and—as a subdiscipline—cariology, are due to progress in three areas: (1) freely available software for the development of complex models and a community for the free exchange of ideas and code (open access philosophy), (2) sufficient memory and data processing (compute) capacity, e.g., through powerful modern graphics cards, and (3) availability and usability of large amounts of data. The latter, data, is the critical foundation for developing AI—and conversely, AI is just one tool for making efficient use of data. AI can be considered the engine of a car—the real fuel is the data. Today, data is already considered a key resource and fulfils several characteristics that can trigger a technological revolution: The cost of using data is low and decreases over time; data is inexhaustible, as it can be used as often as necessary and by as many actors as technologically possible; data is essential for a wide range of applications in different industries and markets; the intelligent use of data increases the efficiency of processes and procedures. Data and computing are now considered the fourth scientific paradigm (along with experimental and theoretical science and simulation) and could also serve to ensure the quality, accessibility, and affordability of healthcare in

F. Schwendicke (✉)
Conservative Dentistry and Periodontology, LMU Klinikum, LMU Munich, Munich, Germany
e-mail: falk.schwendicke@med.uni-muenchen.de

S. E. Uribe
Department of Conservative Dentistry and Oral Health, Riga Stradins University, Latvia/Conservative Dentistry and Periodontology, LMU Klinikum, LMU Munich, Munich, Germany
e-mail: sergio.uribe@rsu.lv

F. Schwendicke et al. (eds.), *Artificial Intelligence for Oral Health Care*,
https://doi.org/10.1007/978-3-031-84047-0_7

the coming decades. For our field, we are entering an era which we have termed "data dentistry" before [1].

7.2 Dental Caries and AI

Dental caries is the most prevalent condition of humankind [2]. For a long time, caries was understood as an infectious disease, with carious tissue (mainly bacterially contaminated and demineralized dentin) to be completely removed for "cure." In contrast, the current understanding of caries defines it as an ecological imbalance within the dental biofilm, whereby cariogenic, i.e., acidogenic (acid-producing) and aciduric (acid-resistant), bacteria produce relevant amounts of organic acids under sufficient frequent carbohydrate intake, which in turn allows them to eventually dominate the dental biofilm (termed "ecological plaque hypothesis") [3].

Based on this understanding, caries management now spans not only from detecting a caries lesion using our eyes (visual detection) and managing it invasively by placing restorations but includes a wide range of detection strategies like radiography (the most common type of adjunct detection method besides visual assessment), optical coherence tomography, quantitative light-induced fluorescence, intraoral scanning, or near-infrared light transillumination [2–4] and then a similar wide range of non-, micro- or invasive treatment approaches. Overall, dentistry has seen significant advancements in caries management since the 1980s, marked by a decrease in prevalence of up to 90% reported in certain high-income countries. The pivotal role of public health policies in these triumphs is a testament to their importance. However, the profession faces ongoing challenges, including the rise in caries rates in specific regions globally and among certain population subgroups, not to mention the persistent prevalence of early childhood caries [4]. Against this backdrop, AI holds the potential to revolutionize the field further. The emerging AI tools could equip dentists with the capacity to shift their focus from merely technical-restorative measures to more biological, noninvasive treatments, thereby expanding their role in caries management [5].

Evaluating imagery for caries detection is a challenge for practitioners; dentists miss a substantial proportion of early caries lesions in radiographs [6] but also other image types and show considerable variability in their diagnostic findings and treatment decisions. Similarly, choosing between the available interventions [7] is challenging and currently performed arbitrarily involving the provider's experience, but also patients' wishes and healthcare system determinants.

The usage of AI, specifically deep learning, may support practitioners in caries lesion detection and diagnosis on imagery, but also treatment decision. It may further foster more regular supportive caries management and enhanced engagement with patients when it comes to self-management.

7.3 Fields of Application

7.3.1 Image Analysis

AI can be used to automatically read, analyze, and merge patient information. A classic example here is image analytics, where patient images such as photographs or radiographs are analyzed by AI. This takes only a few seconds; a standardized evaluation of AI algorithms allows reliable accuracy here.

The most advanced field of application is the automated evaluation of radiographs. Here, carious lesions are detected on single images, bitewing images, or panoramic slice images and visually highlighted either by boxes or pixel masks (Fig. 7.1).

Some software systems already on the market usually also offer to interact with these suggested findings (to correct, add, or delete them); likewise, the automatic generation of a findings report is common. In this regard, such AI-assisted assessment offers dentists a number of advantages:

1. Improvement of diagnostic accuracy. For caries detection on bitewing images, it has been shown that dentists become significantly more

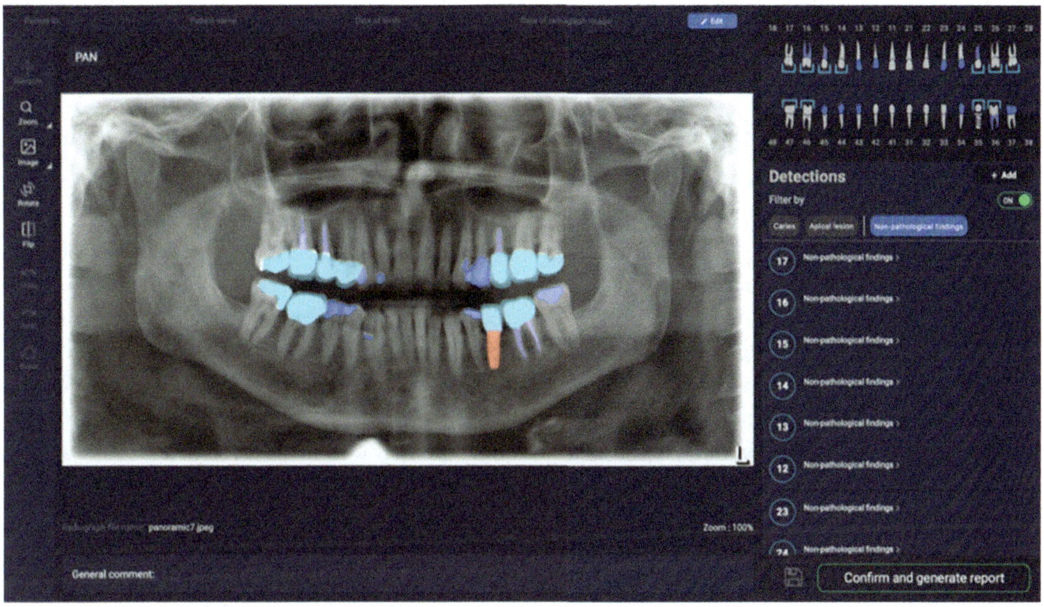

Fig. 7.1 Exemplary AI-based application to analyze 2-D dental radiographs. Findings are displayed as pixel blobs on the radiograph as well as tooth map and findings list

sensitive in detecting early caries through the use of this technology—it is the detection of these early stages that often causes difficulties for dentists, and the majority of lesions have been shown to be missed [8]. However, since modern tooth-preserving approaches focus on detecting caries at this early stage and actively arresting it (i.e., preventing its progression), this early detection is of great importance. The described diagnostic advantage of AI-assisted caries diagnosis has been demonstrated in retrospective as well as prospective controlled studies [9]: If this early diagnosis is combined with adequate non- or micro-invasive therapy (i.e., fluoridation, sealing, infiltration), the use of such an AI assistant is also more cost-effective in the long term [10]. Further gains in accuracy have also been located in the diagnosis on photographs (e.g., differential diagnosis of various white spot lesions on anterior teeth) or other image formats (e.g., near-infrared transillumination images) [11].

2. Automated generation of a report of findings. Within seconds, this is generated by the system; in the process, various AI models are combined in the background to eventually record tooth- or even surface-based findings. This saves time and allows systematic and comprehensive documentation. The next logical step is to use this data for therapy planning with the help of an AI-based assistant. Notably, recent advances in existing software have allowed to automatically discriminate lesions of different depths on radiographs, fostering lesion-specific management, as recommended (see Fig. 7.1).
3. Communication. AI-based systems that visually highlight caries on a radiograph support patient communication: In a recent study, we showed that patients understand significantly better why the dentist is making a particular finding on the basis of such augmented image—especially as they can "see" the affected areas themselves [12]. In this context, it should also be emphasized that AI will generally support patients in better understanding their state of health: AI-based photo analysis apps will enable not only the dentist but also the patient to generate an initial diagnosis for certain conditions (e.g., carious white spots described above) on their smartphone. We

present an in-depth overview on current applications in cariologic image analysis later in this chapter.

7.3.2 Speech Analysis and Generation

The analysis of speech data (conversation, written language) is another field of application. Natural Language Processing could, for example, be used to document important information from a conversation between dentist and patient. Similarly, speech-based therapy planning or automated recording of clinical findings would be possible without the need for another person (e.g., dental assistant) to make separate entries using a mouse and keyboard. In addition, transmission errors are minimized, and significantly more comprehensive documentation is possible.

Similarly, AI-based text processing can easily read existing patient records retrospectively (i.e., over the last 10 years). In the future, the information obtained in this way could be made available to the dentist in the form of a dashboard, presenting caries risk profile, past restorative or other cariologic interventions, and images. Easier access to data, systematizing it, and making it available at a glance should enable more comprehensive, rapid transmission of information to each individual patient. It can also enable better predictions about each patient's health status.

7.3.3 Predictive Dentistry

Predicting events is another field of application for AI. This involves predicting the future based on (past) data—a notoriously difficult undertaking! So far, dentists are already doing this without AI, for example, by using the caries experience (often the most important parameter), the nutritional behavior, or the oral hygiene of a patient to predict the probability of future disease events such as caries. Critically, the accuracy of these predictions is extremely limited [13]. The improved processing of even large amounts of data outlined above (the AI does not care whether it searches through 10, 100, or 1000 pages of patient records or analyzes 5, 50, or 500 x-rays) should make these predictions significantly better. Using data that has been little used so far (e.g., app-based food diaries, digitally recorded health profiles, social media data), it could be possible to arrive at significantly more accurate predictions. Recent advances using microbiomic data to predict early childhood caries have successfully demonstrated that better data will allow better predictions [14]. One goal in cariology should be to dispense with using caries experience parameter for prediction—after all, this can only predict a high caries risk once it is already present (Fig. 7.2).

7.3.4 Teledentistry and Automated Monitoring

Another application of AI is teledentistry. AI can help derive information from telemedicine-derived images, partially eliminating the need for a specialist to be involved: Indeed, if the AI is trained on a dataset created by specialists, it has an accuracy similar to that of the specialist: it does not replace the specialist, but it can help the generalist or even the layperson (e.g., patient) to make an initial "pre-diagnosis." This is helpful where medical specialists are a rare commodity and waiting times are long: AI could prioritize the assessment of urgent problems by specialists and leave less urgent problems in the hands of generalists. For instance, such teledentistry could be useful to assess root caries lesions in care homes, or to monitor lesion arrest under non-restorative cavity control in children, without the older or younger patients needing to attend the practice.

AI-based telecare is also conceivable. It is now clear, for example, that caries prevention carried out exclusively in the dentist's chair (individual prophylaxis) is not suitable for preventing caries equally in all patients—especially as high-risk individuals do not regularly attend dental offices. This conversely means that dentistry must come where these individuals are, for example, via a setting-based approach using teledental

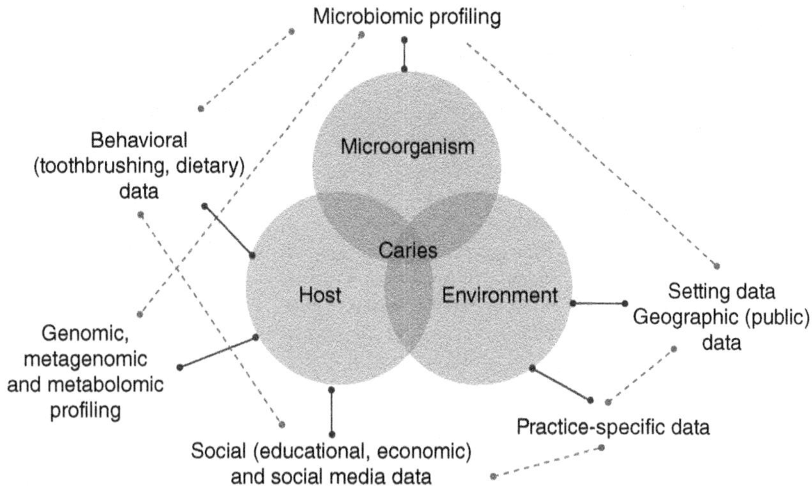

Fig. 7.2 Along the traditional pillars of caries pathogenesis, a wide range of new data can be gathered, connected, and leveraged to yield a better understanding of the disease and to make individual predictions towards future caries risk of lesion activity. Various data sources collected from the host, the oral microbiome, or the environment (slid lines) are intertwined and related (dotted lines), resulting in a complex data lake which could be submitted to advanced data analytics for prediction modeling [15]

interventions. For example, it is conceivable to support dental diagnostics with AI in schools or daycare centers, but also nursing homes. In the latter, for instance, fluoride varnish application could be performed by nursing staff after telediagnostics and teleinstructions by a dental professional as needed.

AI can also revolutionize follow-up and monitoring procedures in dental care. AI systems can be programmed to automatically track the oral health status of patients over time, alerting dentists to any changes that might indicate the onset or progression of caries. This includes reminding patients of their regular check-ups and necessary dental care procedures, facilitating timely intervention and better oral health management, and other administrative tasks.

7.3.5 Patient Engagement and Education

AI can be utilized to improve patient engagement and education. AI-based chatbots and interactive platforms could be designed to educate patients about dental caries and preventive measures tailored to their specific needs. They can also send personalized reminders and advice based on individual patient data, thereby playing a crucial role in promoting better oral health habits.

7.3.6 Research and Discovery

AI also holds promise for research and discovery in the field of cariology. With its capacity to analyze large datasets, AI can facilitate research into dental caries, potentially uncovering novel insights about the causes, progression, and effective interventions for the disease. This could lead to the development of improved prevention and treatment strategies for dental caries [1].

A summary is provided in Table 7.1.

Table 7.1 Summary of potential AI applications in cariology

Applications of AI in cariology	Description
Caries detection	AI algorithms can be trained to analyze dental radiographs or photographs for signs of dental caries. They may identify patterns not easily noticeable to the human eye
Caries risk prediction	AI could be used to predict a patient's risk of developing caries based on various factors such as age, dietary habits, genetic factors, and oral hygiene practices
Treatment planning	AI could be used to devise optimal treatment plans based on the specifics of a patient's caries lesions, including their size, location, severity, and other individual patient factors
Patient engagement and education	AI chatbots and interactive platforms could be used to educate patients about dental caries and encourage preventative measures. They can provide personalized advice and reminders based on individual patient data
Automated follow-up and monitoring	AI systems can automatically monitor patients' oral health over time and alert dentists to changes that may signal the development or progression of caries. They can also remind patients about regular check-ups and necessary dental care
Teledentistry	AI can aid and triage in the pre-diagnosis of dental issues through the analysis of telemedicine-derived images, reducing immediate dependence on specialists. This could prove invaluable in rural places and care homes or for children where in-person visits are challenging
Research and discovery	AI can be used to analyze large datasets for research into dental caries, potentially uncovering new insights about the disease's causes, progression, and effective interventions

7.4 Current State of Affairs in Image Detection

In a recent systematic review, we systematically appraised studies using deep learning (specifically, NNs) for caries detection on dental imagery [11]. Of 252 identified studies, 48 studies were assessed in full text, additional ones identified using hand search, and eventually 42 studies were included. Overall, seven different types of imagery were employed; intraoral photographs (n = 12), periapical radiographs (n = 12), bitewing radiographs (n = 8), optical coherence tomography images (n = 4), panoramic radiographs (n = 3), near-infrared light transillumination images (n = 2), and cone-beam computed tomography (n = 1). A number of datasets for cariology used in these studies were publicly available; the international symposium on biomedical imaging (ISBI) 2015 challenges dataset of bitewing radiographs (used by n = 4 studies), a dataset of periapical radiographs (n = 6 studies), and a dataset of intraoral photographs used in a Kaggle competition (n = 1).

As the standard of current AI and machine learning involves supervised learning, a reference test was needed and established in most studies via expert opinions (n = 37). Specifically, one human expert (n = 8), two (n = 7), three, or more (n = 6) experts were involved in defining the reference test; 16 studies did not mention the number of experts involved. Two studies used other image modalities for establishing the reference test, namely, fluorescent imaging and micro-CT. Four studies did not mention how the reference test was established. Notably, a very recent study employed an alternative to fully supervised learning, self-supervised learning [16], where labels to train on are not provided by experts, and found this strategy useful, too.

The most frequent machine learning task in cariology so far was image classification (n = 26), followed by segmentation (n = 10) and object detection (n = 6). Various deep learning models were used, e.g., customized CNN structures (n = 8), transfer learning models (n = 8), or multilayer perceptron (n = 7) for classification; autoencoders (e.g., U-net) (n = 8) for segmentation;

and one-stage object detectors (e.g., YoLo) or two-stage object detectors (e.g., Faster R-CNN) ($n = 4$) in detection.

Among the included studies, 11 (26.2%) were found to have low risk of bias, 13 studies (31.0%) as low risk for concerns regarding applicability. The most problematic domain was "Reference Standard," where only 20 studies (47.6%) and 22 studies (52.4%) were classified as low risk of bias and low risk of applicability concern, respectively.

The accuracy of the developed models varied widely. In meta-analysis, only focusing on classification tasks, 17 studies were pooled; the range of the reported sensitivity was 25% to 99.8% and specificity 17.2% to 100%, respectively.

Overall, a wide range of image material and AI or clinical tasks are currently investigated, and most studies showed promising results. Notably, the high heterogeneity in study designs and outcomes or outcome measures makes any comparison across studies hard and limits to synthesize the data in a meaningful way. Moreover, data towards the true usefulness of AI for cariology is extremely limited [17].

A whole range of further reviews on the matter have been published. An overview of the most recent systematic reviews is presented in Table 7.2.

Table 7.2 Overview of the latest systematic reviews focusing on AI's role in dental caries detection

Review title	Journal	Year	DOI	Main focus	Main results (numerics)	Conclusion
Detecting dental caries on oral photographs using artificial intelligence: a systematic review	Oral Dis	2023	10.1111/odi.14659	Review of AI models in detecting dental caries on oral photographs	F1-scores for classification were 68.3–94.3% and detection tasks were 42.8–95.4%. For professional cameras, F1-scores were 68.3–95.4%, for intraoral cameras 78.8–87.6%, and for smartphone cameras 42.8–80%	AI could enhance diagnostic objectivity and aid in teledentistry. Future studies should prioritize robust designs, standard metrics, and caries severity assessment
Machine learning in the diagnosis and prognostic prediction of dental caries: a systematic review	Caries Res	2022	10.1159/000524167	Evaluation of machine learning algorithms in dental caries diagnosis and prediction	AUC values ranging from 0.745 to 0.987	Promising potential but limited general applicability due to high bias and non-clinical development settings
Application and performance of artificial intelligence technology in detection, diagnosis and prediction of dental caries (DC): a systematic review	Diagnostics (Basel)	2022	10.3390/diagnostics12051083	Diagnostic accuracy and performance of AI-based models for dental caries	Diagnostic studies: AUC value ranged from 0.740 to 0.987; mean set size of the reports was 1873 images; 9 out of 10 studies utilized variants of ANNs * prognostic prediction studies: Mean set size of the studies was 4061 units; sensitivity of the ML models ranged from 0.000 to 0.971 (mean 0.669, SD 0.420) and the specificity ranged between 0.679 and 0.993 (mean 0.866, SD 0.121)	Artificial intelligence models for the diagnosis and prognostic prediction of dental caries demonstrate promising outcomes, but a notable risk of bias in some studies underlines the necessity for additional high-quality research
Deep learning for caries detection: a systematic review	J Dent	2022	10.1016/j.jdent.2022.104115	Review of deep learning studies on caries detection	Accuracy ranged between 68–99%. Diagnostic odds ratios varied from 2.27 to 32,767	Increasing number of studies with promising accuracy but low study and reporting quality
Deep learning convolutional neural network algorithms for the early detection and diagnosis of dental caries on periapical radiographs: a systematic review	Imaging Sci Dent	2021	10.5624/isd.20210074	Review of deep learning convolutional neural networks for early-stage dental caries detection	Out of 248 reports, only 5 met the inclusion criteria, demonstrating high accuracy (ranging from 63.60 for box-wise to 81.90 for image-wise) in detecting caries	Clinical applications showed significant accuracy in detecting and diagnosing dental caries
Dental caries diagnosis and detection using neural networks: a systematic review	J Clin Med	2020	10.3390/jcm9113579	State of the art of neural networks in caries detection and diagnosis	The image databases ranged from 87 to 3000 images, with a mean of 669 images	Variability in studies complicates the conclusions that can be made about the reliability of a neural network to detect and diagnose caries

7.5 Challenges

Cariology may benefit from the possibilities of digital diagnostics and therapy and the use of AI technology—and the first AI applications have also already reached market maturity. However, there are a number of challenges that need to be overcome before AI can be widely deployed. These often revolve around the data with which the AI has been trained; central to the assessment of an AI is the evaluation of the underlying data material. Only high-quality data will allow for reliable quality at the specialist level (otherwise the "garbage in, garbage out" principle familiar in data science applies). Similarly, only AI that has been trained on the broadest possible data (different populations, ethnicities, dental findings, devices) will work reliably across all possible practices. Manufacturers of AI applications are encouraged to disclose their data source, how the data were evaluated, and how representative they are. For instance, an AI model that was trained using data from German patients has shown high precision for diagnosing conditions within that population. However, its diagnostic efficacy significantly diminishes when applied to a different demographic, such as Indian patients [18].

AI must also be reproducible. Only if it is clear how an AI application was developed and if it can be traced how the reported results of an AI (its accuracy, its generalizability) have come about, should it be used medically. The International Telecommunications Union (ITU) and the WHO are jointly developing a dataset on which medical AI software can be tested—and such "benchmarking" is also the declared goal for dentistry. Only in this way can it then be measured comparably on a representative dataset how good various AI applications are (e.g., for detecting caries lesions on bitewings).

Finally, it must be understood how an AI application works and what decision criteria are used. As described, it is often not clear what exactly an AI has learned (AI systems are black boxes). For medical applications, it is imperative to make the inner logic of the AI explainable when making a decision; only in this way can it be understood whether the decision criteria of the AI are consistent with medical knowledge or whether the recognition of artifacts was learned from biased data [19].

7.6 Conclusions

For cariology, AI harbors a wide range of applications and promises. Current focus of the last years was mainly in image analysis, particularly caries detection on radiographs, where AI has demonstrated to boost sensitivity while supporting reporting and communication. Notably, the clinical impact of such AI on treatment pathways, providers, or healthcare costs is so far not explored well. Further challenges of generalizability, explainability, and reliability of AI for cariology need to be resolved, too.

References

1. Schwendicke F, Krois J. Data dentistry: how data are changing clinical care and research. J Dent Res. 2022;101(1):21–9.
2. Bernabe E, et al. Global, regional, and national Levels and trends in burden of oral conditions from 1990 to 2017: a systematic analysis for the global burden of disease 2017 study. J Dent Res. 2020;99(4):362–73.
3. Marsh PD. Microbial ecology of dental plaque and its significance in health and disease. Adv Dent Res. 1994;8(2):263–71.
4. Uribe SE, Innes N, Maldupa I. The global prevalence of early childhood caries: a systematic review with meta-analysis using the WHO diagnostic criteria. Int J Paediatr Dent. 2021;31(6):817–30.
5. Innes NPT, et al. A century of change towards prevention and minimal intervention in cariology. J Dent Res. 2019;98(6):611–7.
6. Walsh T, et al. Imaging modalities to inform the detection and diagnosis of early caries. Cochrane Database Syst Rev. 2021;3:CD014545.
7. Watt RG. Oral health inequalities—developments in research, policy and practice over the last 50 years. Community Dent Oral Epidemiol. 2023;51(4):595–9.
8. Cantu AG, et al. Detecting caries lesions of different radiographic extension on bitewings using deep learning. J Dent. 2020;100:103425.
9. Mertens S, et al. Artificial intelligence for caries detection: randomized trial. J Dent. 2021;115:103849.
10. Schwendicke F, et al. Cost-effectiveness of artificial intelligence for proximal caries detection. J Dent Res. 2021;100(4):369–76.

11. Mohammad-Rahimi H, et al. Deep learning for caries detection: a systematic review. J Dent. 2022;122:104115.
12. Kosan E, et al. Patients' perspectives on artificial intelligence in dentistry: a controlled study. J Clin Med. 2022;11(8):2143.
13. Fontana M, et al. Improving caries risk prediction modeling: a call for action. J Dent Res. 2020;99(11):1215–20.
14. Blostein F, et al. Evaluating the ecological hypothesis: early life salivary microbiome assembly predicts dental caries in a longitudinal case-control study. Microbiome. 2022;10(1):240.
15. Schwendicke F, Krois J. Precision dentistry-what it is, where it fails (yet), and how to get there. Clin Oral Investig. 2022;26(4):3395–403.
16. Taleb A, et al. Self-supervised learning methods for label-efficient dental caries classification. Diagnostics (Basel). 2022;12(5):1237.
17. Arsiwala-Scheppach LT, et al. Machine learning in dentistry: a scoping review. J Clin Med. 2023;12(3):937.
18. Krois J, et al. Generalizability of deep learning models for dental image analysis. Sci Rep. 2021;11(1):6102.
19. Ma J, et al. Towards trustworthy AI in dentistry. J Dent Res. 2022;101(11):1263–8.

Artificial Intelligence in Endodontics

8

Sascha Herbst
and Mohammad-Rahimi Hossein

8.1 Introduction

Artificial intelligence (AI) and deep learning have been making significant strides in various fields, including healthcare and dentistry [1]. AI has its roots in the 1950s when researchers began exploring the possibility of creating machines that could mimic human intelligence. Decades later, the first application of AI in endodontics was developed: a computer-based system that was used for endodontics decision-making, introduced by Hyman et al. [2]. Since the first AI-based system for endodontics was developed, there has been a growing body of research on the use of AI for various endodontic tasks (Fig. 8.1).

In endodontics, AI has the potential to enhance the complex decision-making process by dental professionals in diagnosing, treating, and managing patients. This could help to improve the accuracy, efficiency, and effectiveness of endodontic treatments [3]. The application of AI is motivated by several factors. First, there is a close link between the radiographic and clinical data gathered during treatment steps. Second, AI enables analyzing technical outcomes through the vast amount of data generated over endodontic procedures. Finally, AI can facilitate the identification of rare conditions in dentistry that may be overlooked due to subject bias. Overall, AI-based tools can reduce bias and assist dental professionals in making better-informed decisions, streamline treatment planning, and ultimately improve patient outcomes.

In recent research, deep learning-based systems have shown promise in detecting and diagnosing periapical radiolucencies compared to evaluations by human clinicians alone [3]. However, more studies are needed to conclusively determine if these systems can outperform human clinicians in a clinical setting. Deep learning approaches are also being explored to detect various other conditions like vertical root fractures [4], fractured instruments in root canals [5], and unobturated second mesiobuccal canal on maxillary molars [6]. Furthermore, AI may contribute to the improvement of treatment and hopefully lead to an increase in the success of endodontic treatment outcomes [7, 8]. While initial study results are encouraging, real-world clinical validation is still required. If proven effective, AI may contribute to improvements in endodontic treatment and outcomes. However, it is important not to overstate current capabilities,

S. Herbst (✉)
Department of Oral Diagnostics, Digital Health and Health Services Research, Center for Dental and Craniofacial Sciences, Charité—Universitätsmedizin Berlin, Berlin, Germany

Clinic for Conservative Dentistry and Periodontology, LMU Klinikum, Munich, Germany
e-mail: sascha.herbst@med.uni-muenchen.de

M.-R. Hossein
Topic Group Dental Diagnostics and Digital Dentistry, ITU/WHO Focus Group AI on Health, Berlin, Germany

F. Schwendicke et al. (eds.), *Artificial Intelligence for Oral Health Care*,
https://doi.org/10.1007/978-3-031-84047-0_8

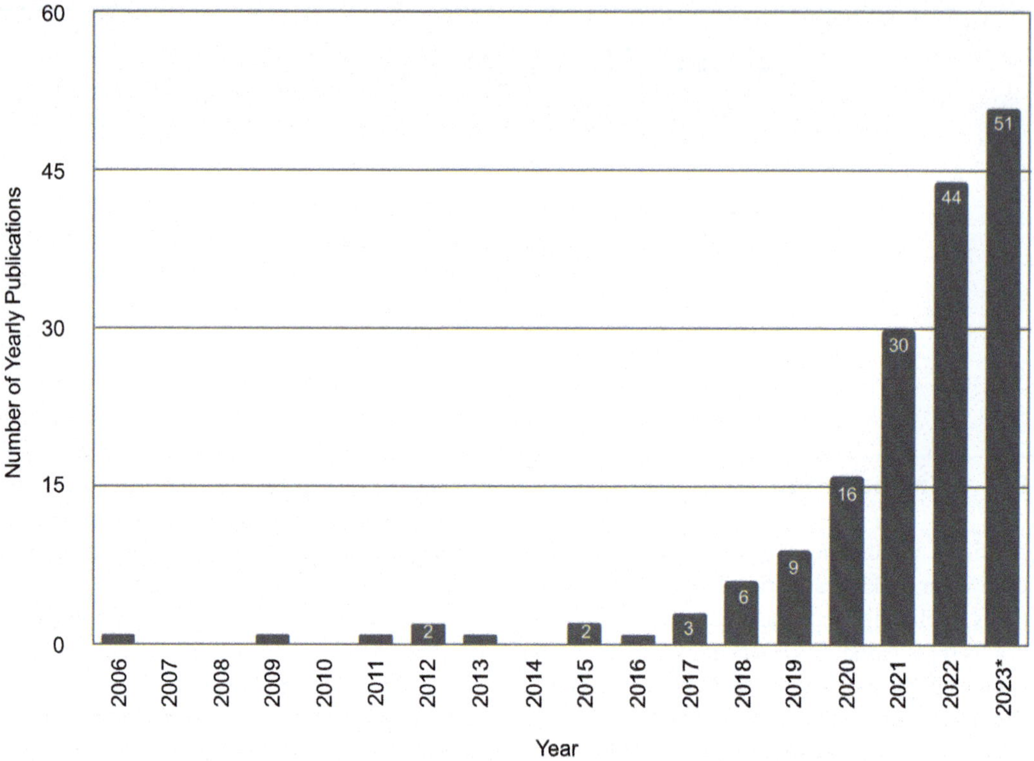

Fig. 8.1 Trends in AI publications in endodontics, yearly search result for ("deep learning" or "artificial intelligence" or "machine learning" or "neural network") and (endodontics or "root canal" or "periapical periodontitis") in PubMed (* year 2023 results is up to 21st October 2023)

Table 8.1 Selected list of startups and businesses focuses on AI application dentistry and endodontics

Name	Website	Year founded	Country of origin	Application in endodontics
Diagnocat	https://diagnocat.com/	2017	Russia	CBCT segmentation, 2D radiography report (including PA lesion detection)
Orca dental AI	https://orca-ai.com/	2001	USA	CBCT segmentation, root resorption diagnosis
DentalXrai	https://www.dentalxr.ai/	2020	Germany	2D radiography report (including PA lesion detection)
Pearl	https://www.hellopearl.com/	2019	USA	2D radiography report (including PA lesion detection), image quality enhancement
Overjet	https://www.overjet.ai/	2018	USA	2D radiography report (including PA lesion detection)
Dental intelligence	https://www.dentalintel.com/	2011	USA	AI-based clinical management

as more research is needed to determine the true impact AI can have in enhancing decision-making and success rates. AI should be seen as a potential aid, rather than a replacement, for the specialized expertise of endodontists.

This chapter will discuss the importance of AI in endodontics, focusing on its potential benefits, techniques employed, and its role in the bigger picture of dentistry. As part of this chapter, we will first review the current applications of AI in endodontics, both at the research and the industry level (Tables 8.1 and 8.2). Then, we will discuss some of the challenges associated with incorporating AI in endodontics. Finally, we are going to discuss current research gaps and how AI is going to play a major role in this field in the future.

Table 8.2 Overview of all included studies

Application	Study	Setting	Results
Periapical lesion detection	Ekert et al. 2019 [16]	Detecting PARL (classification) on 2597 OPG with CNN	Sensitivity: 65 ± 12% Specificity: 87 ± 4% AUC: 0.85 ± 0.04
	Li et al. 2021 [17]	Detecting PARL (classification) on 460 PAR with AlexNet	Sensitivity: 94.9% Specificity: 90.0%
	Li et al. 2022 [19]	Detecting PARL (classification) on 4129 PAR with ResNet-18	Sensitivity: 82% Specificity: 84% F1 score: 82.8%
	Ngoc et al. 2022 [111]	Detecting PARL (classification) on 1400 PAR with RESNET 34	Sensitivity: 96.7% Specificity: 93.9%
	Sajad et al. 2019 [21]	Detecting PARL (classification) on 534 PAR with AlexNet	Accuracy: 97% (single performance metric)
	Bayrakdar et al. 2022 [112]	Detecting PARL (segmentation) on 470 OPG with U-net	Sensitivity: 92% Precision: 84% F1 score: 88%
	Endres et al. 2020 [113]	Detecting PARL (segmentation) on 2902 OPG with U-net	Sensitivity: 51 ± 5% Precision: 0.67 ± 5% F1 score: 58 ± 4%
	Ezhov et al. 2021 [114]	Detecting PARL (segmentation) on 2800 CBCT with U-net	Sensitivity: 83.8% Specificity: 99.5%
	Huang et al. 2021 [115]	Detecting PARL (segmentation) on 40 CBCT with U-net	Accuracy: 86% (single performance metric)
	Khan et al. 2021 [116]	Detecting PARL (segmentation) on 206 PAR with U-net/Xnet//SegNet/U-net + Densenet121	Range dice coefficient: 0.36–0.45
	Kirnbauer et al. 2022 [117]	Detecting PARL (segmentation/classification) on 144 CBCT with U-net	Sensitivity: 97 ± 3% Specificity: 88 ± 4% Dice coefficient: 0.67 ± 0.33
	Krois et al. 2021 [27]	Detecting PARL (segmentation) on 1300 OPG with U-net	Sensitivity: 48 ± 1% Specificity: 99.9% F1 score: 54.1 ± 0.8%
	Moidu et al. 2022 [25]	Detecting PARL (segmentation) on 2200 PAR with YOLO v.3	Sensitivity: 89% Precision: 90% Dice coefficient: 89%
	Orhan et al. 2020 [24]	Detecting PARL (segmentation) on 4009 CBCT with U-net	Sensitivity: 95% Precision: 89% F1 score: 92.8%
	Setzer et al. 2020 [26]	Detecting PARL (segmentation) on 20 CBCT with U-net	Sensitivity: 93% Specificity: 88% Dice coefficient: 0.52
	Zheng et al. 2021 [118]	Detecting PARL (segmentation) on 20 CBCT with U-net	Sensitivity: 78–84% Precision: 81–90% Dice coefficient: 0.74
	Chen et al. 2021 [22]	Detecting PARL (object detection) on 2900 PAR with R-CNN	Sensitivity: 53.5 ± 2.56% Precision: 53.5 ± 2.56% IoU: 0.7 ± 0.02
	Ngoc et al. 2021 [20]	Detecting PARL (object detection) on 1130 PAR with R-CNN	Sensitivity: 89.5% Specificity: 97.9% Accuracy: 95.6%

(continued)

Table 8.2 (continued)

Application	Study	Setting	Results
Vertical root fracture	Johari et al. 2017 [35]	Detecting vertical root fracture in premolars (PAR/CBCT) with a probabilistic neuronal network ex vivo (n = 240)	PAR Sensitivity: 97.8% Specificity: 67.7% Accuracy: 70% CBCT Sensitivity: 93.3% Specificity: 100% Accuracy: 96.6%
	Kositbowornchai et al. 2013 [34]	Detecting vertical root fracture in premolars (PAR) with a probabilistic neuronal network ex vivo (n = 200)	Sensitivity: 97.2–98% Specificity: 60.0–90.5% Accuracy: 88.3–95.7%
	Fukuda et al. 2020 [4]	Detecting vertical root fracture in premolars (OPG) with a CNN in vivo (n = 200)	Recall: 75% Precision: 93% F1 score: 83%
Segmentation of root canal structures	Duan et al. 2021 [40]	Pulp cavity and tooth segmentation on CBCT images using threshold-based segmentation, FCN and U-net (single/multi rooted teeth; n = 20 CBCT)	Single-rooted Dice coefficient: 0.58–0.96 Multi-rooted Dice coefficient: 0.56–0.96
	Lin et al. 2021 [41]	Pulp cavity and tooth segmentation on CBCT images using U-net and micro-CT ground truth (n = 30 sound extracted premolars)	Dice coefficient: 0.74–0.96 Precision: 59.79–97.31% Recall: 81.14–95.11%
	Wang et al. 2023 [8]	Tooth and root canal segmentation on CBCT using Vnet and DentalNet (n = 67 teeth)	Dice coefficient: 0.86–0.88
	Zheng et al. 2021 [50]	Pulp chamber segmentation on CBCT using a custom deep learning model (n = 402 teeth)	Dice coefficient: 0.88
Prediction of root canal anatomies	Hiraiwa et al. 2019 [38]	Predicting second distal roots in mandibular first molars on PSA (CBCT ground truth) with AlexNet and GoogleNet (n = 760 teeth)	Sensitivity: 74.4–77.3% Specificity: 82–95.9% ROC-AUC: 0.85–0.87
	Yang et al. 2022 [39]	Predicting c-shaped root canal anatomies on PAR and OPG (CBCT ground truth) with EfficientNet (n = 370 cases); grad-CAM	PAR/OPG Sensitivity: 93/72% Specificity: 87/93% ROC-AUC: 0.95/0.93
	Jeon et al. 2021 [62]	Predicting c-shaped root canal anatomies on OPG (CBCT ground truth) with Xception (n = 1020 cases); grad-CAM	Sensitivity: 92.7% Specificity: 97% ROC-AUC: 0.98
	Sherwood et al. 2021 [61]	Segmentation of c-shaped root canal anatomies on 135 CBCT with 3 different CNN architectures (U-net, residual U-net, Xception)	Sensitivity: 72–78.6% Positive predictive value: 77.6–80% Dice coefficient: 0.77–0.81
	Duman et al. 2023 [65]	Segmentation of taurodont teeth on OPG (n = 348 with 1090 taurodont teeth) with U-net	Sensitivity: 87% Precision: 79% F1 score: 83%
	Buyuk et al. 2023 [5]	Detecting fractured instruments on OPG (n = 905; 417 showed a fractured instrument) with CNN (long short-term memory network)	Sensitivitiy: 81.3 ± 4.8% Specificity: 87.2 ± 2.8% ROC-AUC: 0.89
	Albitar et al. 2022 [6]	Detection of unobturated mb2 on CBCT (n = 58/102 mb roots) in the presence of root canal fillings and coronal restorations with U-net	Sensitivity: 80% Specificity: 100% Accuracy: 90%

(continued)

Table 8.2 (continued)

Application	Study	Setting	Results
Preoperative working length estimation	Saghiri et al. 2012 [69]	Classifying PAR (single rooted extracted teeth in vitro; $n = 50$) with inserted endodontic instruments 'short', 'exact', and 'long' to the apical foramen with multi-layer perceptron artificial neuronal network; ground truth: Stereomicroscope	Accuracy: 93%
	Saghiri et al. 2012 [70]	Classifying PAR (single rooted teeth in cadavers; $n = 50$ from 19 male cadaver) with inserted endodontic instruments 'short', 'exact', and 'long' to the apical foramen with multi-layer perceptron artificial neuronal network; ground truth: Stereomicroscope	Accuracy: 96%
	Qiao et al. [73]	Neuronal network trained on several combinations of multifrequency signals for improving locating the apical foramen in 21 extracted teeth in vitro	Accuracy: 95%
Preoperative risk assessment	Herbst et al. 2023 [79]	Predicting the technical outcome of a root canal treatment (obturation length) of 555 cases with logistic regression, random forest, support vector machine, decision tree, gradient boosting machine and extreme gradient boosting based on several preoperative risk factors	Sensitivity: 50–77.8% Specificity: 60.8–88.2% ROC-AUC: 0.54–0.62
Outcome prediction	Herbst et al. 2022 [82]	Predicting the healing outcome of root canal treatments (changes in lesion size) of 591 cases with logistic regression, random forest, gradient boosting machine and extreme gradient boosting based on several preoperative risk factors	Sensitivity: 11.6–21.0% Specificity: 87.6–94.3% ROC-AUC: 0.59–0.63
	Lee et al. 2023 [83]	Predicting the healing outcome of endodontically treated single-rooted premolars ($n = 598$) based on preoperative radiographs using a custom 17-layer CNN and ResNet 18	Mean accuracy: 63.4–67% ROC-AUC: 0.59–0.64
	Nosrat et al. 2023 [84]	Predicting the occurrence of an flare-up after non-surgically retreatment based on patient- and tooth-level covariates with a random forest	Sensitivity: 49% Specificity: 83% ROC-AUC: 0.7

8.2 Current Application of Endodontics in Literature

8.2.1 Periapical Lesions

On dental radiographs, apical periodontitis appears as a periapical radiolucency (PARL) due to the mineral loss in the distinct area. Periapical radiographs (PR), panoramic views (OPG), and cone-beam computed tomography are conventional imaging techniques to detect PARL. By comparing these techniques, there is an almost inversely proportional relation between diagnostic accuracy (sensitivity and specificity) and radiation dose: CBCT offers the highest sensitivity and specificity (95% and 90%, respectively) compared to PR (50% and 83%, respectively) [9] but offers the highest effective dose of 5–652 μSv [10] compared to 1–5 μSv for PR [11]. For patient screening, OPG is the most frequently used technique due to the full representation of the dentition [12], despite showing the least sensitivity of 28% when it comes to PARL detection [13].

Detecting PARL depends not only on the used imaging modality but also on the individual analyzing the radiograph. Confounding factors are years of experience, training, and specialty [14]. Additionally, the quality assessment of PARL depends on the utilized scoring system and the calibration between the raters [15]. So, there is a need to overcome this form of rater bias and to objectify the detection process of PARL on radiographs to raise the diagnostic certainty level.

Several neuronal network algorithms have been employed in current research to detect PARL on radiographs. Different architectures were tested for classification, object detection, and segmentation tasks (Fig. 8.2). Classification

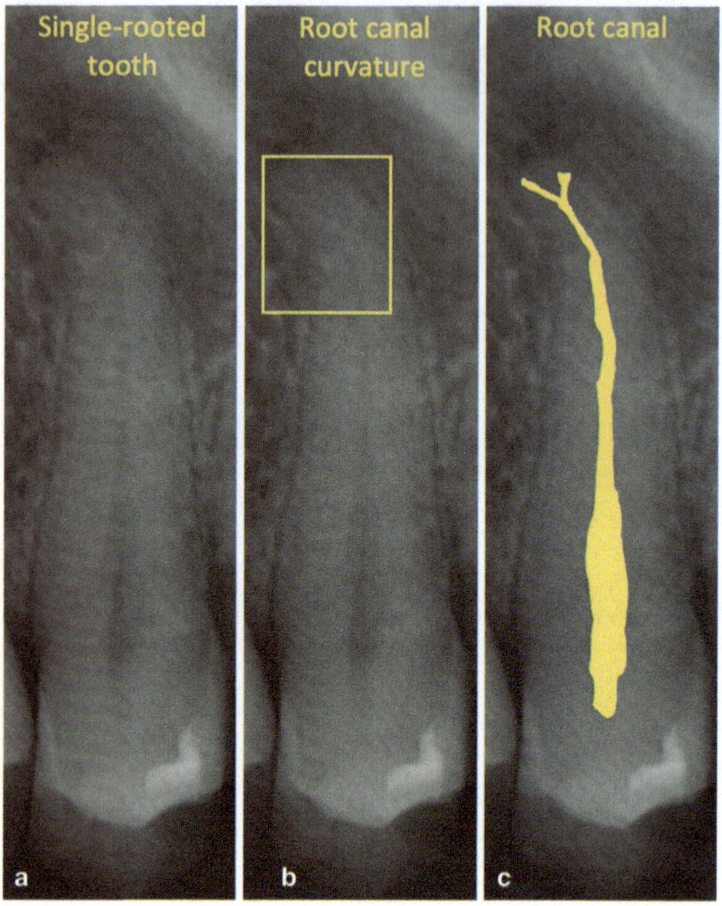

Fig. 8.2 Visualization of classification (**a**), detection (**b**), and segmentation (**c**) tasks

means to label the specific data subject with a diagnosis, e.g., PARL "present" or "not present" on a radiograph. For example, in the study of Ekert et al. [16], six experienced dentists assigned in a gradual majority process a diagnosis PARL condition of teeth on 2579 OPG [16]. After digitally preprocessing, the image data were fed into a convolutional neuronal network (CNN). A similar methodology, but with different CNN architectures, was employed by other studies for the classification of PARL on datasets ranging from 460 to 4129 PR. In these studies, the sensitivity and specificity range between 0.65 to 0.97 and 0.87 to 0.94, respectively [16–21].

Other architectures of CNN-like region-based convolutional neuronal networks allow for boxing out the region of interest, like PARL. This object detection allows for more precise support during the diagnostic process because the region of interest is highlighted through a bounding box instead of labeling the tooth in classification CNN. Two studies investigated the performance of R-CNN for detecting PARL on 1130 to 2900 PR, and sensitivity and specificity ranged between 0.54 to 0.81 and 0.54 to 0.98, respectively [20, 22]. For evaluating the performance of R-CNN regarding the quality of the drawn bounding boxes, only Chen et al. [23] reported the intersection over union (IoU) of 0.7 ± 0.02.

Most studies investigated the automated detection of PARL on radiographs with image segmentation models. Here the PARL on the input images was annotated pixel-wise by the rater and fed to the CNN, which U-Net is the most famous architecture here. Accordingly, the trained model creates a pixel-wise mask for the

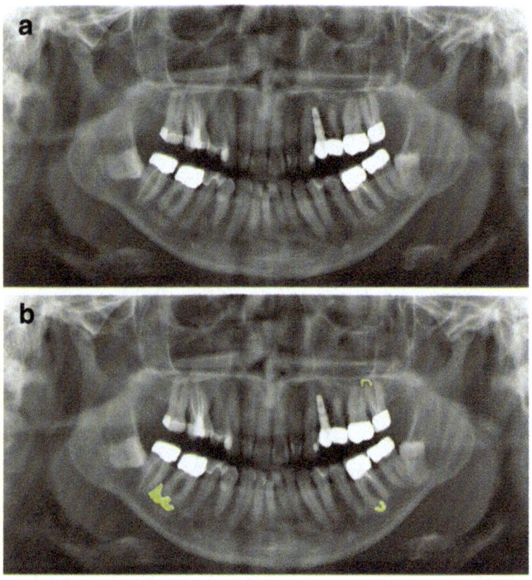

Fig. 8.3 Detection of periapical radiolucencies (**a**) panoramic view without automated detection (**b**) the same panoramic view with automated detected periapical radiolucencies (segmentation)

detected PARL and highlights them on the radiograph, so identifying the potential PARL in a clinical scenario would be more straightforward (Fig. 8.3). PR, OPG, and CBCT were used for image segmentation with varying performances: The highest sensitivity and precision could be found on 3900 CBCT (U-Net) with 0.95/0.89 [24] and on 2200 PA (YOLO v3) with 0.89/0.9 [25]. In general, specificity was relatively high among the studies with values ranging from 0.88 to 0.99 [26, 27]. From a clinical viewpoint, the segmentation and object detection models are more beneficial for clinical application compared to classification models because of their capability to visually highlight the suspicious area.

Furthermore, the staging of PARL by existing scoring systems is a clinically relevant task, especially for outcome assessment in clinical studies [25]. Most classical studies in endodontics used the periapical index (PAI) introduced by Ørstavik [28] for staging periapical conditions on PR. The major drawback of these scoring systems is the susceptibility to observer bias [25] which could have an impact on the results of the outcome studies. To overcome human bias, AI could be implemented for PAI score assignments. One study investigated on a dataset consisting of 2200 PR with 3540 periapical regions of mandibular molars the performance of a CNN (YOLOv.3) [25]. The true predictions varied from 30% to 90% indicating a high variability among the different PAI scores. In an experiment, the authors simplified the PARL staging to a binary decision which led to more accurate predictions with a true prediction value of 92%. The authors evaluated these findings as promising but advocated for further development of an automated system for staging PARL to overcome human bias [25].

8.2.1.1 How to Interpret These Results?

The reported measurements give an estimate of the possible clinical performance of these models. A recent systematic review and meta-analysis focusing on deep learning for the detection of periapical radiolucent lesions performed a subgroup analysis based on the image modality [18]. They found out that in PR, the diagnostic odds ratio was 64.8 and the pooled sensitivity and specificity were 0.9 and 0.87, respectively. Based on these findings, CNNs were able to detect PARL on PR with high sensitivity and specificity. Due to the limited number of studies investigating the performance of OPG and CBCT, no conclusion could be made. There are hints that these models performed less accurate on OPGs. A reason could be the overall reduced diagnostic value when it comes to detecting PARL in general on OPG. The models were trained on reference standards, meaning labeled input data by humans, so there might be an annotator bias irrespective of the used model. As mentioned earlier, the inter-rater and intra-rater agreement on OPG is considerably low compared to PR [29], as well as PR compared to CBCT [30], wherefore the ground truth provided by an expert board might come with higher uncertainty compared to PR or CBCT.

Besides that, these models are trained to detect PARL and not a final diagnosis. The used ground truth is merely based on radiographical annotations and not on histological data, which remains the gold standard for classifying the PARL. Additionally, the staging of PARL remained overall insufficient and highlighted the current obstacles in staging PARL on radiographs and the need for further elaboration on this topic [25].

In general, the final interpretation of the detected PARL with its treatment implications belongs to the dentist. Despite the promising results for automated detection of suspicious apical regions and possible integration in diagnostic tools, the benefit for the patient remains unclear. Studies investigating the cost-effectiveness of automated detection of PARL are still lacking.

8.2.2 Vertical Root Fracture

A vertical root fracture (VRF) is defined as an axial fracture involving the hard tissues and the root canal system of a root. More than 90% of VRF occurs in root-filled teeth [31], and the prevalence ranges from 4% to 32% [31, 32]. An early detection of VRF may prevent further damage to the surrounding tissue. The correct diagnosis of VRF remains a challenge based on radiographic examination and clinical findings. A clinical pilot study assessing the effectiveness of CBCT in identifying VRF reported sensitivity and specificity rates of 88% and 75%, respectively [33]. On two-dimensional radiographs, the sensitivity for detecting VRF was just 5% in an ex vivo study [33]. To support the diagnostic process, especially on two-dimensional radiographs, some research groups employed deep learning algorithms for the detection of VRF on radiographs, whereby two studies used an in vitro setting [34, 35] and one study used real-life OPG for model training and evaluation [4].

Both in vitro studies used probabilistic neuronal networks to investigate VRFs in premolars. Johari et al. [35] used PR and CBCT to compare root canals treated with untreated teeth, whereas Kositbowornchai et al. [34] utilized solely PR to assess untreated teeth. The sensitivity ranged from 67.7% to 90.5%, while the specificity was about 98%, in the PR assessment. In Johari et al. study, the sensitivity was slightly lower at 93.3%, but the specificity was higher at 100%, utilizing CBCT. The in vitro studies found comparable results in detecting VRFs compared to the results of a clinical pilot study with CBCT. However, the in vitro settings are not comparable to a clinical scenario due to several reasons including the absence of surrounding anatomical structures and the use of one distinct tooth type.

Fukuda et al. [4] used 300 OPG from real cases with 330 teeth showing a VRF to train a CNN model. All teeth with VRF showed a clearly visible fracture line and were diagnosed on the OPG during clinical routine. The recall, precision, and F1-score were 0.75, 0.93, and 0.83, respectively, and the authors concluded that the model performance was insufficient for clinical application.

8.2.2.1 How to Interpret the Results?

A meta-analysis considered CBCT to be the most reliable imaging method when it comes to VRF detection [36]. On the other hand, Patel et al. [37] concluded that CBCT and PR were not accurate for detecting VRF in an in vitro setting due to imaging artifacts. To date, deep learning techniques have not been beneficial for detecting VRF on dental radiographs. For future research, a higher accuracy might be achieved by taking further characteristics of VRF into the automated diagnostic process like the presence of an "halo"-lesion, clinical findings (e.g., periodontal probing), and patient reports.

8.2.3 Analyzing of Endodontic Structures

For further treatment planning and patient education, knowledge about the endodontic structures of the particular tooth is crucial. The radiographical analysis comprises the evaluation of the number and type of roots and root canals [38, 39], the appearance of the pulp chamber [40, 41], and in cases of retreatments possibly missed canals [6] or separated instruments [5]. The potential use of AI algorithms in these planning steps was investigated by several research groups.

8.2.3.1 Segmentation of Root Canal Structures

Anatomical structures can be evaluated on two- and three-dimensional radiographs. Although two-dimensional radiographs are generally considered the go-to imaging modality for such assessments in daily practice [42], research on their use for segmentation techniques has been limited. Most existing studies focus on using these radiographs for filling out dental charts rather than for detailed treatment planning [43, 44].

On the other hand, CBCT with a limited field of view is the preferred imaging option when dealing with complex root structures, ambiguous clinical symptoms, or dental anomalies [42]. CBCT provides detailed information about the tooth anatomy and the surrounding tissues. However, the complex endodontic structures are represented in multiple two-dimensional planes, and the three-dimensional imagining of the endodontic structures depends highly on the clinical experience of the observer, so true 3D reconstruction remains a problem for clinicians [40]. Besides the 3D nature of the image modality, low tissue contrast in low-dose CBCT and image noise due to artifacts diminish the interpretability of CBCTs. As a result, not all relevant information could be retrieved from the CBCT for encompassing treatment planning.

Over the past decade, several attempts were undertaken to automate and optimize the 3D reconstruction and segmentation of CBCT data. In general, image segmentation is a post-processing method to split images into regions. The pixels of a region show similarities regarding a characteristic or computed property, so distinct regions differ significantly based on these defined properties [45]. Deep learning techniques were investigated in recent studies for segmentation tasks in CBCT and intended to overcome the shortcomings of the traditional methods [46]. The segmentation of tooth and endodontic structures by employing deep supervised neuronal networks is also a demanding task [40]: Teeth are highly individual and show a varying shape in CBCT irrespective of the viewed axis. The axial view in the crown-to-root direction exhibits changing anatomies per slice as compared to the sagittal view. So, a high number of teeth in the training data set is necessary because the slices in the axial direction offer too many variations in terms of pattern recognition. However, the creation of ground truth for algorithm training with manual labeling of the tooth structures slice-by-slice requires time and highly calibrated raters. However, most studies showed promising results with different convolutional neuronal networks like U-Net [40, 47] or V-Net [48].

Due to the abovementioned reasons, some studies only focused on simple anatomical structures like single-rooted teeth without restorations or root canal fillings, including Lin et al. [41]. and Wang et al. studies [8]. In both studies, the dice score ranged from 0.87 to 0.88 for pulp chamber segmentation. Lin et al. [41] found in single-rooted teeth for pulp chamber and root canal segmentation a dice score of 0.87 and for tooth segmentation 0.96. Duan et al. [40] used single- and multi-rooted teeth for segmentation with U-Net and found a mean dice scores for pulp segmentation in single- and multi-rooted teeth of 0.89 and 0.88, respectively; for tooth segmentation, they found a mean dice score of 0.96 for single- and multi-rooted teeth, which is similar to the findings of Li et al. [49] for root and crown segmentation (dice score 0.96). Zheng et al. [50] found similar results for pulp chamber segmentation in molars (dice score: 0.88) and could positively correlate the pulp chamber volume to the age of the patient (correlation coefficient $r = 0.74$). These data show that segmentation of the endodontic structures is a more challenging task compared to the more straightforward segmentation of the entire tooth.

Most studies used manually labeled CBCT data as the ground truth and model validation, so the accuracy of the data for model training depends highly on the rater's experience and the recognition of the radiographs. However, histology remains the gold standard for defining tissues, but these data are mostly not available in high numbers.

Lin et al. [41] emphasized the lack of high-quality training samples in previous studies and aimed for a more precise ground truth. Micro-computed tomography (micro-CT) is known as the most accurate tool for analyzing root canal anatomy by providing micron-scale resolution and 3D visualization [51]. The dataset in this study comprised matched CBCT and micro-CT data of single-rooted premolars. Micro-CT allows for a more detailed representation of the endodontic structures and may reduce the uncertainty generated by manually labeling the lower-resolution CBCT. Lin et al. [41] compared micro-CT with manually labeled CBCT (control group) ground truth data and found that the use of micro-CT as the ground truth resulted in more accurate predictions: the control group achieved for pulp chamber segmentation a dice score of 73.6% compared to micro-CT 86.8%. This pilot study demonstrates a more reliable training of the CNN, but limitations are that teeth scanned by micro-CT were extracted (CBCT scans were performed in vivo) and micro-CT is not applicable in clinical dentistry, so data cannot be acquired from vivid individuals. Most studies used a comparatively small sample size ranging from 29 [49] to 80 [52], only one study used 180 CBCT [50]. Besides that, all studies used data from one single center, so the generalizability remains questionable.

Studies on tooth segmentation and endodontic structures achieved good results, whereby the recognition of more sophisticated endodontic structures was less accurate compared to segmenting the whole tooth. Future research should focus on establishing a reliable ground truth and investigate the generalizability of the proposed models.

8.2.3.2 Prediction of Root Canal Anatomies

Rare or special anatomies are difficult to identify on 2D radiographs for general dentists and even specialists. Utilizing 3D radiographs like CBCT can facilitate the diagnostic process and increase the treatment confidence [53], but obtaining a preoperative CBCT scan is not always feasible or cost-effective for every case. On the other hand, preoperative knowledge about clinical obstacles may drive the treatment outcome. Assuming that there are hidden patterns in 2D radiographs indicating the special anatomy, deep learning models could be able to learn these patterns and highlight the suspicious regions on the 2D radiograph. Then, the case could be reevaluated by the clinician, and further radiographs could be more precisely recommended by avoiding both unnecessary radiation and costs. Current applications of AI for detecting anatomies are as follows:

Second Distal Roots in the Mandibular First Molars

Second distal roots in the mandibular first molars are in general a rare condition but show a high prevalence in local populations, up to 22% among Asians [54]. So, there might be a varying awareness of this type of anatomy among dentists worldwide accompanying the risk of leaving untreated. Hiraiwa et al. [38] investigated the performances of two CNN architectures (AlexNet and GoogleNet) on 760 mandibular first molars without root canal treatments on OPG. The ground truth was defined by analyzing the matched CBCT of the respective tooth (163 teeth with extra roots). Their study determined that the CNN achieved slightly superior performance compared to the radiologist, with significant differences in specificity and ROC-AUC values. Specifically, the radiologist achieved an ROC-AUC of 0.74, sensitivity of 80.2%, and specificity of 82%. In contrast, the GoogleNet model achieved an ROC-AUC of 0.85, sensitivity of 74.42%, and specificity of 95.9%, while the AlexNet model achieved an ROC-AUC of 0.87, sensitivity of 77.3%, and specificity of 97.1% for the image classification.

C-Shaped Root Canals

C-shaped anatomies show a varying prevalence depending on the geographic region, whereby the prevalence among Asians is reported to be the highest from 8.9% to 44.5% in second molars [55–57]. The American Association of Endodontists categorized c-shaped root canals to be of the highest difficulty to treat [58]. The most frequent reasons for treatment failure were a leaky canal and a present isthmus [59]. Diagnosing c-shaped root canals on 2D radiographs can be challenging due to image superimposition and the bony structure of the mandible, so CBCT can be indicated for further treatment planning [60].

Three studies investigated the application of deep learning in identifying c-shaped root canals on PRs, panoramic views, and CBCT [39, 61,

62]. Two studies used CNN models with application of the gradient-weighted class activation mapping (Grad-CAM) technique [39, 62]. This technique is also an AI explainability approach, because it visualizes class activation maps highlighting regions that are decisive for the model decision on the radiograph [63].

For model training, all studies used CBCT for ground truth evaluation. Jeon et al. [62] used a CNN-based Xception model on second molars from 1020 OPGs, which were manually cropped; so each of the 2040 images shows one sound second molar. They compared the predictive performance of the Xception model to a radiologist and an endodontist and found that the AUC values were 0.98, 087, and 0.89 respectively; the Xception model performed significantly better compared to the endodontist and offered a sensitivity and specificity of 92.7 and 97.0 (endodontist: 91.5% and 85.5%).

Yang et al. [39] developed a CNN (EfficientNet) for OPG and PR (370 cases) and compared EfficientNet to a general practitioner and a specialist; the EfficientNet outperformed the general practitioner, but not the specialist. Additionally, the authors cropped the 2D radiographs in two different ways: one group contains the crown and the root and the second the root only. They found that a reduction in information leads to an overall increase in performance measures (e.g., AUC PR: crown and root 0.95, root only 0.98; AUC OPG: crown and root 0.93, root only 98%).

Grad-CAM analysis in Jeon et al. [62] revealed that the Xception model focused on root canal shapes converging into the apex to predict c-shaped canals and on the furcation for predicting the non-c-shaped canals. Grad-CAM and guided Grad-CAM were applied by Yang et al. and support the findings of Jeon et al. that in most class activation maps highlighted the root portion area, especially in the apical third [39, 62]. Misinterpretations occurred more frequently in the crown and root group with a focus on the cementoenamel junction which is in line with the findings of increased prediction performance in the root-only group. Misclassified heat maps were associated with radiographic c-shaped canals which are hard to distinguish from a non-c-shaped case on 2D radiographs.

Sherwood et al. tested three different CNN architectures for segmentation in 135 CBCT showing different types of c-shaped canals: U-Net, residual U-Net, and Xception. They used U-Net in combination with contrast-limited adaptive histogram equalization (CLAHE) for enhancing the local contrast of each slice. They found that Xception U-Net with its more sophisticated architecture showed significantly better performance with a dice coefficient of 0.81 compared to residual U-Net 0.78 and U-Net 0.77. Enhancing the local contrast via CLAHE increased the performance of each architecture by a mean of 4.6% [61].

Taurodont Teeth

Taurodontism is a developmental condition where the pulp chamber of the tooth is significantly expanded and the furcation is displaced towards the apex [64]. The most commonly affected teeth are the molars. The possibility of additional root canals, narrowed root canals, and canal configurations increases the risk of complications in root canal treatments in taurodontism. Preoperative knowledge of this rare condition and degree may facilitate endodontic treatment planning or hint toward a systemic condition.

Duman et al. [65] investigated the segmentation performance of a U-Net architecture on OPG (whole teeth); the training dataset comprised 348 OPG with 1080 taurodont teeth which were increased by the image augmentation technique to 1392 images with 4320 labels. The segmentation performance of the U-Net was evaluated on a test set of 43 OPG with 126 positive labels; sensitivity, precision, and F1 scores were 0.87, 0.79, and 0.83. The authors concluded that the model performed well concerning the segmentation of taurodont teeth. Future research should focus on taurodontism classification on different image modalities to specify the respective treatment needs. Additionally, Duman et al. found upper molars to be more difficult to automatically segment because of the proximity to the maxillary sinus.

Identification of Previous Treatment Complications

Besides rare and difficult anatomies, previous treatment complications are also difficult to identify on radiographic images and can have a huge clinical impact on the treatment planning and prognosis in both primary and secondary treatment cases. Common complications are separated instruments, perforations, ledge formation, and untreated anatomies. Several factors play a role in identifying these complications in the treatment planning process: level of experience/knowledge and time spent assessing the radiographs. Experienced endodontists can identify most of these complications by studying potentially revealing details like different radiopacities in the root canal filling or double contours of the root.

Two studies tried to transfer this expert knowledge into deep learning applications. Buyuk et al. [5] focused on detecting separated root canal instruments on OPG by comparing a CNN with a long short-term memory network. In total, 905 OPG were used, 417 of them showed a fractured instrument, and 498 did not. The dataset was artificially augmented and copied twice; one copy was used with a Gabor filter for image enhancement and the other one without. The authors found that Gabor-filtered models, in general, showed higher performance measures and that the Gabor-filtered CNN (sensitivity 81.26 ± 4.79; specificity 87.16 ± 2.82; ROC-AUC 0.89) showed slightly better performance measures, but without statistical significance. The authors concluded that the tested models could improve the diagnostic accuracy for separated instruments in daily practice on OPG. One major drawback is the exclusion of post or pin restorations from the dataset, which might be misinterpreted as a separated instrument.

CBCT is considered to be the most reliable image modality when it comes to preoperative anatomy evaluation. However, metallic restorations or radio-opaque root canal filling can cause significant artifacts which impede the full examination. Albitar et al. [6] analyzed a potential solution for this problem and tried to develop a U-Net for detecting unobturated second mesiobuccal canals (mb2) in CBCT in the presence of root canal fillings and coronal restorations. They used 58 CBCT with 102 mesiobuccal roots, whereby 51 roots showed obturated and unobturated root canals, respectively. The original scans were manually cropped, so only one root was visible for each element of the dataset. After model training, the performance was evaluated on a test set comprising 10 roots with equal numbers of obturated and unobturated mb2. The model achieved a sensitivity of 0.8 and a specificity of 1, the accuracy was 0.9. However, these performance measures were evaluated on ten elements, so the generalizability is questionable. In general, this study is highly relevant, because the authors addressed the problem of non-standardized training data with artifacts and in consequence algorithm training on different background qualities. One major drawback is also the definition of a ground truth: of the 102 cases, in 44 a tiebreaker (third observer) was needed for a final decision on whether mb2 was present or not. Between the two main observers, the Kappa score was 0.35 for the mb2 cases. So, the U-Net learned on a questionable ground truth, which is not an insufficiency in the study design, but rather the effect of using real-world CBCT. Handling artifacts, varying anatomical configurations, and calcifications is a major challenge for automated CBCT evaluation and needs huge amounts of input data with reliable ground truth.

Additional and challenging anatomies can be successfully detected by CNN and are in most cases of similar performance compared to specialists or experienced dentists. As highlighted by Yang et al. [39], the performance of the algorithms can be increased by reducing the unnecessary information from the radiograph. Future attempts should focus on combining segmentation algorithms with algorithms for image classification. Besides that, enhancing image parameters like contrast via CLAHE can improve the overall performance of CNN [61]. Nevertheless, one has to emphasize that these studies lack generalizability and external validation.

8.2.3.3 Preoperative Working Length Estimation

Determining the apical foramen for working length estimation is a crucial step in endodontic treatment, and root canal-relative-impedance measuring devices (known as electronic apex locators (EAL)) in combination with PR are considered to be the most reliable method to identify the apical foramen [66]. Despite a recent systematic review indicating that EAL is more precise than PR [67], some concerns arise from the underlying study designs [68]; hence radiographic control of the measured working length is still indicated, especially for forensic reasons. The evaluation of PR depends, as described above, on the experience of the observer. Therefore, some studies investigated the application of deep learning techniques for improving the accuracy of radiographic length evaluation.

Saghiri et al. [69] investigated the application of a multilayer perceptron artificial neuronal network (ANN). They used 50 extracted single-rooted mandibular incisors and second premolars and positioned them in a dried skull. Further, a K-file was placed in the root canal and a radiograph was taken; as a ground truth, two endodontists evaluated the apical region with the placed K-file under a stereomicroscope and labeled the position either as “short,” “exact,” and “long.” Thirty-six radiographs were used for ANN training, and the remaining 14 radiographs were used for model testing. The authors found that only one radiograph was misclassified and accordingly the accuracy was 93% and concluded that ANN could act as a second opinion to locate the apical foramen.

The same research group investigated the performance of the proposed model in a cadaver setting [70]. They used 50 single-rooted teeth placed in a K-file in each root canal system and performed a PR afterwards. The radiographs were classified by two endodontists according to the abovementioned scheme: “short,” “exact,” and “long.” Additionally, the radiographs were fed to the ANN as test data for classification. All examined teeth were extracted, and for ground truth evaluation, two endodontists evaluated the apical areas under a stereomicroscope and classified the position of the K-file as mentioned above. The performances of the endodontists (for the radiographic evaluation) and the ANN were compared to the ground truth; the accuracy of the endodontists was significantly lower (76%) compared to the ANN (96%). There was no statistically significant difference between the ground truth and the ANN.

Despite technical improvements in EAL, studies found no benefit of [71] or even inferior performance [72] multifrequency-based methods compared to dual frequency-based EAL. Qiao et al. [73] proposed using a neural network trained on multifrequency impedance measurements to account for the complex environment in root canals. In an in vitro study on 21 extracted teeth, they found this approach improved accuracy in identifying the apical foramen compared to dual-frequency EAL. While limited by sample size and lack of statistical analysis, this pilot study indicates that AI-based multifrequency analysis may enhance EAL performance by reducing confounding measurement factors in root canals. Further research is needed to confirm clinical viability. Overall, it demonstrates the potential of AI approaches to improve accuracy of working length determination.

The presented studies exhibit promising approaches to enhance the robustness of determining the apical foramen for working length estimation. The drawbacks of these studies in general are the in vitro setting; it is well known that body parameters like temperature, blood pressure, and electric potential influence the measurement accuracy of EAL. However, these studies show the potential of deep learning techniques to facilitate the process of determining the apical foramen.

8.2.3.4 Preoperative Risk Assessment

Endodontic treatments are in general demanding procedures, and the skills needed to accomplish a certain case and to avoid mishaps depend on several preoperative factors. Endodontic societies have published several paper-based and online risk assessment tools for assigning a case either a “low,” “moderate,” or “high” difficulty with implications on the referral decision [58, 74–76].

Some studies support the usefulness of these forms [77, 78], but the criteria for assigning a case to a certain difficulty level are preponderantly not evidence-based and the impact of single risk factors remains unclear [76]. Essam et al. [76] proposed an online tool based on the best evidence available and the thorough evaluation of 75 real-life cases by 35 specialists. The authors also emphasized the subjective nature of risk assessment by showing that the assignment of a case to moderate difficulty resulted in the highest disagreement among specialists. AI could play a crucial role in identifying certain risk factors. With the ability to find patterns within datasets or radiographs, these algorithms could be an auxiliary tool to understand the risk assessment process from a different perspective and to gain different insights. Additionally, the individual experience could be considered for a holistic case evaluation.

Only one research found on AI and risk assessment exists. Herbst et al. [79] employed different machine learning algorithms for predicting the technical outcome of root canal treatments ("adequate" or "inadequate" root canal filling). They analyzed 555 retrospective endodontic treatments first with logR to find significant associations between discussed risk factors from the risk assessment form of the AAE. In a second step, they trained machine learning algorithms (random forest, support vector machine, decision tree, gradient boosting machine, and extreme gradient boosting) on a training dataset and tested their predictive. They found out that achieving an adequate obturation quality depends mainly on the operator's experience and several risk factors (e.g., canal visibility or retreatment cases). But the predictive performance of all models was considerably low (AUC 0.63–0.71 and accuracy 63.4–78.9%).

8.2.3.5 Outcome Prediction

Precise outcome prediction of an endodontic treatment would be the top goal of implementing AI in endodontics. Some of the previously cited studies can be seen as a valuable part of the entire process meaning that outcome prediction can be understood as an orchestra of different AI algorithms. However, some studies tried to approach the outcome prediction based on different types of data. Some studies used features extracted from the patient record and radiographs, and other studies aimed to predict the treatment outcome only based on radiographs. So far, most observational studies in endodontics focused on outcome analysis used descriptive statistics and/or logistic regression models for data analysis [80].

In a study by Signor et al. [81], a decision tree was employed to analyze retrospective retreatment cases using 32 independent variables. However, it is worth noting that the decision tree was primarily used to describe the data and conduct association analysis, rather than evaluating the predictive value of the trained algorithm. The main purpose of this type of study is to gain insights into the underlying patterns within the data by utilizing a machine learning algorithm.

Herbst et al. [82] employed machine learning algorithms for analyzing their retrospective data of 591 orthograde endodontic treatments with a mean follow-up of 15.2 months. They first performed a multivariate analysis via logistic regression and several machine learning (random forest, gradient boosting machine, extreme gradient boosting) to identify significant associations between tooth-, patient- and treatment-level covariates and the healing outcome ("healing" or "no healing"). In the second step, they used the same dataset for predictive modeling, aiming to predict the healing outcome. The predictive value of the trained models on the test dataset was low; the ROC-AUC-values on the test dataset ranged from 0.59 (random forest) to 0.63 (logistic regression). Limitations of this study were the lack of long-term recalls and the size of the dataset. However, this study highlights the complexity of predicting the healing outcome even based on several covariates.

Lee et al. [83] aimed to forecast the outcome of endodontically treated single-rooted premolars ($n = 598$) based on preoperative radiographs using a custom 17-layer CNN and ResNet-18 network. The reported mean accuracy of their model (67.0%) was significantly higher compared to ResNet-18 (63.4%) and the no-information rate (majority class). The authors state that the AUC value is difficult to interpret because no other studies on CNN for endodontic prognosis exist so far. However, this pilot study involving solely periapical radiographs for predicting the treatment outcome shows promising results for future research.

The abovementioned studies aimed to predict the clinician-centered outcome "periapical healing" after an endodontic treatment. One study intended to predict the patient-reported outcome "occurrence of flare-up" after orthograde endodontic retreatments [84]. An endodontic flare-up is defined by a postoperative exaggeration of intense pain after an endodontic treatment. Predicting the likelihood of a flare-up could be helpful in treatment planning and patient education because a flare-up is a disruptive event which could negatively alter the relationship between patient and clinician resulting in an unscheduled appointment. Nosrat et al. [84] analyzed 2846 cases retrospectively; all patients reported their pain level in a 4-point verbal rating system, comprising the following levels: "none," "mild," "moderate," and "severe." The levels "moderate" and "severe" indicated the need for an additional visit and were defined to be a "flare-up." Conversely, "none" and "mild" pain were defined to be "no flare-up." In a multivariate analysis, they could identify significant associations between several covariates and the occurrence of a flare-up. In a second step, the dataset was split in a train and test dataset (70/30%) and a random forest was trained on the test dataset. The predictive performance was evaluated on the test dataset, and the sensitivity, specificity, and ROC-AUC were reported with 49%, 83%, and 69.8%. Despite having a large sample size and a complex machine learning algorithm, the trained random forest and the used covariates (several patient-level covariates like clinical findings and medical history) were not sufficient to make valuable predictions, and a further understanding is needed.

How to Interpret the Results?

AI has the potential to be a powerful tool in the future for diagnosis and treatment planning (Fig. 8.4). To date, algorithms are suitable for detecting patterns in clear-cut and homogenous datasets (especially image data) with low variance (Fig. 8.5). High variance is given in datasets, when human activities are involved, like predicting the technical outcome of a root canal treatment or the treatment outcome. Neither extracted clinical and radiographic data nor radiographs only were yet able to predict the outcome of endodontic treatments precisely. The outcome of an endodontic treatment depends on several independent factors including the clinical

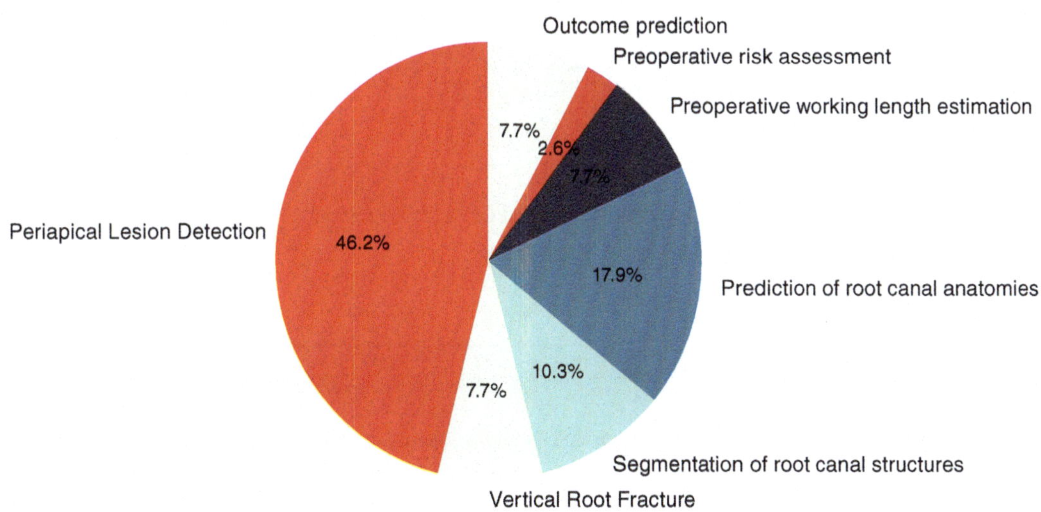

Fig. 8.4 Distribution of studies based on application

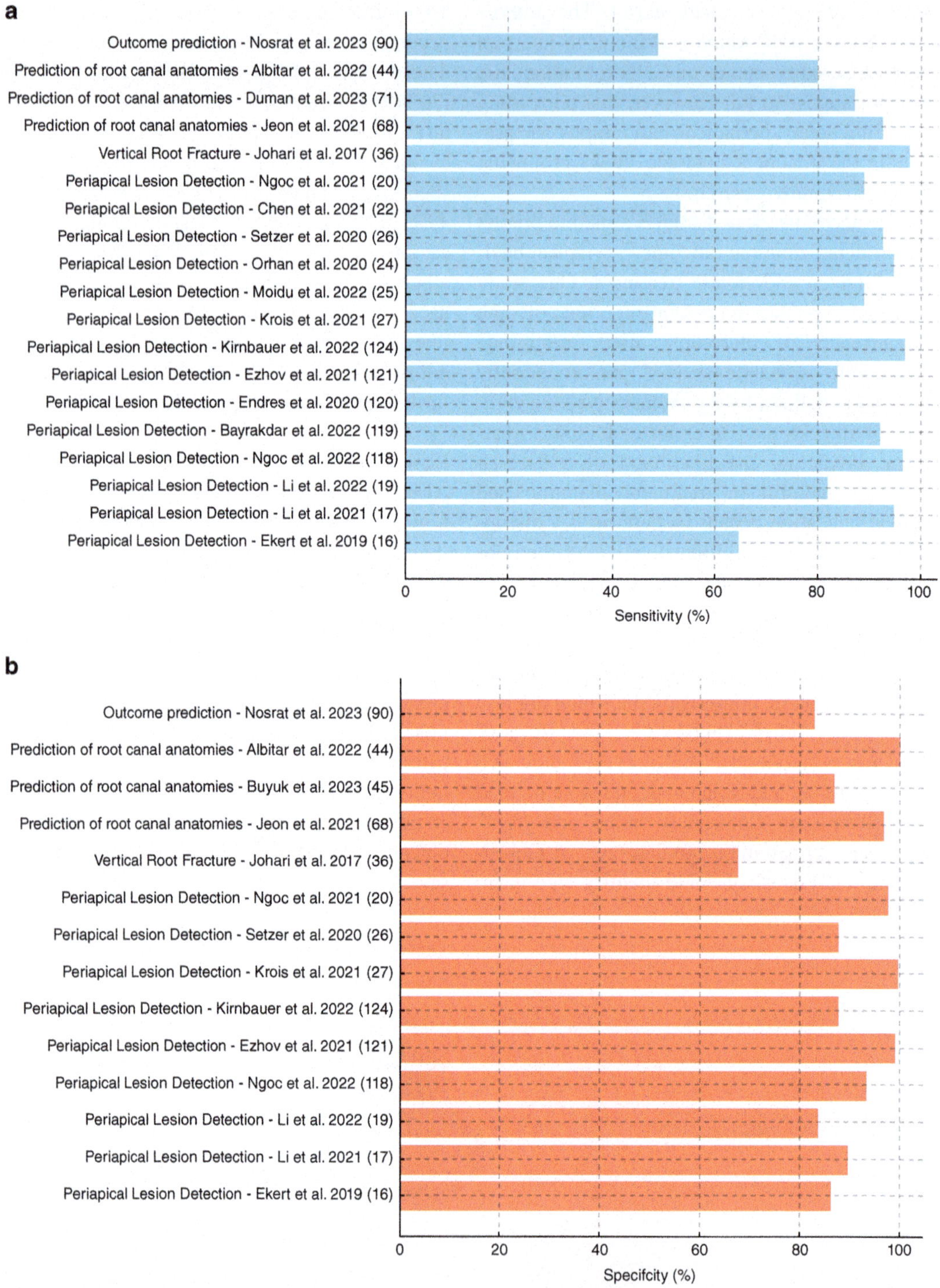

Fig. 8.5 Sensitivity (**a**) and specificity (**b**) of each study with corresponding application

situation, tooth anatomy, diagnosis, medical history, and operator training.

The high variance could be compensated by increasing the datasets. Without exception, the main drawback of all recent AI studies in endodontics is the limited dataset and/or the non-real-life scenario. All mentioned studies provided a valuable contribution to the knowledge of AI in endodontics and proved the concept accordingly. Future endeavors should focus on collaboration to achieve larger datasets.

8.3 AI and Endodontics in Industry/Real-World Practice and Education

AI also has made its way into the industry and has started to influence real-world practices and education in endodontics. This section explores how AI is impacting endodontics at industry-level through imaging software and tools, chatbots, and dental education.

8.3.1 Imaging Software and Tools

AI has been integrated into various imaging software and tools in endodontics, including radiographic analysis software and CBCT analysis software. These tools help dental professionals analyze and interpret dental images more accurately and efficiently. For example, most of the current tools only focus on reporting and segmentation of dental and structure. A list of AI solutions that can be used in the field of endodontics is provided in Table 8.1.

8.3.2 Role of Chatbots

Due to deep learning advancements, chatbots like ChatGPT, Google Bard, and Bing have gained a lot of attention among the population. AI-powered chatbots in dentistry and more specifically endodontics can improve patient interaction and clinical decision-making. These chatbots can provide patients with information about dental procedures, answer frequently asked questions, and even help schedule appointments. In addition, chatbots can assist dental professionals in making clinical decisions by providing relevant information and suggestions based on the patient's dental history and current condition [85, 86]. However, recent research by Suárez et al. [87] indicates that while ChatGPT shows promise, it is not yet capable of fully replacing dentists in clinical practice. They evaluated ChatGPT's performance in answering dichotomous endodontic questions found 85% consistency but only 57% accuracy compared to endodontic experts. Significant differences were seen in accuracy based on question difficulty. The authors concluded that ChatGPT cannot currently replace dentists in endodontic decision-making, though its performance may improve over time with further training.

8.3.3 Dental Education

AI has also started to play a role in dental education, particularly in endodontics. With the integration of AI in radiographic and CBCT analysis software, dental students can now receive real-time feedback on their image interpretations, thereby improving their diagnostic skills. Additionally, through the use of AI-driven simulation tool and emerging virtual reality platforms like Virtual Endo, students can practice endodontic procedures in a risk-free environment, which helps in honing their clinical skills. Such virtual reality simulators allow students to repeatedly perform procedures and receive feedback without risk to patients. AI systems can also be used to create personalized learning paths for students, by analyzing their performance and learning styles [88].

8.4 Challenges of Using AI in Endodontics

As it has been seen, AI has shown immense potential in the field of endodontics, promising to transform practices from diagnostics to treatment planning and execution. However, the path to full-scale integration is not without its hurdles. This section discusses the key challenges associated with the application of AI in endodontics.

8.4.1 Model Explainability

Model explainability, also known as interpretability, refers to the degree to which a human can understand and interpret the process and outcomes of a machine learning model [89]. AI algorithms, particularly those based on deep learning, are often described as "black box" models due to their complex and nonlinear nature. These models can generate predictions based on thousands, if not millions, of parameters, and their decision-making process is not easily interpretable by humans. In other words, while these models can generate accurate predictions or classifications, they do not readily reveal the reasoning or rules behind these decisions [90].

In a clinical setting, such as endodontics, this lack of transparency can be problematic. When a clinician makes a diagnosis or suggests a treatment, they base their decision on a clear understanding of the patient's condition, established medical knowledge, and clinical guidelines. The decision-making process can be explained and justified. However, with a "black box" AI model, it becomes hard to understand why the model arrived at a particular diagnosis or treatment recommendation. This makes it difficult to trust the decision made by the model [91]. Moreover, clinicians are obligated to obtain informed consent from patients before any procedure. This includes explaining the diagnosis and the proposed treatment. If the decision is based on the recommendations of a "black box" AI model, it could be challenging to provide a comprehensive explanation to the patient, which might compromise the process of obtaining truly informed consent [92].

In response to these issues, there is an increasing interest in developing more interpretable AI models or creating methods to make existing models more interpretable. Techniques such as feature importance ranking, partial dependence plots, and local interpretable model-agnostic explanations (LIME) are being employed to provide more insight into the decision-making process of AI models [93]. In endodontics, some studies detecting c-shaped anatomies have implemented Grad-CAM [39, 62], which generates heat maps to visualize the regions of the image most relevant to the model's predictions. This provides a representative example of how AI model decisions can be explained. Nevertheless, making complex AI models truly interpretable remains an open challenge and is an active area of research in the field.

8.4.2 Rare Conditions

AI algorithms, particularly those based on machine learning, rely heavily on large quantities of data for their training. They learn by identifying patterns and correlations in these large datasets and applying those learned patterns to new, unseen data. However, when it comes to diagnosing rare conditions, the data can often be sparse, leading to a significant challenge known as the "rare event" or "class imbalance" problem [94, 95].

Rare conditions in endodontics, such as complex root canal morphologies, atypical presentations of periapical pathologies, or external cervical resorption, occur infrequently in the general population. As a result, they are underrepresented in the datasets used to train AI models. This underrepresentation can lead to suboptimal performance of the AI models when it comes to detecting and diagnosing these conditions. AI models trained predominantly on common conditions can be "biased" towards these conditions and may struggle to identify rare conditions accurately, leading to a high false-negative rate. This means the model might overlook or incorrectly classify these rare conditions, which can have serious implications for patient care [96].

To mitigate these issues, several strategies can be employed. One common approach is data augmentation, where techniques such as synthetic minority over-sampling (SMOTE) are used to artificially increase the instances of rare conditions in the training dataset [97]. Another approach is to use advanced machine learning techniques designed to handle class imbalance, such as cost-sensitive learning or anomaly detection algorithms. However, even with these strategies, diagnosing rare conditions using AI remains a significant challenge, highlighting the importance of ongoing research and development in this area [98].

8.4.3 Ethical Consideration and Regulation

AI in dentistry, including endodontics, ushers in a new wave of ethical considerations and regulatory challenges. Here are a few primary areas of concern [99]:

1. *Data Privacy and Security*: AI models often require vast amounts of data to learn and make accurate predictions. In endodontics, these data might include patient images, clinical notes, or personal health information. Therefore, ensuring data privacy and security is paramount. Ethical considerations revolve around how data is collected, stored, and used. Proper consent must be obtained, and de-identification techniques should be used to protect patient privacy. However, even anonymized data can sometimes be re-identified, posing additional privacy risks.
2. *Accountability and Liability*: Who is responsible when an AI makes a mistake? Is it the clinician, the AI developer, or someone else? As AI models increasingly contribute to decision-making in endodontics, the question of who is accountable when things go wrong becomes more complex. Regulatory bodies have yet to create comprehensive rules for liability in AI-assisted healthcare. Currently, the clinician remains ultimately responsible when an AI makes a mistake, as AI is viewed as an assistive tool rather than an independent practitioner.
3. *Regulation*: Existing regulatory frameworks (e.g., "Artificial Intelligence and Machine Learning in Software as a Medical Device" by US Food and Drug Agency [100]) are struggling to keep pace with the rapid advancement of AI in healthcare. Regulators face the challenging task of ensuring safety and efficacy without stifling innovation. Standardized validation and testing procedures need to be established, and a balance must be struck between pre-market and post-market regulation.

8.4.4 Model Generalizability

Generalizability in machine learning is the ability of a model to apply its learning from one context to new and unseen contexts. In other words, the model can perform well not just on the data it was trained on but also on new data it has never encountered. Generalizability is a critical aspect when considering the application of AI in endodontics. An AI model used in this domain might be trained on a large dataset of radiographic images and associated diagnoses, with the expectation that it should perform well on images it has not seen before [101].

However, achieving high generalizability is a significant challenge. The AI model's performance can degrade if the new data differ substantially from the data used for training. For instance, the new data may originate from a different patient population, or the images may be captured using different radiography machines or protocols. This concept is known as distribution shift or dataset shift, and managing it is an ongoing research problem [102].

One main strategy to improve model generalizability is that data from various sources [27]. Despite the efforts, ensuring that AI models in endodontics generalize well across various settings remains a significant challenge, emphasizing the need for external validation studies that test the model on independent data from different sources and populations. For example, a study by Krois et al. [27] showed that training deep learning models on panoramic radiographs from multiple centers improved the generalizability for detecting apical lesions compared to single center training.

8.4.5 Lack of Public Standardized Dataset

Data plays a crucial role in the development of AI models. Standardized datasets are collections of data that have been processed and formatted consistently. They are essential for several reasons [103, 104]:

1. They allow different AI models to be trained and tested on the same data, providing a fair basis for comparison. Without standardized datasets, it is challenging to objectively assess and compare the performance of different models.
2. They facilitate the reproduction of research results. If a study uses a proprietary or private dataset, other researchers cannot reproduce or verify the findings. This situation impedes scientific progress.
3. Publicly available, standardized datasets promote collaboration among researchers and drive innovation by providing data resources to those who might not otherwise have access.

In conclusion, the availability of public, standardized datasets can significantly accelerate the development and deployment of AI in endodontics. Therefore, while there are various datasets in other healthcare domains, one of the significant challenges in the development of AI in endodontics is the lack of public and standardized datasets.

8.5 Current Gaps and Future Direction of AI in Endodontics

8.5.1 AI-Based Robotics and AI-Guided Endodontic Instrumentation

The integration of AI and robotics has immense potential to transform endodontic treatment but remains an underexplored area needing further research. One promising approach is reinforcement learning (RL), a machine learning technique where agents learn by interacting with an environment [105]. In endodontics, as an example, RL could allow robotic systems to optimize procedural skills like access cavity preparation through repetitive simulated practice. RL-based training of robot-assisted endodontics should be prioritized in future work. It addresses the need for automated and consistent skill development, while avoiding risks to patients. This could enhance precision, reduce errors, democratize expertise, and improve patient outcomes [106, 107].

On the other hand, AI-guided endodontic instrumentation is an emerging concept that could enhance procedural accuracy and minimize risks like perforations or instrument separation. Further research is needed to realize this potential. Intelligent robotic systems could analyze root canal anatomy and then autonomously prepare canals while avoiding errors. Alternatively, AI could provide real-time guidance during manual instrumentation by dentists.

Developing clinically viable solutions poses significant technical challenges involving subtle motor skills, complex anatomy, and dynamic visual/haptic feedback. High-fidelity canal morphology simulation and advanced RL algorithms will be critical. Extensive validation using phantoms and cadavers is required before human trials. Thoughtful integration into clinical workflows while keeping the dentist "in-the-loop" will also be essential. If these hurdles can be overcome, AI-guided instrumentation could make procedures safer and more precise. It may reduce dependency on operator expertise and lead to more predictable outcomes. However, more multidisciplinary research is imperative to translate this emerging technology into patient benefit.

8.5.2 Clinical Management (Referral Systems, Treatment Duration Prediction)

Integrating AI into the clinical management of endodontics is a promising yet underutilized application needing further research. Areas like intelligent referral systems and treatment duration prediction could optimize workflows and improve quality of care.

AI-driven referral prioritization and scheduling systems would allow dental clinics to triage patients, allocate resources, and expedite access to endodontic specialists. AI could evaluate the difficulty of performing nonsurgical root canal therapy and guide clinicians for better case selection and referral to specialists. Meanwhile, treatment duration forecasting models trained on procedural data could provide more accurate appointment booking and patient expectations. However, substantial research is required to develop and validate these AI tools. Challenges include data scarcity, algorithmic biases, and integration with practice workflows. Thoughtful implementation could significantly enhance efficiency, transparency, and patient-centricity.

8.5.3 Drug Interaction Analysis

Utilizing AI for the examination of drug-drug interactions (DDIs) and implications in patients receiving specific medications within the field of endodontics presents a promising and relatively unexplored avenue for future research. The realm of dentistry and endodontic pharmacotherapy is intricate, as patients frequently take multiple medications which have the potential to interact. Ensuring safe and efficacious treatment planning is of utmost importance in this context [108].

Advanced AI techniques like natural language processing and graph neural networks hold immense potential for extracting DDIs from dental records and predicting risks [109, 110]. The benefits could be transformative. AI-assisted DDI analysis at chairside could alert dentists to potential adverse events, prompting modifications to medication or treatment regimens. This could significantly improve the precision and safety of pharmacotherapy in endodontics. Overall, DDI detection represents a clinically valuable and technologically promising application area for AI in endodontics warranting greater research focus.

8.5.4 AI-Powered Microscopes

Integrating AI capabilities into dental operating microscopes represents an exciting innovation in endodontics needing further research. Intelligent microscopes could analyze the operating field in real-time and provide guidance to the clinician. For instance, AI could help detect cracks or secondary canals, assess preparation geometry, and alert surgeons about procedural errors or potential mishaps.

If done well, AI-powered microscopes could act as invaluable co-pilots during complex procedures. They could enhance situational awareness, reduce risks, and improve the accuracy and safety of treatment. This technology remains largely conceptual but offers tremendous potential. Concerted research efforts are needed to assess clinical needs, prototype solutions, and evaluate feasibility. AI-powered microscopes exemplify an exciting frontier in augmented endodontics that could profoundly benefit patients in the years ahead.

8.6 Conclusion

AI is poised to transform endodontics, offering new capabilities to enhance diagnosis, treatment planning, clinical procedures, and outcomes. As outlined in this chapter, AI has already shown promise in areas like radiographic analysis, anatomy evaluation, risk assessment, and instrumentation guidance. However, realizing the full potential of AI in endodontics still faces significant hurdles, including model interpretability, handling of rare conditions, ethical considerations, generalizability issues, and lack of standardized datasets. Addressing these challenges through ongoing multidisciplinary research and thoughtful integration into clinical practice will be crucial. If these obstacles can be overcome, AI-enabled tools have immense potential to improve the precision, accessibility, and patient-centricity of endodontic care. Emerging frontiers like intelligent endodontic robotics and augmented analytics using AI-powered microscopes exemplify exciting possibilities. Ultimately, AI should be seen as enabling clinicians, not replacing them. Thoughtful co-development of human expertise and AI capabilities, while keeping patients' best interests at the center, will help drive the next evolution in endodontic treatment.

References

1. Mohammad-Rahimi H, Rokhshad R, Bencharit S, Krois J, Schwendicke F. Deep learning: a primer for dentists and dental researchers. J Dent. 2023;130:104430.
2. Hyman JJ, Doblecki W. Computerizd endodontic diagnosis. J Am Dent Assoc. 1983;107(5):755–8.
3. Sadr S, Mohammad-Rahimi H, Motamedian SR, Zahedrozegar S, Motie P, Vinayahalingam S, et al. Deep learning for detection of periapical radiolucent lesions: a systematic review and meta-analysis of diagnostic test accuracy. J Endod. 2023;49(3):248–61.e3.
4. Fukuda M, Inamoto K, Shibata N, Ariji Y, Yanashita Y, Kutsuna S, et al. Evaluation of an artificial intelligence system for detecting vertical root fracture on panoramic radiography. Oral Radiol. 2020;36(4):337–43.
5. Buyuk C, Arican Alpay B, Er F. Detection of the separated root canal instrument on panoramic radiograph: a comparison of LSTM and CNN deep learning methods. Dentomaxillofac Radiol. 2023;52(3):20220209.
6. Albitar L, Zhao T, Huang C, Mahdian M. Artificial intelligence (AI) for detection and localization of unobturated second mesial buccal (MB2) canals in cone-beam computed tomography (CBCT). Diagnostics (Basel). 2022;12(12):3214.
7. Aminoshariae A, Kulild J, Nagendrababu V. Artificial intelligence in endodontics: current applications and future directions. J Endod. 2021;47(9):1352–7.
8. Wang Y, Xia W, Yan Z, Zhao L, Bian X, Liu C, et al. Root canal treatment planning by automatic tooth and root canal segmentation in dental CBCT with deep multi-task feature learning. Med Image Anal. 2023;85:102750.
9. Mostafapoor M, Hemmatian S. Evaluation of the accuracy values of cone-beam CT regarding apical periodontitis: a systematic review and meta-analysis. Oral Radiol. 2022;38(3):309–14.
10. Ludlow JB, Timothy R, Walker C, Hunter R, Benavides E, Samuelson DB, et al. Effective dose of dental CBCT-a meta analysis of published data and additional data for nine CBCT units. Dentomaxillofac Radiol. 2015;44(1):20140197.
11. Patel S, Puri T, Mannocci F, Navai A. Diagnosis and management of traumatic dental injuries using intraoral radiography and cone-beam computed tomography: an in vivo investigation. J Endod. 2021;47(6):914–23.
12. Tiburcio-Machado CS, Michelon C, Zanatta FB, Gomes MS, Marin JA, Bier CA. The global prevalence of apical periodontitis: a systematic review and meta-analysis. Int Endod J. 2021;54(5):712–35.
13. Estrela C, Bueno MR, Leles CR, Azevedo B, Azevedo JR. Accuracy of cone beam computed tomography and panoramic and periapical radiography for detection of apical periodontitis. J Endod. 2008;34(3):273–9.
14. Meusburger T, Wülk A, Kessler A, Heck K, Hickel R, Dujic H, et al. The detection of dental pathologies on periapical radiographs-results from a reliability study. J Clin Med. 2023;12(6):2224.
15. Cotti E, Schirru E. Present status and future directions: imaging techniques for the detection of periapical lesions. Int Endod J. 2022;55(S4):1085–99.
16. Ekert T, Krois J, Meinhold L, Elhennawy K, Emara R, Golla T, et al. Deep learning for the radiographic detection of apical lesions. J Endod. 2019;45(7):917–22.e5.
17. Li C-W, Lin S-Y, Chou H-S, Chen T-Y, Chen Y-A, Liu S-Y, et al. Detection of dental apical lesions using CNNs on periapical radiograph. Sensors (Basel). 2021;21(21):7049.
18. Sadr S, Mohammad-Rahimi H, Motamedian SR, Zahedrozegar S, Motie P, Vinayahalingam S, et al. Deep learning for detection of periapical radiolucent lesions: a systematic review and meta-analysis of diagnostic test accuracy. J Endod. 2023;49(3):248–261.e3.
19. Li S, Liu J, Zhou Z, Zhou Z, Wu X, Li Y, et al. Artificial intelligence for caries and periapical periodontitis detection. J Dent. 2022;122:104107.
20. Ngoc VT, Viet DH, Anh LK, Minh DQ, Nghia LL, Loan HK, et al. Periapical lesion diagnosis support system based on X-ray images using machine learning technique. World J Dentistry. 2021;12(3):189–93.
21. Sajad M, Shafi I, Ahmad J, editors. Automatic lesion detection in periapical X-rays. 2019 International conference on electrical, communication, and computer engineering (ICECCE). Swat: IEEE.
22. Chen H, Li H, Zhao Y, Zhao J, Wang Y. Dental disease detection on periapical radiographs based on deep convolutional neural networks. Int J Comput Assist Radiol Surg. 2021;16(4):649–61.
23. Chen H, Li H, Zhao Y, Zhao J, Wang Y. Dental disease detection on periapical radiographs based on deep convolutional neural networks. Int J CARS. 2021;16(4):649–61.
24. Orhan K, Bayrakdar IS, Ezhov M, Kravtsov A, Özyürek T. Evaluation of artificial intelligence for detecting periapical pathosis on cone-beam computed tomography scans. Int Endod J. 2020;53(5):680–9.

25. Moidu NP, Sharma S, Chawla A, Kumar V, Logani A. Deep learning for categorization of endodontic lesion based on radiographic periapical index scoring system. Clin Oral Investig. 2022;26(1):651–8.
26. Setzer FC, Shi KJ, Zhang Z, Yan H, Yoon H, Mupparapu M, et al. Artificial intelligence for the computer-aided detection of periapical lesions in cone-beam computed tomographic images. J Endod. 2020;46(7):987–93.
27. Krois J, Garcia Cantu A, Chaurasia A, Patil R, Chaudhari PK, Gaudin R, et al. Generalizability of deep learning models for dental image analysis. Sci Rep. 2021;11(1):6102.
28. Orstavik D, Kerekes K, Eriksen HM. The periapical index: a scoring system for radiographic assessment of apical periodontitis. Endod Dent Traumatol. 1986;2(1):20–34.
29. Saunders MB, Gulabivala K, Holt R, Kahan RS. Reliability of radiographic observations recorded on a proforma measured using inter- and intra-observer variation: a preliminary study. Int Endod J. 2000;33(3):272–8.
30. Patel S, Wilson R, Dawood A, Foschi F, Mannocci F. The detection of periapical pathosis using digital periapical radiography and cone beam computed tomography—part 2: a 1-year post-treatment follow-up: outcome of endodontic treatment part 2. Int Endod J. 2012;45(8):711–23.
31. Yoshino K, Ito K, Kuroda M, Sugihara N. Prevalence of vertical root fracture as the reason for tooth extraction in dental clinics. Clin Oral Investig. 2015;19(6):1405–9.
32. von Arx T, Maldonado P, Bornstein MM. Occurrence of vertical root fractures after apical surgery: a retrospective analysis. J Endod. 2021;47(2):239–46.
33. Edlund M, Nair MK, Nair UP. Detection of vertical root fractures by using cone-beam computed tomography: a clinical study. J Endod. 2011;37(6):768–72.
34. Kositbowornchai S, Plermkamon S, Tangkosol T. Performance of an artificial neural network for vertical root fracture detection: an *ex vivo* study. Dent Traumatol. 2013;29(2):151–5.
35. Johari M, Esmaeili F, Andalib A, Garjani S, Saberkari H. Detection of vertical root fractures in intact and endodontically treated premolar teeth by designing a probabilistic neural network: an *ex vivo* study. Dentomaxillofac Radiol. 2017;46(2):20160107.
36. Patel S, Bhuva B, Bose R. Present status and future directions: vertical root fractures in root filled teeth. Int Endod J. 2022;55(S3):804–26.
37. Patel S, Brady E, Wilson R, Brown J, Mannocci F. The detection of vertical root fractures in root filled teeth with periapical radiographs and CBCT scans. Int Endod J. 2013;46(12):1140–52.
38. Hiraiwa T, Ariji Y, Fukuda M, Kise Y, Nakata K, Katsumata A, et al. A deep-learning artificial intelligence system for assessment of root morphology of the mandibular first molar on panoramic radiography. Dentomaxillofac Radiol. 2019;48(3):20180218.
39. Yang S, Lee H, Jang B, Kim K-D, Kim J, Kim H, et al. Development and validation of a visually explainable deep learning model for classification of C-shaped canals of the mandibular second molars in periapical and panoramic dental radiographs. J Endod. 2022;48(7):914–21.
40. Duan W, Chen Y, Zhang Q, Lin X, Yang X. Refined tooth and pulp segmentation using U-net in CBCT image. Dentomaxillofac Radiol. 2021;50(6):20200251.
41. Lin X, Fu Y, Ren G, Yang X, Duan W, Chen Y, et al. Micro-computed tomography-guided artificial intelligence for pulp cavity and tooth segmentation on cone-beam computed tomography. J Endod. 2021;47(12):1933–41.
42. Special Committee to Revise the Joint AAE/AAOMR Position Statement on use of CBCT in Endodontics. AAE and AAOMR joint position statement: use of cone beam computed tomography in endodontics 2015 update. Oral Surg Oral Med Oral Pathol Oral Radiol. 2015;120(4):508–12.
43. Vinayahalingam S, Goey R-S, Kempers S, Schoep J, Cherici T, Moin DA, et al. Automated chart filing on panoramic radiographs using deep learning. J Dent. 2021;115:103864.
44. Rohrer C, Krois J, Patel J, Meyer-Lueckel H, Rodrigues JA, Schwendicke F. Segmentation of dental restorations on panoramic radiographs using deep learning. Diagnostics (Basel, Switzerland). 2022;12(6):1316.
45. Michetti J, Georgelin-Gurgel M, Mallet JP, Diemer F, Boulanouar K. Influence of CBCT parameters on the output of an automatic edge-detection-based endodontic segmentation. Dentomaxillofac Radiol. 2015;44(8):20140413.
46. Tian S, Dai N, Zhang B, Yuan F, Yu Q, Cheng X. Automatic classification and segmentation of teeth on 3D dental model using hierarchical deep learning networks. IEEE Access. 2019;7:84817–28.
47. Hsu K, Yuh D-Y, Lin S-C, Lyu P-S, Pan G-X, Zhuang Y-C, et al. Improving performance of deep learning models using 3.5D U-net via majority voting for tooth segmentation on cone beam computed tomography. Sci Rep. 2022;12(1):19809.
48. Wang L, Li J-p, Ge Z-p, Li G. CBCT image based segmentation method for tooth pulp cavity region extraction. Dentomaxillofac Radiol. 2019;48(2):20180236.
49. Li Q, Chen K, Han L, Zhuang Y, Li J, Lin J. Automatic tooth roots segmentation of cone beam computed tomography image sequences using U-net and RNN. XST. 2020;28(5):905–22.
50. Zheng Q, Ge Z, Du H, Li G. Age estimation based on 3D pulp chamber segmentation of first molars from cone-beam–computed tomography by integrated deep learning and level set. Int J Legal Med. 2021;135(1):365–73.
51. Wolf TG, Stiebritz M, Boemke N, Elsayed I, Paqué F, Wierichs RJ, et al. 3-dimensional analysis and literature review of the root canal morphology and

physiological foramen geometry of 125 mandibular incisors by means of micro-computed tomography in a German population. J Endod. 2020;46(2):184–91.
52. Deleat-Besson R, Le C, Al Turkestani N, Zhang W, Dumont M, Brosset S, et al. Automatic segmentation of dental root canal and merging with crown shape. In: 2021 43rd Annual International Conference of the IEEE Engineering in Medicine & Biology Society (EMBC). Mexico: IEEE; 2021.
53. Patel S, Patel R, Foschi F, Mannocci F. The impact of different diagnostic imaging modalities on the evaluation of root canal anatomy and endodontic residents' stress levels: a clinical study. J Endod. 2019;45(4):406–13.
54. Zhang X, Xiong S, Ma Y, Han T, Chen X, Wan F, et al. A cone-beam computed tomographic study on mandibular first molars in a Chinese subpopulation. PLoS One. 2015;10(8):e0134919.
55. Jin G-C, Lee S-J, Roh B-D. Anatomical study of C-shaped canals in mandibular second molars by analysis of computed tomography. J Endod. 2006;32(1):10–3.
56. Zhang R, Wang H, Tian YY, Yu X, Hu T, Dummer PMH. Use of cone-beam computed tomography to evaluate root and canal morphology of mandibular molars in Chinese individuals. Int Endod J. 2011;44(11):990–9.
57. Helvacioglu-Yigit D, Sinanoglu A. Use of cone-beam computed tomography to evaluate C-shaped root canal systems in mandibular second molars in a Turkish subpopulation: a retrospective study. Int Endod J. 2013;46(11):1032–8.
58. American Association of Endodontists. AAE endodontic case difficulty assessment form and guidelines. American Association of Endodontists; 2022.
59. Kim Y, Lee D, Kim D-V, Kim S-Y. Analysis of cause of endodontic failure of C-shaped root canals. Scanning. 2018;2018:2516832.
60. Jafarzadeh H, Wu Y-N. The C-shaped root canal configuration: a review. J Endod. 2007;33(5):517–23.
61. Sherwood AA, Sherwood AI, Setzer FC, Devi KS, Shamili JV, John C, et al. A deep learning approach to segment and classify C-shaped canal morphologies in mandibular second molars using cone-beam computed tomography. J Endod. 2021;47(12):1907–16.
62. Jeon S-J, Yun J-P, Yeom H-G, Shin W-S, Lee J-H, Jeong S-H, et al. Deep-learning for predicting C-shaped canals in mandibular second molars on panoramic radiographs. Dentomaxillofac Radiol. 2021;50(5):20200513.
63. Selvaraju RR, Cogswell M, Das A, Vedantam R, Parikh D, Batra D. Grad-CAM: visual explanations from deep networks via gradient-based localization. Int J Comput Vis. 2020;128(2):336–59.
64. Weckwerth GM, Santos CF, Brozoski DT, Centurion BS, Pagin O, Lauris JRP, et al. Taurodontism, root dilaceration, and tooth transposition: a radiographic study of a population with nonsyndromic cleft lip and/or palate. Cleft Palate Craniofac J. 2016;53(4):404–12.
65. Duman S, Yılmaz EF, Eşer G, Çelik Ö, Bayrakdar IS, Bilgir E, et al. Detecting the presence of taurodont teeth on panoramic radiographs using a deep learning-based convolutional neural network algorithm. Oral Radiol. 2023;39(1):207–14.
66. Dummer PM, McGinn JH, Rees DG. The position and topography of the apical canal constriction and apical foramen. Int Endod J. 1984;17(4):192–8.
67. Tsesis I, Blazer T, Ben-Izhack G, Taschieri S, Del Fabbro M, Corbella S, et al. The precision of electronic apex locators in working length determination: a systematic review and meta-analysis of the literature. J Endod. 2015;41(11):1818–23.
68. ElAyouti A, Connert T, Dummer P, Löst C. A critical analysis of research methods and experimental models to study working length determination and the performance of apex locators—a narrative review with recommendations for the future. Int Endod J. 2022;55(S2):281–94.
69. Saghiri MA, Asgar K, Boukani KK, Lotfi M, Aghili H, Delvarani A, et al. A new approach for locating the minor apical foramen using an artificial neural network. Int Endod J. 2012;45(3):257–65.
70. Saghiri MA, Garcia-Godoy F, Gutmann JL, Lotfi M, Asgar K. The reliability of artificial neural network in locating minor apical foramen: a cadaver study. J Endod. 2012;38(8):1130–4.
71. Stöber EK, Duran-Sindreu F, Mercadé M, Vera J, Bueno R, Roig M. An evaluation of root ZX and iPex apex locators: an in vivo study. J Endod. 2011;37(5):608–10.
72. Welk AR, Baumgartner JC, Marshall JG. An in vivo comparison of two frequency-based electronic apex locators. J Endod. 2003;29(8):497–500.
73. Qiao X, Zhang Z, Chen X. Multifrequency impedance method based on neural network for root canal length measurement. Appl Sci. 2020;10(21):7430.
74. Canadian Academy of Endodontics. Standards of practice—treatment classification. Canadian Academy of Endodontics; 1998.
75. Ree MH, Timmerman MF, Wesselink PR. An evaluation of the usefulness of two endodontic case assessment forms by general dentists: endodontic case difficulty assessment. Int Endod J. 2003;36(8):545–55.
76. Essam O, Boyle EL, Whitworth JM, Jarad FD. The endodontic complexity assessment tool (E-CAT): a digital form for assessing root canal treatment case difficulty. Int Endod J. 2021;54(7):1189–99.
77. Alsulaimani RS, Al-Manei KK, Alsubait SA, AlAqeely RS, Al-Shehri SAM, Al-Madi EM. Effects of clinical training and case difficulty on the radiographic quality of root canal fillings performed by dental students in Saudi Arabia. Iranian Endod J. 2015;10(4):268–73.
78. Haug SR, Solfjeld AF, Ranheim LE, Bårdsen A. Impact of case difficulty on endodontic mishaps in an undergraduate student clinic. J Endod. 2018;44(7):1088–95.

79. Herbst SR, Herbst CS, Schwendicke F. Preoperative risk assessment does not allow to predict root filling length using machine learning: a longitudinal study. J Dent. 2023;128:104378.
80. Marquis VL, Dao T, Farzaneh M, Abitbol S, Friedman S. Treatment outcome in endodontics: the Toronto study. Phase III: initial treatment. J Endod. 2006;32(4):299–306.
81. Signor B, Blomberg LC, Kopper PMP, Augustin PAN, Rauber MV, Rodrigues GS, et al. Root canal retreatment: a retrospective investigation using regression and data mining methods for the prediction of technical quality and periapical healing. J Appl Oral Sci. 2021;29:e20200799.
82. Herbst CS, Schwendicke F, Krois J, Herbst SR. Association between patient-, tooth- and treatment-level factors and root canal treatment failure: a retrospective longitudinal and machine learning study. J Dent. 2022;117:103937.
83. Lee J, Seo H, Choi YJ, Lee C, Kim S, Lee YS, et al. An endodontic forecasting model based on the analysis of preoperative dental radiographs: a pilot study on an endodontic predictive deep neural network. J Endod. 2023;49(6):710–9.
84. Nosrat A, Valancius M, Mehrzad S, Dianat O, Verma P, Aminoshariae A, et al. Flare-ups after nonsurgical retreatments: incidence, associated factors, and prediction. J Endod. 2023;49(10):1299–1307.e1.
85. Aggarwal A, Tam CC, Wu D, Li X, Qiao S. Artificial intelligence-based Chatbots for promoting health Behavioral changes: systematic review. J Med Internet Res. 2023;25:e40789.
86. Safi Z, Abd-Alrazaq A, Khalifa M, Househ M. Technical aspects of developing Chatbots for medical applications: scoping review. J Med Internet Res. 2020;22(12):e19127.
87. Suárez A, Díaz-Flores García V, Algar J, Gómez Sánchez M, Llorente de Pedro M, Freire Y. Unveiling the ChatGPT phenomenon: evaluating the consistency and accuracy of endodontic question answers. Int Endod J. 2024;57(3):371–2.
88. Thurzo A, Strunga M, Urban R, Surovková J, Afrashtehfar KI. Impact of artificial intelligence on dental education: a review and guide for curriculum update. Educ Sci. 2023;13(2):150.
89. Rudin C. Stop explaining black box machine learning models for high stakes decisions and use interpretable models instead. Nat Mach Intell. 2019;1(5):206–15.
90. Castelvecchi D. Can we open the black box of AI? Nature News. 2016;538(7623):20.
91. Gilpin LH, Bau D, Yuan BZ, Bajwa A, Specter M, Kagal L. Explaining explanations: an approach to evaluating interpretability of machine learning. arXiv preprint arXiv:180600069. 2018:118.
92. Vayena E, Blasimme A, Cohen IG. Machine learning in medicine: addressing ethical challenges. PLoS Med. 2018;15(11):e1002689.
93. van der Velden BHM, Kuijf HJ, Gilhuijs KGA, Viergever MA. Explainable artificial intelligence (XAI) in deep learning-based medical image analysis. Med Image Anal. 2022;79:102470.
94. Sun Y, Wong AKC, Kamel MS. Classification of imbalanced data: a review. Int J Pattern Recognit Artif Intell. 2009;23(4):687–719.
95. Tajbakhsh N, Jeyaseelan L, Li Q, Chiang JN, Wu Z, Ding X. Embracing imperfect datasets: a review of deep learning solutions for medical image segmentation. Med Image Anal. 2020;63:101693.
96. Haixiang G, Yijing L, Shang J, Mingyun G, Yuanyue H, Bing G. Learning from class-imbalanced data: review of methods and applications. Expert Syst Appl. 2017;73:220–39.
97. Chawla NV, Bowyer KW, Hall LO, Kegelmeyer WP. SMOTE: synthetic minority over-sampling technique. J Artif Intell Res. 2002;16:321–57.
98. Krawczyk B. Learning from imbalanced data: open challenges and future directions. Prog Artif Intell. 2016;5(4):221–32.
99. Rokhshad R, Ducret M, Chaurasia A, Karteva T, Radenkovic M, Roganovic J, et al. Ethical considerations on artificial intelligence in dentistry: a framework and checklist. J Dent. 2023;135:104593.
100. U.S. Food and Drug Administration. Artificial intelligence/machine learning (AI/ML)-based software as a medical device (saMD) action plan. 2021. 2023.
101. Liang X, Nguyen D, Jiang SB. Generalizability issues with deep learning models in medicine and their potential solutions: illustrated with cone-beam computed tomography (CBCT) to computed tomography (CT) image conversion. Mach Learn Sci Technol. 2020;2(1):015007.
102. Quinonero-Candela J, Sugiyama M, Schwaighofer A, Lawrence ND. Dataset shift in machine learning. Mit Press; 2008.
103. Pooch EHP, Ballester P, Barros RC. Can we trust deep learning based diagnosis? The impact of domain shift in chest radiograph classification. In: Thoracic image analysis. Cham: Springer International Publishing; 2020.
104. Stodden V, Seiler J, Ma Z. An empirical analysis of journal policy effectiveness for computational reproducibility. Proc Natl Acad Sci. 2018;115(11):2584–9.
105. Ibarz J, Tan J, Finn C, Kalakrishnan M, Pastor P, Levine S. How to train your robot with deep reinforcement learning: lessons we have learned. Int J Robot Res. 2021;40(4–5):698–721.
106. Jiang J, Guo Y, Huang Z, Zhang Y, Wu D, Liu Y. Adjacent surface trajectory planning of robot-assisted tooth preparation based on augmented reality. Eng Sci Technol Int J. 2022;27:101001.
107. Wu Y, Wang F, Fan S, Chow JK-F. Robotics in dental implantology. Oral Maxillofac Surg Clinics. 2019;31(3):513–8.
108. de Oliveira MLR, Nery GO, Torresan TT, Arcanjo RA, Ferreira MBC, Montagner F. Frequency and characterization of potential drug interactions in dentistry-a cross-sectional study. Clin Oral Investig. 2022;26(11):6829–37.

109. Basile AO, Yahi A, Tatonetti NP. Artificial intelligence for drug toxicity and safety. Trends Pharmacol Sci. 2019;40(9):624–35.
110. Machado J, Rodrigues C, Sousa R, Gomes LM. Drug–drug interaction extraction-based system: an natural language processing approach. Exp Syst. 2025;42:e13303.
111. Ngoc VTN, Viet DH, Tuan TM, Hai PV, Thang NP, Tuyen DN, et al. VNU-diagnosis: a novel medical system based on deep learning for diagnosis of periapical inflammation from X-rays images. J Intell Fuzzy Syst. 2022;43(1):1417–27.
112. Bayrakdar IS, Orhan K, Çelik Ö, Bilgir E, Sağlam H, Kaplan FA, et al. A U-net approach to apical lesion segmentation on panoramic radiographs. Biomed Res Int. 2022;2022:1–7.
113. Endres MG, Hillen F, Salloumis M, Sedaghat AR, Niehues SM, Quatela O, et al. Development of a deep learning algorithm for periapical disease detection in dental radiographs. Diagnostics (Basel, Switzerland). 2020;10(6):430.
114. Ezhov M, Gusarev M, Golitsyna M, Yates JM, Kushnerev E, Tamimi D, et al. Clinically applicable artificial intelligence system for dental diagnosis with CBCT. Sci Rep. 2021;11(1):15006.
115. Huang J, Yan H, Li J, Stewart HM, Setzer F, editors. Combining anatomical constraints and deep learning for 3-D CBCT dental image multi-label segmentation. 2021 IEEE 37th International Conference on Data Engineering (ICDE); 19–22 Apr 2021.
116. Khan HA, Haider MA, Ansari HA, Ishaq H, Kiyani A, Sohail K, et al. Automated feature detection in dental periapical radiographs by using deep learning. Oral Surg Oral Med Oral Pathol Oral Radiol. 2021;131(6):711–20.
117. Kirnbauer B, Hadzic A, Jakse N, Bischof H, Stern D. Automatic detection of periapical osteolytic lesions on cone-beam computed tomography using deep convolutional neuronal networks. J Endod. 2022;48(11):1434–40.
118. Zheng Z, Yan H, Setzer FC, Shi KJ, Mupparapu M, Li J. Anatomically constrained deep learning for automating dental CBCT segmentation and lesion detection. IEEE Trans Autom Sci Eng. 2021;18(2):603–14.

9 A Primer on Artificial Intelligence Research in Dentistry

Sergio E. Uribe and Falk Schwendicke

9.1 Role of AI in Scientific Discoveries

Artificial Intelligence (AI) could significantly expand research horizons. A recent review [1] revealed the integration of AI into scientific discovery, demostrating how AI augments and accelerates research across scientific disciplines. For instance, self-supervised learning, a form of AI that trains models on large amounts of unlabeled data, allows dental researchers to analyze extensive datasets, such as dental imaging and patient records. This approach can reveal patterns and insights previously hidden with traditional methods, potentially leading to breakthroughs in areas like dental disease prediction and treatment. Geometric deep learning, another promising development in AI, could considerably enhance dental research. AI models can enhance their understanding of intricate multimodal dental data from large and complex datasets, leading to more precise dental image analysis, diagnosis, and prediction, ultimately improving patient outcomes.

AI also facilitates the transformation and analysis of input data, enabling dimensionality reduction to discover patterns hidden in the data's complexity or size. Additionally, AI is becoming invaluable in automating the literature review process, employing large language models (LLMs) to facilitate dynamic, context-aware search capabilities. AI also assists in brainstorming research directions, enhancing writing, and detecting gaps in existing studies.

Lastly, AI, particularly robotics, helps automate low-value-added but accuracy-intensive lab tasks, enhancing efficiency. Generative AI methods, which produce new designs by analyzing various data types, could open up new possibilities in dental research. For instance, they could contribute to the creation of novel drug compounds or the design of advanced dental materials, potentially improving treatment options and procedures in the field. AI and simple robotics can enhance the efficiency of laboratory tasks such as sample preparation or pipetting, allowing researchers to focus more on high value-added tasks.

Despite these potential advancements, challenges persist. Data quality and stewardship issues must be addressed to integrate AI into scientific research successfully. The performance of AI models heavily depends on the quality and handling of data; hence, reliable and ethical data

S. E. Uribe (✉)
Department of Conservative Dentistry and Oral Health, Riga Stradins University, Latvia/Conservative Dentistry and Periodontology, LMU Klinikum, LMU Munich, Munich, Germany
e-mail: sergio.uribe@rsu.lv

F. Schwendicke
Conservative Dentistry and Periodontology, LMU Klinikum, LMU Munich, Munich, Germany
e-mail: falk.schwendicke@med.uni-muenchen.de

F. Schwendicke et al. (eds.), *Artificial Intelligence for Oral Health Care*,
https://doi.org/10.1007/978-3-031-84047-0_9

practices are essential for generating dependable AI-driven insights in dental research.

Finally, developing foundational algorithmic approaches that enable AI to contribute to scientific understanding autonomously could be pivotal: AI systems capable of independently understanding and generating scientific insights. Such AI systems could actively contribute to discoveries in dental research, potentially revolutionizing oral health practices and research.

Currently, AI can enhance various processes in dental research, including the following:

1. *Hypothesis Generation*: AI can assist scientists in generating hypotheses by analyzing large datasets, identifying patterns, and suggesting potential research directions.
2. *Experimental Design*: AI can help design experiments by optimizing experimental parameters and outcomes, increasing their efficiency.
3. *Data Collection and Interpretation:* AI can automate the collection and interpretation of large datasets, enabling researchers to extract valuable insights more efficiently.
4. *Image and Sequence Analysis*: AI techniques, such as deep learning, can analyze complex data, facilitating tasks like image recognition, pattern detection, and DNA sequence analysis.
5. *Self-Supervised Learning:* AI models trained using self-supervised learning can use vast amounts of unlabeled data, leading to a more robust and comprehensive understanding of scientific phenomena.
6. *Geometric Deep Learning:* AI can use knowledge about scientific data structure to enhance model accuracy and efficiency, particularly in complex systems with intricate relationships.
7. *Generative AI for Design:* AI can create designs, such as small-molecule drugs and proteins, by analyzing diverse data modalities, opening new opportunities for innovative solutions and discoveries.
8. *Insights Beyond Human Capability:* AI can uncover insights that might not have been possible using traditional scientific methods alone, accelerating the pace of scientific discovery.
9. *Cross-Disciplinary Applications:* AI can be applied across various scientific disciplines, providing solutions and approaches cutting traditional boundaries.
10. *Autonomous Scientific Understanding:* AI has the potential to contribute to scientific understanding autonomously, leading to discoveries and insights beyond human capabilities.
11. *Error Detection and Quality Control:* AI can be utilized to identify errors in data and ensure data quality and stewardship, improving the reliability of scientific research.
12. *AI-Augmented Decision Making:* Researchers can use AI systems to assist decision-making processes, combining human expertise with AI insights for more informed choices.

9.2 Where to Start?

If you are reading this, it means you have already set foot in the exciting world of Artificial Intelligence in dentistry. Congratulations! Like you, many others around the globe share this interest. As a result, research in AI for health has surged in recent years, a trend we can expect to continue. The best way to get started and familiarize yourself with research topics, designs, and common terms is by reviewing systematic reviews. These offer a synthesis of the evidence and are also helpful for identifying gaps in knowledge that future research should address. To find such studies in health, PubMed[1] is your go-to database. Here, AI-related terms like machine learning, deep learning, and neural networks are grouped under a parent term, or Medical Subject Heading (MeSH),[2] "Artificial Intelligence." So, when you search for this MeSH term, you can find all associated terms, as shown in Fig. 9.1.

[1] https://pubmed.ncbi.nlm.nih.gov/

[2] https://www.ncbi.nlm.nih.gov/mesh/

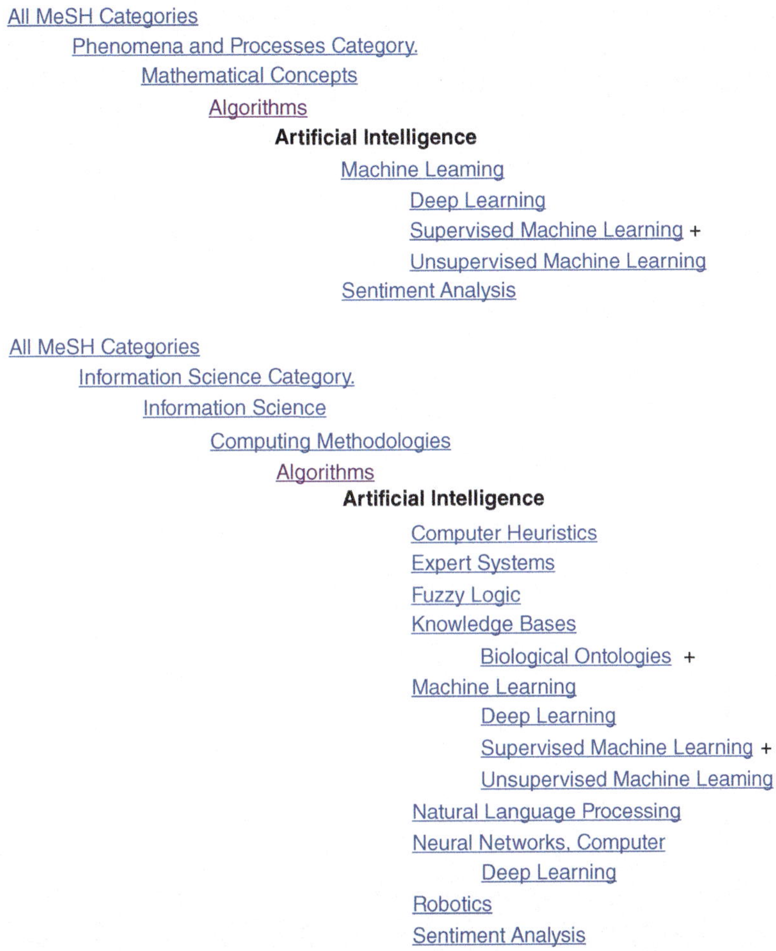

Fig. 9.1 Artificial intelligence with medical subject heading in PubMed. (Courtesy of the National Library of Medicine)

Fig. 9.2 Option for advanced search in PubMed. (Courtesy of the National Library of Medicine)

Next, you can combine the term "systematic review" with the condition of your interest and your preference's focus (diagnosis, prognosis, treatment). We recommend searching each term separately using the ADVANCED SEARCH option, as shown in Fig. 9.2, and then combining them.

In Fig. 9.3, we show an example of a search for systematic reviews related to the diagnosis of caries using Artificial Intelligence. Feel free to replicate this search for practice!

A systematic review provides a synthesis of evidence, giving you an idea of current research topics, what is known, and what remains to be explored. You can then search for a particular study cited in any reviews that caught your eye and read the article in more detail.

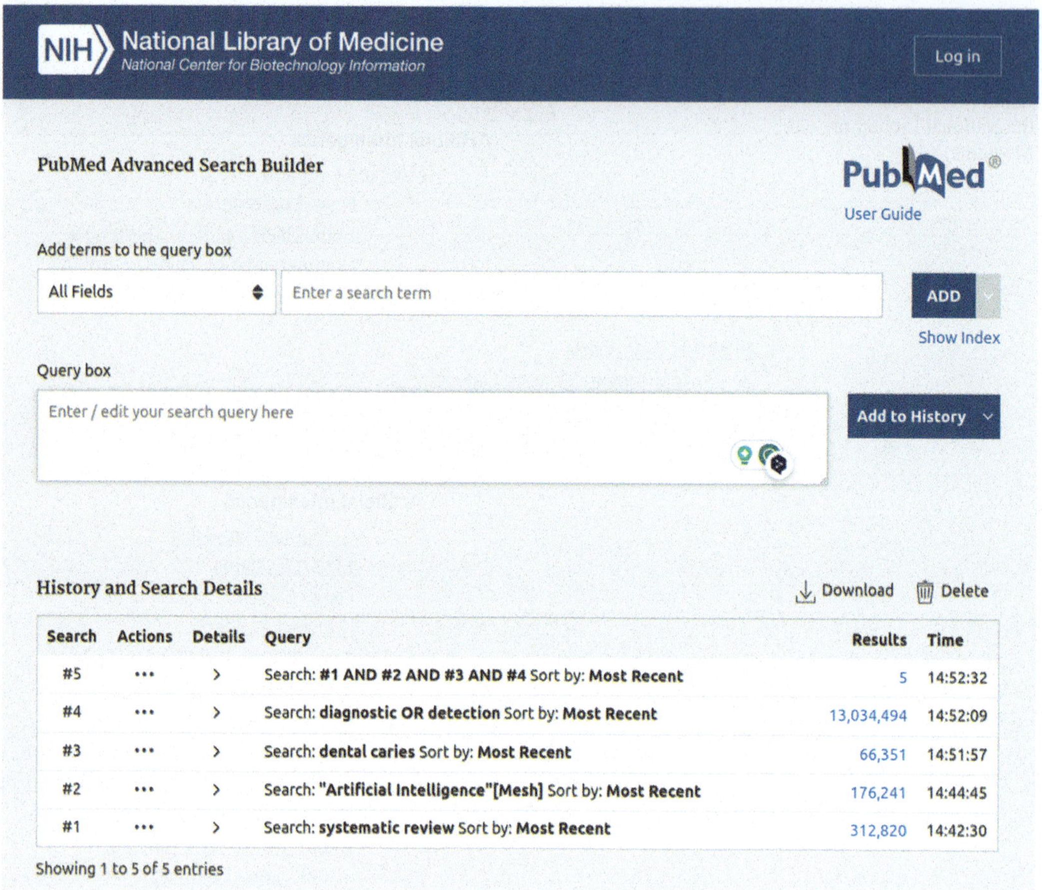

Fig. 9.3 PubMed's advanced view enables the combination of different search strategies. (Courtesy of the National Library of Medicine)

9.3 Which Questions Are Relevant for Artificial Intelligence Research in Dentistry?

For simplicity, questions in Dental AI can be divided into two broad groups: (a) those designed to solve a technical problem, develop and test a new AI model, or (b) those aiming for a clinical outcome. As for technical questions, these overlap with engineering, data science, and computer science. Some examples of such questions are as follows:

- Can we develop an AI model that predicts dental implant success rate based on patient data?
- Under controlled conditions similar to in vitro studies, how does the performance of a deep learning model for detecting dental caries in bite-wing radiographs compare to other methods using data from a single or few clinics?
- Using our data, is there a significant difference in accuracy when comparing multiple algorithms designed to predict orthodontic treatment durations?
- Can we engineer a novel algorithm that adjusts dental treatment plans based on continuously updated patient data?

Now, for the clinical relevant questions, three fundamental issues can be addressed, representing the conventional research methodologies in medicine: case-control, cohort, and randomized controlled trials. These studies form the corner-

Table 9.1 Essential AI research clinical questions in dentistry: study design and key metrics

Research question	Basic study type	Key elements of the study design	Usual metrics reported and terms associated
How accurate is the AI system in detecting caries from dental X-rays?	Diagnostic study	AI model training and validation on labeled dental X-rays. Differentiating between images with caries and without caries	Sensitivity, specificity, AUC-ROC, accuracy, % change in diagnostic decisions
Does AI-assisted treatment planning improve patient outcomes in implant dentistry?	Intervention study	Randomized control trial design. Comparing patient outcomes between AI-assisted treatment planning and traditional methods	Success rate, survival rate, complications, number needed to treat, Kaplan-Meier plot, cox regression, % change in treatment decisions, costs
Can AI accurately predict the progression of periodontal disease over time?	Prognostic study	Cohort study design. The AI model is trained to predict disease progression based on initial input variables	Incidence rate, hazard or rate ratio, calibration slope, C (concordance) statistics, goodness of fit, decision curves, calibration plot, net benefit

stone of evidence-based medicine. For dental research, the questions addressed are as follows:

1. Can AI improve the detection of oral pathologies?
2. Can AI optimize their treatment?
3. Can AI improve patient prognostic outcomes?

Each question is associated with a specific research study design, allowing for a valid methodology to answer it. Table 9.1 provides examples and a summary of the essential research designs, their main components, and the metrics they typically report.

9.4 What to Measure in Dental AI Research?

There is a distinction between technical and clinical questions in dental AI research. To understand the effectiveness and value of AI in dentistry, it is essential to consider not only technical performance metrics but also, more importantly, the impact on clinically oriented outcomes and overarching healthcare goals.

Research with AI introduces some unique challenges. Unlike a conventional intervention, such as a drug or a new implant, AI systems interact with the clinician, and this dynamic must be considered when assessing the impact of AI use. For instance, imagine a study involving a new AI diagnostic model where you have expert radiologists (with over 10 years of experience) and junior ones. The effect of the AI model could be measured both at the subclinician level (effect by expertise), clinician level (changes in their diagnostic decisions, for example) and the patient level (enhancement in diagnostic accuracy) or societal (decrease in healthcare cost, increase in health coverage). Any study should not only aim to gauge the performance of the AI system but also understand how it impacts clinical practice and patient outcomes. In Table 9.2, you will see some key technical and clinical metrics and their predominant applications, and we also provide example metrics for each application. This information will enhance your understanding of what measurements to focus on in AI dental research, facilitating better data analysis and interpretation.

Table 9.2 AI metrics framework for dental research applications

Metric outcome	Main impact	Application	Example metrics
Technical	AI development	Detection	Intersection over Union (IoU), dice score
			Sensitivity (recall)
			Specificity
		Segmentation	IoU, dice score
		Classification	Receiver operating characteristics (ROC) curve
			Accuracy
			Sensitivity
			Specificity
		Prediction	ROC curve
			Accuracy
			R-square
			Root mean squared error
Clinical (modified from [2])	AI deployment	Diagnostic process	Percentage of diagnostic decisions changed AI assistance
		Therapeutic process	Percentage of therapeutic decisions changed with AI assistance
			Percentage of dental procedures avoided due to the use of AI
		Patient outcomes	Percentage of patients improved with the use of AI
			Cost per QALY[a] saved with the use of AI
			Percentage decrease in incidence or prevalence of Oral diseases
		Societal outcomes	Cost-benefit analysis of the use of AI from a societal point of view
			Cost-effectiveness analysis of the use of AI from a societal point of view
			Percentage increase in dental healthcare coverage for population

[a] QALY, or Quality-Adjusted Life Year, is a measure used in health economics to evaluate the value of health interventions. For example, imagine a periodontal treatment preventing tooth loss. Without treatment, a patient with 10 years to live and a quality of life rated 0.7 would have 7 QALYs (10 years × 0.7). The treatment improves their quality of life to 0.9, yielding 9 QALYs (10 years × 0.9). Hence, the treatment adds 2 QALYs, indicating a significant health benefit and helping policymakers decide whether to fund the treatment

9.5 Specific Considerations for AI Dental Research

However, when planning, evaluating, or using AI in dental research, there are three specific aspects to consider: (1) data, (2) labeling or annotations, and (3) benchmarking of AI models.

Data forms the backbone of AI research, and its quality is instrumental in determining the efficacy and applicability of AI models. Therefore, creating large, diverse, and representative datasets is crucial to develop robust AI models. The data should be devoid of biases or discrimination to ensure the outcomes' precision, validity, and fairness. However, a significant challenge is that most current research tends to rely on existing data, which often overlooks underrepresented populations. Consequently, the results derived from such models may only partially represent these diverse groups, raising issues about the fairness and inclusivity of AI applications. Thus, proactively investing in generating datasets that capture the broad spectrum of population diversity is critical for the comprehensive utilization of AI in dental research.

Next in line is the **labeling or annotation** process, a crucial but often underemphasized aspect of AI research. Clear guidelines and protocols for labeling AI datasets are essential, regardless of whether the data are in images, text, or speech. Important considerations include who should annotate the data, the criteria used for labeling, and how differences or disagreements should be resolved. This step necessitates a thoughtful selection of the labeling criteria as it significantly impacts the training of AI models. The transparent and accurate labeling of data ensures a reliable ground truth for AI models, contributing to their performance and reliability.

Lastly, **benchmarking** forms an integral part of AI research [3]. Benchmarks serve as common, recognized, and accepted standards against which AI models can be measured. The need for benchmarks extends to different technical, clinical, patient, and societal levels and objectives, such as diagnosis, treatment, prognosis, or decision-making. Benchmarks allow for comparisons between AI models, aiding in selecting the best solution for a given problem. Moreover, benchmarks drive innovation by setting performance goals, promoting accountability, and facilitating adopting effective AI solutions in dentistry. You will find more details in the Chap. 10.

While data, annotations, and benchmarks are important, external and independent testing (formerly known as external validation) remains crucial in confirming the efficacy and trustworthiness of AI models. A primary concern that underscores the need for this external and independent testing is *data leakage*. This means the model is tested on the same or similar data it is trained on. This overlap can produce overly optimistic accuracy estimates. When applied in real-world scenarios, these models tend to underdeliver, much like students who only study exam-specific questions or, even worse, have been given the answers beforehand. Thus, consistent external and independent evaluations are essential to genuinely affirm the efficacy of AI tools in clinical practice and counter potential pitfalls like data leakage.

9.6 How to Read and Plan AI Research in Dentistry

The primary purpose of any scientific article is to share findings about a sound scientific question so that other scientists can independently replicate and validate them. With the explosion of dental research publications related to AI, ensuring that research is reported clearly and systematically is more critical than ever. This is where you, as a researcher, come into play. Your AI research publications should provide crucial information that upholds high scientific standards and enables others to reproduce your results independently. Remember that reproducibility and validation are cornerstones for the practical application and acceptance of AI algorithms in healthcare—without them, your results may be purely theoretical and of limited clinical impact.

Once you have defined your research question, the next step is to draft the study protocol. This protocol allows you to plan and anticipate potential problems. Moreover, creating a research protocol provides (1) a clear framework for the research and (2) the ability to identify and prepare for possible challenges and (3) ensures methodological consistency. It is advisable to publish the protocol for the following reasons: (1) to promote transparency, (2) to allow feedback from the scientific community, and (3) to prevent duplication in research. Consider publishing it on platforms like Open Science Foundation (osf.io), Zenodo, the ISRCTN registry for clinical studies, or specialized journals that accept protocols for publication. When drafting the protocol, it is recommended to follow a reporting guide, which we will address next.

Various tools and guidelines have been established to foster comprehensive reporting of AI research, which supports research reproducibility, strengthens adherence to ethical standards, enhances the comprehensibility of research manuscripts, and encourages the publication of scientifically valid results. Many scientific journals have either recommended or imposed these guidelines, making it easier for research output to be appropriately evaluated during the review process. You can access these guides or view more specific ones and guidelines for writing and revising an article on Equator-Network website.[3] A detailed comparison of these guidelines can be found in Table 9.3.

[3]https://www.equator-network.org/

Table 9.3 Available reporting guidelines for AI research

Acronym	Purpose	Format	Salient features
Dental-AI [4]	Planning and reporting of AI studies in dentistry	Checklist	The primary reporting guideline for AI in dental research can be supplemented with other guides. Table 9.4 Provides more details
CLAIM [5]	AI applications in imaging	Checklist	Distinguishes prospective and retrospective studies, references common data elements
CONSORT-AI [6]/ SPIRIT-AI [7]	Clinical trials involving AI interventions	Checklist	Distinguishes prospective and retrospective studies, references common data elements
FUTURE-AI [8]	Safe, trusted, and ethical solutions for dental imaging	Process map	Outlines principles for fairness, traceability, usability, robustness, and explainability
MI-CLAIM [9]	Minimal items to include in AI research	List of principles	Details data handling, structured vs. unstructured data, and model evaluation metrics
MINIMAR [10]	Minimum items for reporting classification and prediction models	Step-by-step guide	Promotes transparency, nonimaging data inclusion, and socioeconomic status consideration
PROBAST-AI [11]	Risk and applicability assessment for prediction models	Checklist	Geared towards individualized predictions, assesses bias and applicability
REFORMS [12]	Provide clear reporting standards for ML-based science	Checklist/ guideline	Additional guidance to prevent or minimize data leaking
RQS [13]	Quality assessment for radiomics	Set of criteria	Assesses image protocol quality, reproducibility, imaging at multiple time points, cost-effectiveness, clinical applications, and data openness
STARD-AI [14]	Diagnostic and accuracy studies	Checklist	Details on image protocol quality, reproducibility, imaging at multiple time points, cost-effectiveness, clinical applications, and data openness
TRIPOD-AI [11]	Prediction model development/validation	Checklist	Addresses missing data, tailored to developing or validating a prediction model
DECIDE-AI [15]	Early-stage AI decision support in clinical settings	Checklist	Reporting guideline for initial clinical evaluation of AI-driven decision support systems

As we mentioned, the planning and reporting of AI in dental research possess particular characteristics that must be considered to ensure the quality and applicability of the studies. This means that your planning and reporting need to carefully consider these elements to ensure the integrity and applicability of your studies. Think about where your data are coming from and its quality. Consider how you will select and validate AI models, the strategy for annotation, and the clinical relevance of your chosen metrics for optimization. All these elements demand your careful attention. And do not forget about the broader picture—how will your AI solution impact real-world dental health, treatment costs, and service provision?

Recognizing these specific demands, the International Telecommunication Union/World Health Organization (ITU/WHO) focus group on AI for Health (FG AI4H), composed of global experts, researchers, and clinicians, crafted a comprehensive list of necessary items for planning and reporting AI studies in dental research [4]. Consider this list your blueprint—it will help you design, conduct, and report AI studies to enhance their robustness, transparency, reproducibility, and clinical applicability. You will find detailed information about these essential items in Table 9.4.

These guidelines are designed to uphold a reporting standard consistent with scientific rigor, facilitating independent verification of your findings by others. Generally, these core elements are foundational across all such guidelines:

Table 9.4 Items to be considered when planning, conducting, and reporting AI studies in dental research

Item no.	Item	Description
For planning		
1.	Study goal	Consider the AI application's relevance, scope, meaning, and limitations
2.	Study focus	Clarify if developing a new or validating an existing model, or if scope diagnostics or prognostics, technical or clinical aim
3.	Data	Scrutinize the available dataset and mitigate bias, ensuring generalizability
4.	Study aim	Define whether the study is exploratory or hypothesis-testing and consider implications for the conception of the study
5.	Reference test	Decide on a justifiable basis for establishing a reference test, especially when involving multiple annotators
6.	Clustering	Consider clustering of teeth and patients in your dataset, for example, during data partitioning ("data snooping bias")
7.	Test dataset	Report test metrics from an independent test dataset
8.	Computational resources	Consider resources when working with larger datasets or complex models
9.	Comparators	Compare your model against relevant comparators (experts, other models) using meaningful metrics
For reporting		
10.	Title	Define that any kind of AI was used, and specify which one and for which focus and problem
11.	Abstract	Present a structured summary of the study's aim, methods, results, and conclusion
12.	Introduction	Sum up the clinical background and need for AI solution, achievements and limitations so far, goal of the study, hypothesis (if needed)
13.	Study design	Assist the reader in understanding your study by providing an overview of the study goal, data characteristics, modeling techniques, evaluation, and scope.
14.	Data	Provide details on the data source, inclusion/exclusion criteria, sampling method, applicability to target population, heterogeneity, partitioning for training/testing, and data accessibility (or reasons for non-accessibility)
14a.	Sampling	Provide inclusion and exclusion criteria, case definition, image type and quality, data source(s)/centers, sampling strategy, and information towards heterogeneity
14b.	Data protection	Provide information on how data protection requirements were fulfilled
14c.	Missing data	Explain how missing data was handled
14d.	Data processing	Lay out how data processing (extracted, transposed, loaded, preprocessed) was performed
15.	Reference test	Explain how the reference test was generated, including case definition, grading schemes, test thresholds, and unification strategies for multiple labels
16.	Sample size	If your study is hypothesis-testing, provide information on how you arrived at your test dataset sample size
17.	Model	Provide detailed information on model inputs, outputs, intermediate layers, pooling, normalization, regularization, and activation, as well as software packages and hardware used. The structure of the model may be presented
17a.	Model parameters	Describe how the model parameters were initialized

(continued)

Table 9.4 (continued)

Item no.	Item	Description
18.	Training	Describe the training procedures, including data augmentation techniques, criteria for stopping the training, and hyperparameters and search strategy. For neural networks, at least the learning rate schedule, optimization method, batch size, dropout rates, regularization parameters (if any), and number of epochs should be provided
19.	Justify the best-performing model	Describe the method and model metric to select the final model and evaluate it against the hold-out test set
20.	Evaluation	Describe the primary outcome and outcome metric. Consider further outcomes with relevance to your question
21.	Uncertainty	Describe how uncertainties in the model results (comparisons, subgroups) are reflected
22.	Explainability	Lay out how explainability, trustworthiness, and transparency were assessed
23.	Results	Provide information on data flow, including those in and excluded, and data partitions into training, validation, and test dataset. Characterize the dataset
23a.	Performance metrics and data partitions	The final model's performance on the test partition should be detailed and benchmarked against current technical standards. Provide uncertainty estimates. Provide information to understand incorrect predictions and explainability
24.	Discussion	Provide a summary, a strengths and limitations section, a section on findings and their implications, and one on future directions
25.	Other	Provide information about authorship and registration, study protocol, and potential conflicts of interest

Modified from Schwendicke et al. [4]

1. **Computational Reproducibility**: Ensure an independent party can consistently achieve your research results. This fosters credibility and permits other researchers to verify or expand upon your findings. Achieving reproducibility, while fundamental, can be challenging in AI research.

   Example: Provide the code in a GitHub repository or create a minimal viable product.
2. **Data Quality:** Emphasize the importance and relevance of the data you use. Avoid poor or inappropriate data, which can yield irrelevant or distorted outcomes. Understand that the data's integrity directly influences the research results.

   Example: Provide all the details of the dataset as size, demographic composition, type of data, any instrument used to generate the data, as dental radiography equipment details, and preferably provide an example dataset or a synthetic representation.
3. **Data Preprocessing:** Detail the steps taken in data preparation. Minor alterations in the sequence or method of preprocessing can substantially modify the study's outcome. Highlight potential pitfalls like errors from splitting datasets improperly.

   Example: For a dental AI application, document the techniques used for image enhancement, normalization, or segmentation of the teeth from the periodontal tissues.
4. **Model Development:** Detail the entire modeling process, from feature selection to evaluation, to ensure clarity and ease of replication. Not providing exhaustive details can make replication difficult or nearly impossible based on the textual description alone.

   Example: For developing an AI model to detect early signs of oral cancer, describe the machine learning algorithms employed, hyperparameter settings, and the technical/clinical evaluation metrics. Also, explain the feature extraction methods used to capture relevant information from oral images, like texture and shape descriptors.
5. **Addressing Data Leakage:** Highlight and rectify any unintentional correlations between variables resulting from data handling or modeling. Leakage can cause exaggerated results,

jeopardizing the study's credibility. Researchers should explicitly demonstrate that their methodology avoids common leakage sources.

Example: In dental research, when creating a model to predict the outcome of orthodontic treatments, you might have information from both before and after the treatment. First, you would split the data into training and validation sets to prevent data leakage. Then, when preprocessing, such as normalization or scaling, ensure these steps are applied separately to each set. Using posttreatment information from the validation set during preprocessing of the training set can lead to misleadingly positive results.

6. **Metrics and Uncertainty Assessment:** Justify the chosen evaluation metrics, ensuring they align with the study's objectives. Also, discuss any uncertainties in the model's predictions. Proper reporting of metrics and uncertainties bolsters the research's trustworthiness.

   Example: In a study aiming to use AI for predicting the risk of periodontal disease, clearly outline why metrics such as sensitivity, specificity, and the area under the Receiver Operating Characteristic (ROC) curve were chosen. Discuss how these metrics relate to the study's early and accurate disease detection goals. Also, discuss uncertainties like confidence intervals around predictions and the model's limitations in dealing with unbalanced datasets or missing data.
7. **Generalizability and Validation:** Address potential limitations in the external validity of your study, particularly when you have created and tested the model in the same or similar datasets.

   Example: When developing an AI model to identify dental caries from intraoral scans, test its effectiveness not just on your initial dataset (maybe from one clinic) but also on external datasets, perhaps from different regions or demographics, to ensure its broad applicability.

By considering these fundamental considerations for AI research in dentistry and adhering to guidelines for planning and reporting, you ensure that your results have scientific significance and proceed ethically, paving the way for the exciting advancement of this dental field to benefit patients.

9.7 Data: The Key Ingredient for AI Research

Artificial Intelligence (AI) relies on three elements to function effectively:

1. *Data*: This is the raw material the AI system will use to learn, make decisions, or offer predictions. Data can come in many forms, such as text, numbers, images, or more complex structures like time series or graphs.
2. *Algorithm* refers to the rules or models the AI uses to make sense of the data. Algorithms are the "brain" of the AI, dictating how data should be interpreted, sorted, or acted upon. In machine learning, algorithms can learn and improve from data, refining their operations for better outcomes.
3. *Processing Power:* This is the computational capacity required to run the algorithms and manage the data. As AI algorithms can be computationally intensive and may require handling large datasets, sufficient processing power (often provided by high-performance GPUs or specialized hardware) is critical for the efficient functioning of AI systems.

It is crucial to understand that an algorithm's performance depends on the balance between the data used for its training and the adjustments, or tuning, that empower its operation. Given our roles as healthcare professionals, our assessment of AI primarily involves securing its safety and efficacy in patient care. However, as researchers, we have more control and influence over data. In dental AI research, these data should have certain characteristics. These are as follows:

1. *High Quality*: The data should be accurate, complete, and reliable. Data quality can significantly impact the performance of an AI

model. Misclassifications or errors in data collection can lead to misleading results and flawed conclusions.
2. *Relevant*: The data must be relevant to the research question. For instance, if you are creating an AI model to predict the progression of periodontal disease, you will need data about the patient's oral health history, periodontal measurements, genetic factors, lifestyle factors, habits, and so on.
3. *Diverse and Representative:* The data should represent the population for which the model is intended. They should cover different demographics, conditions, and other variables of interest to avoid biases and ensure the model's applicability to a broad range of patients or algorithm fairness [16].
4. *Sufficiently Large:* The volume of data should be large enough to support the creation of an effective AI model. Larger datasets generally improve the model's ability to learn and make accurate predictions. Beware of oversampling, i.e. creating seudoreplications of a small dataset. For instance, three patients (N = 3) can provide three panoramic radiographs and these radiographs can be sliced into thousands of small images (n = 3000). Here, the sample size is still three.
5. *Structured Appropriately:* Depending on the AI method used, the data might need to be structured in a specific way. For example, supervised learning requires input variables (e.g., some potential risk factors for oral cancer prognosis) and the corresponding output or target variable (whether the patient developed oral cancer or not).
6. *Correctly Annotated:* The data must be labeled or annotated for many types of AI, especially supervised learning methods. In dental AI research, this could mean having expert dentists identify and label images of oral conditions using specific criteria.
7. *Compliant with Privacy Regulations*: Data used for AI research should respect individuals' privacy rights. Identifiable information should be anonymized or de-identified in compliance with regulations like the Health Insurance Portability and Accountability Act (HIPAA) or General Data Protection Regulation (GDPR).

You must be particularly cautious when using readily available data, as it may not accurately represent the population to which you intend to apply your model. For instance, if you are using patient records from an urban public hospital to develop a predictive model risk model for oral disease, remember that these patients might differ significantly from those in rural areas or private clinics. The diversity in healthcare access, overall health status, and other socioeconomic factors could influence the applicability of your model. So, always ensure that your dataset accurately represents the population it is intended to model. Specify which population or type of patient your model is expected to perform similarly based on the results obtained during development.

Data are typically divided into a set for training the model, another for testing, and a third for internal testing (formerly known as validation). However, this *internal testing* with the same dataset does not provide robust validation. For that, *external testing* is needed, either temporal (prospective patients to whom neither the model nor the researchers have had access) or geographical (different centers with different patients). Ideally, this external testing should be independent, involving researchers who have not participated in the model's development or internal validation.

9.8 Ensuring Trustworthiness and Transparency for Dental AI Research

Trustworthiness in AI refers to the degree to which an AI system can be relied upon to make accurate, unbiased, ethical, and transparent decisions or recommendations. It encompasses reliability, fairness, accountability, transparency, and ethical considerations. For developing trustworthy dental AI applications, these seven principles summarized in Table 9.5 proposed by the EC's High-Level Expert Group on AI (HLEG-AI) [17], are essential.

Remember that achieving trustworthiness in AI is an ongoing and collaborative effort involving multidisciplinary expertise, ongoing evaluation, and adaptation to evolving ethical, regulatory, and societal considerations.

Table 9.5 Principles and considerations for trustworthy AI in dental research

Principle	Definition	Dental AI implementation
Human agency and oversight	AI systems should empower human beings, fostering their rights and ensuring oversight via human-in-the-loop, human-on-the-loop, and human-in-command approaches	Does the AI system in dental diagnostics primarily assist the dentist? Does the dentist remain the final decision-maker?
Technical robustness & safety	AI must be resilient, secure, accurate, and reliable and have a fallback plan to minimize unintentional harm	How reliable and accurate is the AI system in identifying dental pathologies from X-rays, and what safeguards exist for inaccuracies or misdiagnoses?
Privacy & data governance	Ensure full respect for privacy and data protection, with adequate data governance, considering data quality and integrity and ensuring legitimized access	How does the AI system protect patient dental records, and what measures are in place to ensure data integrity and controlled access?
Transparency and explanaibility	AI and data models should be transparent. Decisions should be explainable to stakeholders. When interacting with AI, knowing its capabilities/limitations is essential	Can the dentist easily understand and trace back the AI system's decision-making process when recommending a dental procedure or treatment?
Diversity, non-discrimination, & fairness	AI systems should avoid unfair bias, be accessible to all, and involve stakeholders throughout their life cycle	How does the AI system ensure consistent diagnostic accuracy/prediction across diverse patient demographics, such as age groups or ethnicities?
Societal & environmental Well-being	AI should benefit all, including future generations, be sustainable and environmentally friendly, and consider their societal impact	How does the AI system promote dental treatments that are both effective for the patient and environmentally sustainable?
Accountability	Ensure responsibility and accountability for AI outcomes. Emphasize auditability, especially in critical applications, and ensure redress	In the event of a diagnostic error by the AI system in dental practice, what mechanisms are in place to determine responsibility and provide rectification?

Modified from [17]

9.9 Ethical Considerations for AI Dental Research

As with any other health research, ethical considerations play a critical role. For dental AI applications, it is essential to consider and apply guidelines like those presented by the HLEG-AI [17]. They have delineated clear guidelines on trustworthy AI. For dental AI research, this translates into creating models that adhere to regulations, are technically and socially sound, and uphold ethical standards.

AI HLEG-AI underscores four core ethical principles: (1) *respect for human autonomy*—ensuring patients maintain control over their dental health decisions; (2) *prevention of harm*—ensuring AI predictions or recommendations do not harm the patient; (3) *fairness*—ensuring equitable treatment and representation in dental outcomes; and (4) *explicability*—ensuring dental professionals and patients can understand AI-driven decisions. Adopting these principles in dental AI research ensures ethical integrity while pushing the boundaries of technological advancement.

9.10 Key Challenges in Dental AI Research and Development

By now, you should have gained a clearer perspective on identifying research interests and interpreting an AI article. You have probably reviewed some AI dental research reports. While technological development often draws our attention to some technical details in AI research, it is time to take a step back and appreciate the broader picture.

Two main challenges confront the field of dentistry when it comes to effectively translating research findings for practical clinical use and finding ways to reduce care costs to improve population coverage. Indeed, rising care costs often leave segments of the population without coverage, a phenomenon not necessarily tied to technological innovations.

Significantly, the escalating costs can be attributed to the various administrative layers added to patient care in recent decades. This highlights an area where AI applications could become more instrumental: improving administrative efficiency in healthcare. An AI application that reduces administrative costs could impact coverage more than one focused solely on diagnosis, which may not be universally accessible.

Given the 2030 WHO's Oral Health objectives [18], these goals can serve as vital benchmarks for determining the effectiveness of an AI application in dentistry. The following critical metrics should be considered:

1. The extent to which the application helps achieve 75% universal health coverage and
2. The effectiveness of the application in aiding the reduction of oral diseases by 10%.

Therefore, anyone involved in developing AI models for healthcare—from developers and engineers to healthcare professionals—should be able to estimate how much their new AI model or application will likely contribute to these goals.

Given this perspective, AI in dentistry may not only enhance diagnostic and treatment procedures but also significantly contribute to broader public health goals, such as expanding access to care and reducing the burden of oral diseases.

So now, the question to you, dear reader, is this: Are you ready to take the leap and contribute to this fascinating, impactful field? Are you prepared to use your skills, knowledge, and passion to develop AI solutions that could improve dental healthcare? There is no better time than now to join this incredible journey. You have the power to create the tools and solutions that will shape the future of dentistry and improve patient care globally. As you move forward, remember every step you take in AI research is a stride towards improving health outcomes and enhancing the quality of life for many. So, buckle up, let your curiosity guide you, and remember to enjoy the journey of discovery, innovation, and impact. Good luck, and happy researching!

9.11 Learn More

Venturing into AI's role in dental research requires proficiency in statistics, algebra, data science, and coding. To help dental professionals like you better grasp these essentials, we have curated a list of resources and courses to start your journey into AI Dental Research.

9.11.1 Books

- The StatQuest Illustrated Guide To Machine Learning: break down complex machine learning concepts into digestible, easy-to-understand visuals and explanations. For beginners, it offers a clear roadmap to navigate the intricate world of machine learning,[4]
- Deep Learning: A Visual Approach: simplifies complex concepts with visuals, making it easier to harness deep learning's potential in healthcare without getting bogged down by technical jargon.[5]
- Introduction to Statistical Learning is an essential read to understand the statistical foundations for machine learning.[6]

9.11.2 Coding

- Understand the basics of code, from Google.[7]
- Python for beginners, from Microsoft.[8]

[4] https://statquest.org/statquest-store/

[5] Glassner A. Deep learning: a visual approach. No Starch Press; 2021.

[6] https://www.statlearning.com/

[7] https://learndigital.withgoogle.com/digitalgarage/course/basics-code

[8] https://learn.microsoft.com/en-us/training/paths/beginner-python/

9.11.3 Courses

- Kaggle courses offer various free online tutorials and guides on key data science skills, including Python, Machine Learning, AI Ethics, and more, with exercises.[9]
- Yann LeCun's Deep Learning Course by a pioneer in the field. Explore the foundations of deep learning from computer vision to speech recognition. Ideal for those with a background in data science or prior machine learning coursework.[10]
- Also check Coursera, edX, Code.org, Stanford, MIT, or FutureLearn for any course on AI for Health course.

9.11.3.1 Machine Learning

- Machine Learning for Beginners - A Curriculum, from Microsoft.[11]
- Understand the basics of machine learning, from Google.[12]

9.11.3.2 Artificial Intelligence

- Elements of AI, from University of Helsinki/Google.[13]
- Artificial Intelligence for Beginners - A Curriculum, from Microsoft.[14]

References

1. Wang H, Fu T, Du Y, et al. Scientific discovery in the age of artificial intelligence. Nature. 2023;620:47–60.
2. Fryback DG, Thornbury JR. The efficacy of diagnostic imaging. Med Decis Mak. 1991;11:88–94.
3. Wiegand T, Krishnamurthy R, Kuglitsch M, Lee N, Pujari S, Salathé M, Wenzel M, Xu S. WHO and ITU establish benchmarking process for artificial intelligence in health. Lancet. 2019;394:9–11.
4. Schwendicke F, Singh T, Lee J-H, Gaudin R, Chaurasia A, Wiegand T, Uribe S, Krois J, IADR e-Oral Health Network and the ITU WHO Focus Group AI for Health. Artificial intelligence in dental research: checklist for authors, reviewers, readers. J Dent. 2021;107:103610.
5. Mongan J, Moy L, Kahn CE. Checklist for artificial intelligence in medical imaging (CLAIM): a guide for authors and reviewers. Radiol Artif Intell. 2020;2:e200029.
6. Liu X, Rivera SC, Moher D, Calvert MJ, Denniston AK, SPIRIT-AI and CONSORT-AI Working Group. Reporting guidelines for clinical trial reports for interventions involving artificial intelligence: the CONSORT-AI extension. BMJ. 2020;370:m3164.
7. Cruz Rivera S, Liu X, Chan A-W, et al. Guidelines for clinical trial protocols for interventions involving artificial intelligence: the SPIRIT-AI extension. Lancet Digit Health. 2020;26:e549–60.
8. Lekadir K, Osuala R, Gallin C, et al. FUTURE-AI: guiding principles and consensus recommendations for trustworthy artificial intelligence in medical imaging. arXiv [cs.CV]. 2021.
9. Norgeot B, Quer G, Beaulieu-Jones BK, et al. Minimum information about clinical artificial intelligence modeling: the MI-CLAIM checklist. Nat Med. 2020;26:1320–4.
10. Hernandez-Boussard T, Bozkurt S, Ioannidis JPA, Shah NH. MINIMAR (MINimum information for medical AI reporting): developing reporting standards for artificial intelligence in health care. J Am Med Inform Assoc. 2020;27:2011–5.
11. Collins GS, Dhiman P, Andaur Navarro CL, et al. Protocol for development of a reporting guideline (TRIPOD-AI) and risk of bias tool (PROBAST-AI) for diagnostic and prognostic prediction model studies based on artificial intelligence. BMJ Open. 2021;11:e048008.
12. Kapoor S, Cantrell E, Peng K, et al. REFORMS: reporting standards for machine learning based science. arXiv [cs.LG]. 2023.
13. Lambin P, Leijenaar RTH, Deist TM, et al. Radiomics: the bridge between medical imaging and personalized medicine. Nat Rev Clin Oncol. 2017;14:749–62.
14. Sounderajah V, Ashrafian H, Aggarwal R, et al. Developing specific reporting guidelines for diagnostic accuracy studies assessing AI interventions: the STARD-AI Steering Group. Nat Med. 2020;26:807–8.
15. Vasey B, Nagendran M, Campbell B, et al. Reporting guideline for the early-stage clinical evaluation of decision support systems driven by artificial intelligence: DECIDE-AI. Nat Med. 2022;28:924–33.

[9] https://www.kaggle.com/learn

[10] https://cds.nyu.edu/deep-learning/

[11] https://microsoft.github.io/ML-For-Beginners/#/?id=machine-learning-for-beginners-a-curriculum

[12] https://learndigital.withgoogle.com/digitalgarage/course/machine-learning-basics

[13] https://learndigital-staging.withgoogle.com/digitalgarage/course/elements-artificial-intelligence

[14] https://microsoft.github.io/AI-For-Beginners/

16. Ricci Lara MA, Echeveste R, Ferrante E. Addressing fairness in artificial intelligence for medical imaging. Nat Commun. 2022;13:4581.
17. EU High-Level Expert Group on AI. Ethics guidelines for trustworthy AI. European Comission; 2019.
18. World Health Organization. Regional Office for Europe. Global oral health status report: towards universal health coverage for oral health by 2030: summary of the WHO European Region. World Health Organization. Regional Office for Europe; 2022.

10 Data Foundations for Trustworthy AI in Dentistry

Sergio E. Uribe and Falk Schwendicke

10.1 Data Foundations for Trustworthy AI in Dentistry

10.1.1 Computer Processing + AI Algorithms + Data = Artificial Intelligence

Artificial intelligence (AI) relies on three fundamental elements for advancements: computing power, algorithms, and data.

The rapid advancement in processing power, often referred to in light of Moore's Law,[1] provides the necessary computational power. This, coupled with algorithms like Convolutional Neural Networks (CNNs), has accelerated AI's application development. However, the data, particularly the vast and diverse datasets used to train these algorithms, truly drive AI's capabilities.

As clinicians, we are familiar with data. Regardless of the sophistication of AI algorithms, their efficacy dependes on the quality of the input data. Hence, data cleaning, preprocessing, and management should precede algorithm development. In this step, dental professionals should be actively involved, ensuring that the data utilized aligns with the clinical complexities of the dental field.

For AI models like machine and deep learning to succeed in healthcare, they require large, well-described, well-curated, and annotated datasets. Therefore, proper data management, incluiding acquisition, cleaning, normalization, augmentation, annotation, and validation sets, is ritical for AI in dental applications. Furthermore, transparent documentation of the data management process contributes to the reproducibility and generalizability of AI studies in dentistry.

[1]The number of transistors on a microchip doubles approximately every 2 years, leading to exponential growth in computing power while reducing the cost of technology over time—Gordon Moore, co-founder of Intel.

S. E. Uribe (✉)
Department of Conservative Dentistry and Oral Health, Riga Stradins University, Latvia/
Conservative Dentistry and Periodontology, LMU Klinikum, LMU Munich, Munich, Germany
e-mail: sergio.uribe@rsu.lv

F. Schwendicke
Conservative Dentistry and Periodontology, LMU Klinikum, LMU Munich, Munich, Germany
e-mail: falk.schwendicke@med.uni-muenchen.de

F. Schwendicke et al. (eds.), *Artificial Intelligence for Oral Health Care*,
https://doi.org/10.1007/978-3-031-84047-0_10

10.2 Data Quality: The Bedrock of Dental AI

In AI and data science, the adage *Garbage in, garbage out* highlights the direct link between the quality of input and output. Given its importance, data is often compared to the new oil [1]. However, like raw oil cannot be used in cars or machines, raw data cannot yield the clinical insights or AI models we seek. It necessitates extensive refinement to become useful. A more fitting analogy might be that data is the new sand [2], abundant like the information in every dental clinic and hospital, yet of limited use in its unprocessed form. It can be transformed into something valuable only through advanced and sophisticated processing—like sand is refined into silicon microprocessors. To help you understand the data management for AI applications, the next section focuses on factors for ensuring data quality.

10.2.1 Structured and Unstructured Data

Data comes in various forms, primarily categorized as *structured* and *unstructured. Structured* data is organized in a predefined manner, typically found in relational databases. For example, in dentistry, patient records containing specific fields like age, gender, or number of dental caries fall under structured data. Machine learning is often trained using structured data. On the other hand, *unstructured* data does not have a specific form or structure. For unstructured data such as radiographic images, handwritten notes from a dentist, or even audio recordings of patient consultations, deep learning is often used.

Structured data, typically in spreadsheets, provides a clear format for training machine learning applications. Conversely, unstructured data, including CBCT scans, radiographs, dentist's notes, and audio files, lacks a set structure. Deep learning applications have traditionally employed various neural networks to decode this data type. They interpret and organize unstructured data to extract valuable information, such as detecting a caries lesion in a bitewing radiograph. Recently, transformer architectures have emerged, offering enhanced capabilities to outperform and replace traditional neural networks, particularly in handling unstructured data complexities.

10.2.2 Data Characteristics

Most datasets reported in dental research papers are small, originating from a single center or population, which can inadvertently introduce biases [3], ompromizing the generalizability and reliability of any AI application. For instance, an assessment of datasets available for machine learning in head and neck cancer identified class imbalance (when one class of data significantly outnumbers another) and data fairness (ensuring equitable representation of different groups to avoid biases) as the predominant limitations in data quality [4]. Understanding the dataset's characteristics provides insights into where we can anticipate the AI model to perform optimally and where not. The better the training dataset matches the patient demographics where the AI will be used, the more accurate and reliable the AI predictions.

10.2.3 Data Aim

AI models aim to emulate human cognition, so they must encounter situations akin to a clinician's experience. When deciding on a treatment, a clinician relies on clinical data from the anamnesis and factors in insights gained from patient interactions. They might consult with peers or obtain additional patient details from their assistants. This information often exists in unstructured forms, like a handwritten note at the edge of a patient's record or even a conversation in thes hallway. Yet, today's healthcare AI models are predominantly trained on electronic health record data—highly structured but tailored mainly for administrative purposes, such as insurance claims. This discrepancy, data generated for administrative purposes being used for clinical purposes, could contribute to why, during the COVID-19 pandemic, over 600 machine-learning predictive models were developed using hospital data for outcomes like hospital admissions or mortality. At the same time, only two demonstrated specific clinical utility, with their application limited to certain centers or locales and not widely adaptable elsewhere [5]. Hence, as AI models aim to mirror human decision-making processes, they should be trained on data that captures clinical complexities.

Dental research has the potential to provide rich data from AI models collected systematically using validated and reproducible methodologies. However, only 1.5% of dental research articles share their datasets and when data is shared, its quality is frequently subpar, scoring 1.0 out of 3 for accessibility, 1.1 out of 4 for interoperability, and 2.4 out of 10 for reusability [6]. This compromised data quality hinders its applicability in machine learning [6]. Solutions such as forming large-scale data consortia or implementing federated learning have been proposed [7], where centers train models independently and combine model attributes. While synthetic data has also been proposed to overcome the scarcity of broad data, recent studies indicate that AI models trained with synthetic data can suffer from Model Autophagy Disorder (MAD), indicating potential unpredictability and unreliability in outcomes [8]. The MAD refers to when AI models trained on synthetic data, start producing nonsense. For example, instead of writing clear sentences, the model might start generating gibberish or incoherent phrases because it's too focused on the fake data patterns. We present a summary in Table 10.1 to further emphasize the distinctions between the data type used for AI technical development and that for clinical application.

Another aspect to consider is the quality of data labeling or annotation. Data annotation or labeling refers to attaching meaningful information to raw data, effectively transforming it into a dataset from which an AI model can learn in the widely common "supervised" way. Annotation is critical because the accuracy and relevance of annotations dictate how well the AI system can understand and interpret new, unseen data. Consider annotations as the teachers guiding an AI student: if the teacher provides incorrect or

Table 10.1 Comparative analysis of data usually available and data likely need to train clinically useful AI

	Datasets	
	Available	Desired
Sources	One or few (>5)	Many
Server type	Central	Federated
Data type	Unimodal	Multimodal
Data preprocessing	Extensive	Minimal (real world data)
Source of annotations	Manual by research members	Cross-annotations, e.g., imaging data cross-referenced with lab exam results
Diversity of data	Limited to specific technical challenges (e.g., data with/without a condition)	Broad to reflect clinical variability
Validation process	Primarily internal testing	External testing
Patients	Homogeneous	Heterogeneous
Diseases or conditions	One or few	Many
Metrics [9]	Technical metricos of accuracy: Accuracy, F1-score, dice coefficient	Impact metrics of value: Impact on diagnosis/treatment decisions, patient- or society-outcome oriented, e.g., QALY[a] gained using AI model

[a] The quality-adjusted life-year (QALY) measures the value of health outcomes. Since health is a function of length of life and quality of life, the QALY was developed as an attempt to combine the value of these attributes into a single index number

ambiguous information, the student will develop a flawed understanding. Inconsistent labeling, such as over-sizing or under-sizing bounding boxes (BBs), can drastically influence AI outcomes [10]. A recent study utilized bitewing radiographs to detect calculus with AI models. When trained on accurate data, the AI models showed a high level of performance. When the AI models were trained on inaccurately labeled data, performance decreased. Interestingly, this drop was not always obvious when tested on imperfect data. The study highlights the need for accurate data labeling and warns dentists about the risks of relying on improperly trained models.

Thus, it is essential to ensure rigorous, transparent, documented quality control for dataset creation and annotations. The introduction of *model cards* [11] detailing dataset composition and annotation procedures, combined with the principles of FAIR data (Findable, Accessible, Interoperable, and Reusable) [11], provides the way for ensuring trustworthiness and transparency.

Using "model cards" in AI applications for health is similar to a nutrition label on food products. It provides essential information about a machine learning model's purpose, performance, training data, and potential biases. Just as a nutrition label helps consumers make informed choices about their food, a model card equips clinicians, researchers, and other stakeholders with key insights about an AI model's capabilities and limitations. Similarly, a "data card" offers detailed information about the datasets used to train these models. It includes descriptions of the dataset's origins, collection methods, composition, preprocessing steps, and any known limitations or biases. A "data card" outlines the number of samples, the distribution of different categories or labels, and the diversity of data sources. This transparency helps users understand the data's reliability and relevance, much like how a nutrition label informs about food ingredients. This transparency helps users understand the data's reliability and relevance, much like how a nutrition label informs about food ingredients. For example, just as you would check a food label to understand its calorie content or ingredient list, in AI, you would consult a model card to understand where the model was trained, its accuracy rate, and any potential biases it might hold.

10.3 Dataset Preparation

Preparing data for AI algorithm development involves several crucial steps. Initially, ethical approval is obtained from the local committee, or an institutional review board may evaluate the potential risks and benefits to patients. After ethical approval, relevant dental data are accessed, de-identified, and securely stored. The data are then structured in standardized and machine-readable formats. Finally, the dental data are linked to respective annotations.

10.3.1 Dataset Sources

Training AI algorithms using data from a single institution or limited geographic areas can introduce sampling bias. If such an AI model is used in a different region, its accuracy may be compromised due to discrepancies between the training data and the new target population. Potential biases stem from variations in age, race, sex, imaging equipment and protocols, and disease prevalence. A global review [12] identified that US and Chinese datasets heavily dominate clinical AI, limiting its applicability in other regions—its generalizability. For instance, an AI model trained on panoramic radiographs from Germany to identify apical lesions saw reduced performance when applied to radiographs from India [13]. This decline in efficacy was attributed to variations in dental treatment experiences in the training dataset, significantly influencing generalizability. Interestingly, factors such as image brightness and contrast did not play a notable role in this performance discrepancy.

10.3.2 Dataset Bias

Potential biases in data may stem from variations in age, race, sex, imaging equipment and protocols, and disease prevalence. Some examples of dataset-induced bias are as follows:

- *Hospital Data Bias:* Relying on data exclusively from a hospital can lead to biased estimations of disease prevalence by an AI model. As hospitals primarily serve individuals with health conditions, the model could overestimate the prevalence of certain diseases in the wider population.
- *Population Bias:* If an AI model for predicting public health outcomes is trained primarily on data from urban populations, it might not account for health issues more prevalent in rural areas, such as those arising from agricultural work or limited access to healthcare.
- *Device and Technique Bias:* If two imaging centers utilize different equipment and serve communities with varying prevalence of conditions, like caries, the AI might mistakenly assign the likelihood of caries based on the device that captured the radiograph rather than actual dental health indicators. For instance, in a COVID-19 study, an AI model trained to assess patient severity mistakenly learned that a specific marking from a gurney in a chest radiograph indicated higher disease severity. The error arose because sicker patients were imaged lying down while those with milder symptoms were standing. Rather than concentrating on lung characteristics, the AI relied on the incidental presence of the gurney to predict disease severity [14].
- *High-End Imaging Equipment Bias:* A specific form of device bias. Training AI on images from state-of-the-art imaging machines might result in it performing suboptimally on images from older or less advanced machines. The AI could become overly accustomed to high-resolution, clear images and struggle with lesser-quality ones. Latent biases, such as those arising from local medical practices, can inadvertently infiltrate datasets. When experts evaluate medical data, inconsistencies can introduce biases, particularly when annotations are done manually. Although having several experts assess the same case might minimize this bias, practical constraints like costs and time often render this solution unfeasible. There are specific guidelines for handling data considering the risk of bias, for example, for radiology [15], which we recommend considering.

10.3.3 Federated Learning

To address clinical data privacy concerns, federated learning (FL) allows data to remain in its original location, such as the hospital or clinic data server, with algorithms trained locally across multiple sites. So in FL, the algorithm comes to learn from the data, rather than the data going to the algorithm, avoiding privacy issues as the data never leaves the original source. Various approaches, including parallel and nonparallel training, have been suggested. Although early evaluations indicate federated learning may outperform models based on single institutions, its widespread clinical adoption is hindered by several challenges. These include standardizing data annotations, ensuring adequate computational resources at each site, data preprocessing difficulties, terminology discrepancies, and potential data sensitivity in gradient information. For federated learning to see extensive use, solutions to data structuring, labeling, and standardization across sites are imperative. In dentistry, federated learning has been applied to automate tooth segmentation on panoramic radiographs from nine global centers, demostrating its potential to enable generalizable dental AI models when central data pooling is not feasible [16].

10.3.4 Dataset Size

Generalizability in AI often requires large training datasets. While niche applications might work with smaller datasets, AI for broader applications, especially in medical imaging, demands 1000 or 10,000 of images. The balance between dataset size and annotation quality is crucial. As datasets grow, the risk of annotation errors also increases. Conversely, while accurately annotated, smaller datasets may not reflect the full spectrum of real-world scenarios. Researchers face a choice between larger datasets with potential annotation errors or smaller, precise datasets with possible limited applicability. A solution might be a hybrid dataset that merges a larger set's diversity with a smaller one's quality control. Semi-supervised learning presents a potential answer here, utilizing labeled and unlabeled data for training. By combining vast amounts of unlabeled data with limited labeled data, this method seeks to enhance learning. Incorporating tools like Reinforced Learning Human Feedback (RLHF), where human insights periodically refine the model, may combine human knowledge and machine efficiency. RLHF improves AI by combining large amounts of unlabelled data with a small amount of labelled data. It uses human feedback to fine-tune the model, bringing it closer to human preferences. For example, instead of a human annotating large amounts of data, a model is created to annotate the data, with some instructions. A human then tests the model's performance by reviewing some of the data annotations, correcting them and giving further instructions until the model improves its performance.

10.3.5 Data Annotations

Understanding and choosing labels is critical for supervised learning in dental AI development. Two terms often come into play: "Ground Truth" and "Gold Standard." These terms are frequently used interchangeably in AI but have distinct medical meanings. Ground truth refers to objective diagnostic confirmation, while the gold standard is the best effort to substitute the ground truth.

A gold standard may, for example, be established by several annotators labeling the same data point (e.g., an image). In this case, a final (unified) label must be constructed. Some strategies include reaching a consensus, involving a third-party evaluator, or using a "dictatorship" system where a lead annotator decides on the correct annotation. Ground truth, on the other hand, is an objective and unquestionable label. For example, the measurement of a laboratory instrument or a dead/alive status.

Confirmatory clinical labels, like those from pathological or surgical reports, might be needed to triangulate any gold standard. Besides imaging, non-imaging data like patient demographics or clinical outcomes, requiring extraction from electronic medical records, are also helpful. Different techniques, including structured labels, image annotations, segmentations, and electronic phenotypes, aid in labeling the data. Undertaking these measures ensures the effective training and testing of dental AI algorithms.

Models trained on such multimodal datasets may eventually even overcome the capacities of humans. A recent example is an AI model trained on chest images to assess the patient's race: Somehow, the AI could identify the patient's race by viewing the chest imaging, a feat impossible for a human [17].

10.3.6 Dataset Partition

After constructing and annotating a dataset, researchers or developers typically divide it into three subsets: training, validation, and test data. This partitioning strategy is illustrated in Fig. 10.1.

Initially, the model is trained on the training data, and the training process is optimized on the internal testing data. The best-developed model is then tested for performance on the test data. However, it is important to note that maintaining a separate test dataset is critical in AI model development to ensure that the model can generalize to unseen data.

10.3.6.1 The Problem with Repeated Testing

Continually using the same test dataset can risk *model overfitting*, where the model becomes overly tuned to that specific dataset

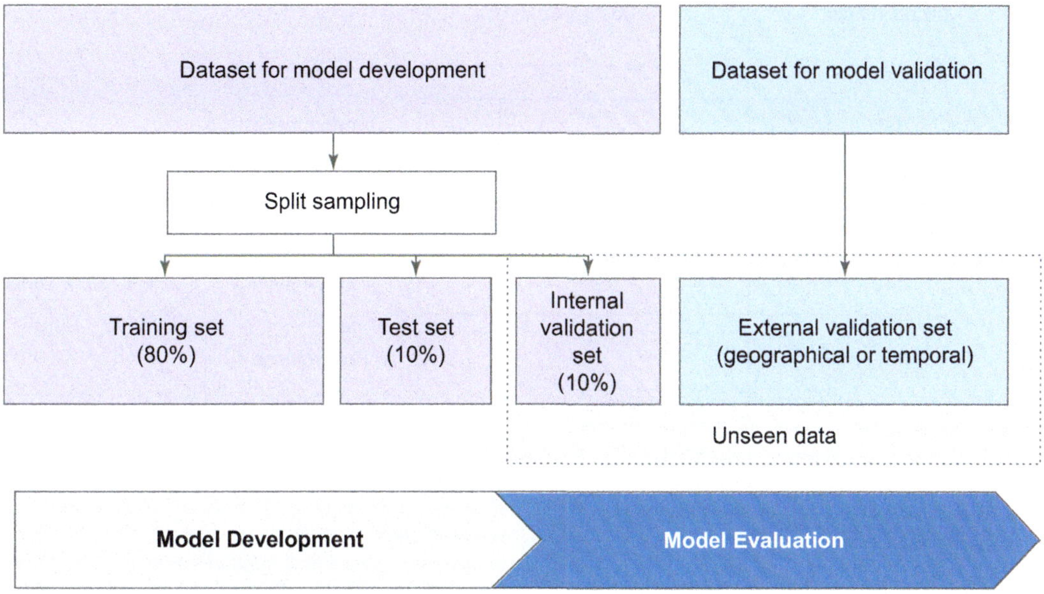

Fig. 10.1 Overview of dataset split for machine learning development and evaluation

and loses its ability to predict new data. An analogy to consider is a classroom scenario: students take a test and then are allowed to retake it multiple times, making corrections based on previous feedback. Over time, the test results no longer accurately reflect their understanding of the subject but their ability to recall the answers on that particular test. This phenomenon, where the model or students adjust their responses based on exposure to the test data, is known in AI as *data snooping or data leaking*.

10.3.6.2 Alternative: *k*-Fold Cross-Validation

To address the limitations of continuous testing on the same dataset, an alternative method for internal testing is *k*-fold cross-validation. Simply, *k*-fold cross-validation involves dividing the dataset into "*k*" subsets. The model is trained on $k - 1$ of these subsets and tested on the remaining one. This process is repeated *k* times, with a different subset serving as the test data each time, ensuring a comprehensive evaluation of the model's performance. Figure 10.2 shows an example of *k*-fold cross-validation.

10.3.6.3 The Downside of Data Splitting and the Benefits of Resampling

Let us examine the problems with data splitting. Data splitting and resampling methods are commonly used for AI model validation in dentistry and other fields. However, data splitting can be unstable, especially for datasets with fewer than 20,000 independent subjects or samples and high signal-to-noise ratios, because it can lead to inconsistent validation results.

10.3.6.4 Resampling Methods for Robust Validation

In contrast, resampling methods, such as repeated cross-validation and bootstrapping, provide more robust validation. They evaluate the entire modeling process, including feature selection, and provide a clearer picture of uncertainty. It is worth noting that researchers sometimes resort to multiple testing attempts with data splitting, reporting multiple iterations without confirmation.

10.3.6.5 The Superiority of Bootstrapping

We recommend using the bootstrapping method for greater accuracy, especially with smaller

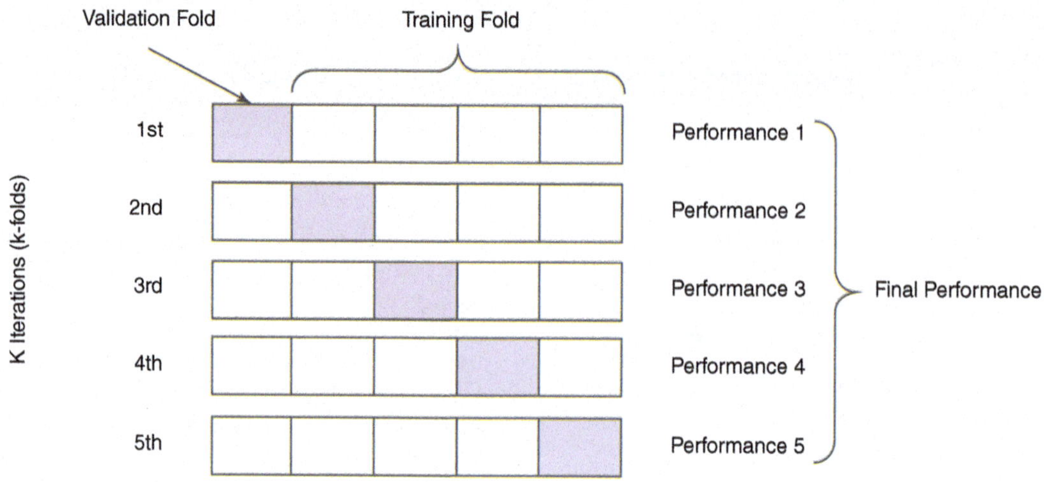

Fig. 10.2 Example of *k*-fold cross-validation ($k = 5$)

datasets. It outperforms data splitting and standard cross-validation by more reliably estimating model performance [18].

10.3.6.6 External Testing: A Better Approach

When external testing is required, it is more effective to incorporate time and location effects into a unified model than to split the data. Internal testing using bootstrapping, while accounting for these effects, can lead to more useful predictive models. For more details, see "Describing, Resampling, Validating, and Simplifying the Model" chapter in Harrell's Regression book [18].

10.4 Data Management

Transparent data management documentation is crucial for enhancing the reproducibility and generalizability of AI studies in dentistry.

The FAIR principles for data management are guidelines that aim to ensure data are Findable, Accessible, Interoperable, and Reusable (FAIR). They were developed to improve the infrastructure supporting the reuse of research data. A cornerstone of these principles is the emphasis on enhancing the ability of machines to automatically find and use data and supporting its reuse by individuals (Fig. 10.3).

This is key in artificial intelligence, where machine learning algorithms rely on large quantities of quality data for internal and external testing. Importantly, FAIR data are not synonymous with open data. While the FAIR principles encourage data sharing, they acknowledge that there are legitimate reasons, such as privacy concerns, to keep certain datasets closed. However, even if the data are closed, the metadata, i.e., data about the data, should still be open. This allows researchers to discover what data exists and decide if it is relevant to their work, even if they cannot access it. Table 10.2 describes the FAIR principles and an example of their application in dental research.

You will find some metadata examples in the supplementary section at the end of this chapter.

10.4.1 Why Use FAIR Data for AI Research Data Management

The FAIR data principles offer a crucial framework for ethical and efficient research data management, promoting collaboration and accelerating scientific advancement. From an ethical standpoint, much research is publicly funded, and thus, the resulting data should be viewed as a public good. Making research data FAIR maximizes its value by allowing it to be used to its full potential. Furthermore, when data

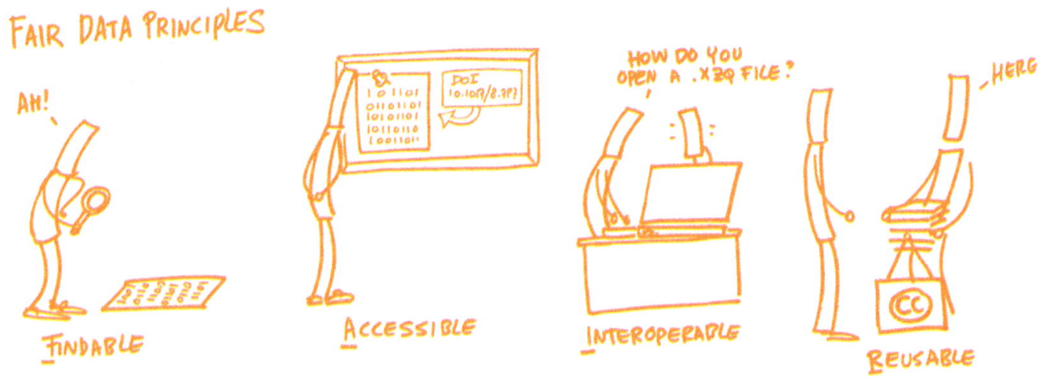

Fig. 10.3 The FAIR data principles. Image: https://book.fosteropenscience.eu (Courtesy of the National Library of Medicine)

are made FAIR, it enables transparency and reproducibility, which are essential for scientific integrity. It allows for the validation of results and provides a basis for further research. Even when data are sensitive and cannot be openly shared, FAIR principles encourage sharing metadata. Metadata is "data about data," providing information about the data's content, quality, condition, and other characteristics. By sharing metadata, valuable insights can be offered without compromising privacy or ethical guidelines.

Adopting FAIR data principles is a step towards responsible and efficient research practices that can drive scientific discovery and innovation while upholding the ethical principles of transparency, accountability, and accessibility.

10.5 Dataset Best Practices

Given that datasets fundamentally shape AI model outcomes, it is vital to recognize that a mismatch between a model's training or evaluation datasets and its real-world application—or the presence of societal biases within the data—can significantly compromise its performance. Furthermore, if a dataset lacks comprehensive description or documentation, the likelihood of experiencing data shift—when the input data during deployment deviates from the data used for training—rises [19]. Although there is significant attention on model development, the importance of thoroughly documenting dataset creation and utilization often goes overlooked. Here are essential factors to consider when creating or leveraging datasets for AI in dental applications [20].

1. *General Characteristics*: Dataset name, access type, link to dataset, sources of data (clinic, hospital, research), numbers of data sources, country of origin, data collection period, year of dataset publication, source of data acquisition, reason for image acquisition, and imaging modality (e.g., photograph, periapical)
2. *Acquisition Details:* Image acquisition device, ethical approval, individual participant consent for image, inclusion or exclusion criteria (for both patient and image), and any image processing or adjustment
3. *Annotation and Ground Truth or Gold Standard:* Segmentations, lesion features or image size annotations, ground truth method described, number of subjects, image format, associated publication, anonymization strategy, metadata details, and data without ground truth
4. *Licensing and Publication*: License availability, license type, and related publications
5. *Image Specifics*: (if applicable) Number of patients and images in the dataset, image size, and resolution.
6. *Disease or Condition Characteristics*: The prevalence at patient, tooth, or lesion level and severity (are all disease stages represented?)

Table 10.2 The FAIR principles for AI dental datasets

Principle	Explanation	Implementation in AI dental development or research
Findable	The data should be easily locatable and identifiable	Publish your dental data and/or metadata in searchable repositories such as Dataverse, Zenodo, Figshare, or your institutional repository. These repositories assign a persistent identifier like a digital object identifier (DOI) that uniquely identifies your data. Include rich, accurate, machine-readable metadata and keywords, adhering to dental or medical community standards (e.g., Dublin Core)
Accessible	The data should be easily retrievable and accessible	Include a data license or clear accessibility statement in your administrative metadata. Use a standard protocol to ensure your dental data are archived for long-term storage and retrievable via its persistent identifier (like a DOI or URI). Even if the data are closed, metadata should remain accessible
Interoperable	The data should be integrated with other datasets and compatible with various applications	Use standardized structural metadata by dental community standards. Utilize common terminologies, vocabularies, ontologies, and taxonomies for the data. Prefer open, long-term viable file formats for your data and metadata
Reusable	The data should be capable of being used for future research	Attach all relevant contextual information required for reuse in the documentation or metadata attached to your dental data. Apply standardized structural metadata and prefer open, long-term viable file formats for your data and metadata. Apply a machine-readable data license

7. *Demographics*: Age, gender, and ethnicity (when available in metadata labels).
8. *Annotation Details:* The number of annotators, annotation type (pixel-wise, box, label), diagnostic criteria, inter-rater reliability (Kappa or ICC), annotators' age and experience, strategies for handling disagreements, software used for annotations, and method for establishing ground truth

Each of these elements plays a critical role in ensuring the dataset's robustness and credibility and its subsequent applications in AI models for dentistry.

10.6 The Future

The volume of available medical data continues to grow daily. Data sources are increasingly diverse, from wearable devices such as mobile phones, smartwatches, and specialized medical gadgets capturing vital statistics to expanding electronic medical records. The rise of smart toothbrushes and future intraoral sensors may provide real-time insights into dietary and toothbrushing habits and wider oral health. Moreover, when analyzed with AI, social media data offers a comprehensive view of a patient's lifestyle, mental well-being, and potential health risks, gauged from online interactions and behaviors. Beyond consumer-generated data, hospitals and clinics produce vast amounts of information daily, including patient records, imaging, and lab tests. Much of this information is safely stored in secured silos to protect individual privacy. The advent of federated servers could mark a significant step in AI's role in dentistry. These servers allow algorithms to learn from diverse data sources without directly accessing the data, preserving patients' privacy. AI models are on the verge of being an integral part of daily dental routines, enhancing professional expertise and potentially amplifying patient care results.

Yet, these models' true value and efficiency largely depend on the detailed curation, annotation, and management of datasets. We will likely shift towards unsupervised learning and human-reinforced learning feedback as we advance. This approach can offer the promise of large datasets without the associated issues of annotation quality deterioration. Additionally, there is potential in cross-annotating datasets, for instance, augmenting dental radiograph images with information from intraoral scanners, further expanding the capabilities of medical devices.

The FAIR (Findable, Accessible, Interoperable, Reusable) principles offer guidance in this evolving landscape. Adopting these principles provides a robust framework ensuring transparency and trustworthiness, both vital in developing reliable AI dental tools.

10.7 Summary

The development and application of AI in dentistry highlights the critical importance of the data in constructing AI models. Understanding the data's role is essential to ensure complete transparency during the model development. This facilitates the identification of patients or communities where the model may be highly effective and those contexts where it might fall short. While an AI model may demonstrate efficacy in controlled environments, its performance in real-world situations can be compromised due to inherent factors in the dataset, such as data quality and annotations. Therefore, special attention must be paid to aspects such as the formation of the dataset, annotation criteria, and data management. Here, the FAIR principles provides a useful framework, ensuring transparency in data handling, enhancing replicability and external validation of AI models, and strengthening the trustworthiness of AI applications in dentistry.

Supplementary Material

Example of Dental Radiograph Dataset and Metadata Specifications for AI Research

General Image Processing

- All submitted files must be fully de-identified to ensure patient privacy. This includes the removal of text overlays and any patient-related metadata within the image files.
- Radiographs should exhibit appropriate contrast and brightness to differentiate hard tissues (bone, enamel, dentin).
- Ensure images are free of sensor, board, or scanner defects.

Metadata

A file, readme.txt, should be included with each image dataset containing the following:

- Author
- Date
- Number of images
- Image format
- Country of origin (if multiple, separated by commas)
- Radiograph type
- Tube specifications
- Sensor specification (digitized film radiograph, sensor-based (CCD, etc.), PSP plate)
- Any postprocessing details

File Types

- Preferred file formats are DICOM, JPEG (or JPG), PNG, GIF, TIFF, RAW. BMP format should be avoided.
- Maximum compression should be 70%.

File Naming

- File name should ideally include the patient's sex and age. If not, a CSV file containing this information for each image should be provided.
- Use hyphens "-" or underscores "_" to seprate the information, e.g., "XQVKXBLZWSON-male-21.JPG."

Image Requirements for 2D Bitewing

- Images should be complete radiographs, not cropped.
- Minimum resolution: 300 dpi.
- Minimum dimensions: 400 px by 300 px.
- Ideal size: >600 px by 400 px.
- Depth: ≥8-bit.
- Images should be taken with a sensor or plate holder.
- Occlusal plane should not deviate more than 40° from the horizontal plane.

Image Requirements for Panoramic

- Ensure the radiograph shows the patient correctly positioned.
- Minimum resolution: 170 dpi.
- Minimum dimensions: 800 px by 400 px.
- Ideal size: > 2000 px by 900 px.
- Depth: ≥8-bit.

Example Metadata Describing a Dental AI Research Dataset

1. *Dataset Title*
2. *Dataset Creator:* The name of the individual, team, or organization that created the dataset.
3. *Dataset Description*: A high-level summary of the dataset, its purpose, and how it was collected.
4. *Data Source*: Information about where the data was obtained, including any relevant institutional affiliations or links to the original data source.
5. *Date of Collection:* The data's collection period. This is particularly important for datasets where the temporal aspect may impact the data's validity or relevance.
6. *Data Dimensions*: Number of instances (samples) and features (variables) in the dataset.
7. *Data and File Types:* The data types included in the dataset and their formats (e.g., .csv, .png, .jpeg, etc.).
8. *Feature Description:* A brief description of each feature, including its data type (e.g., numerical, categorical), its scale (if applicable), and what it represents. These should also be described if the dataset includes target labels for supervised learning.
9. *Labeling and Annotation:* Detailed information about how the data was labeled or annotated, including who did the labeling/annotation, what guidelines or protocols were followed, and any quality checks or verification processes used. This should also cover the explanation of labels and how to interpret them.
10. *Standards and Vocabularies*: Any standards, taxonomies,
11. *Data Collection Process*: Information on how the data was gathered, processed, and cleaned. This should include any potential biases in the data collection process.
12. *Data Accessibility*: Details on how others can access the dataset if it is publicly available. If the dataset is private, provide reasons.
13. *Licenses or Restrictions:* Any legal or ethical considerations associated with using the dataset.
14. *Data Preprocessing:* Details on the steps to preprocess the data for machine learning. This can include data cleaning, normalization, feature extraction, and any other transformation applied to the dataset.
15. *Quality Control:* Information about quality control processes applied to the dataset.
16. *Known Issues or Limitations*: Any known issues, anomalies, or limitations in the data should be acknowledged.
17. *Relevant Publications*: If the dataset has been used in published research, reference these works.
18. *Contact Information*: Name, email, and/or other contact details for the person or team to contact with questions or issues related to the dataset.

References

1. Humby C. Data is the new oil. In: ANA Marketing Maestros. 2006. https://ana.blogs.com/maestros/2006/11/data_is_the_new.html. Accessed 28 Aug 2023.
2. O'Reilly T. Data is the new sand. In: The Information. 2021. https://www.theinformation.com/articles/data-is-the-new-sand. Accessed 28 Aug 2023.
3. Arsiwala-Scheppach LT, Chaurasia A, Müller A, Krois J, Schwendicke F. Machine learning in dentistry: a scoping review. J Clin Med Res. 2023;12(3):937. https://doi.org/10.3390/jcm12030937.
4. Adeoye J, Hui L, Su Y-X. Data-centric artificial intelligence in oncology: a systematic review assessing data quality in machine learning models for head and neck cancer. J Big Data. 2023;10:1–25.

5. Wynants L, Van Calster B, Bonten MMJ, et al. Prediction models for diagnosis and prognosis of covid-19 infection: systematic review and critical appraisal. BMJ. 2020;369:m1328.
6. Uribe SE, Sofi-Mahmudi A, Raittio E, Maldupa I, Vilne B. Dental research data availability and quality according to the FAIR principles. J Dent Res. 2022;101:1307–13.
7. Schwendicke F, Büttner M. Artificial intelligence: advances and pitfalls. Br Dent J. 2023;234:749–50.
8. Alemohammad S, Casco-Rodriguez J, Luzi L, Humayun AI, Babaei H, LeJeune D, Siahkoohi A, Baraniuk RG. Self-consuming generative models go MAD. arXiv [cs.LG]. 2023.
9. Schwendicke F, Samek W, Krois J. Artificial intelligence in dentistry: chances and challenges. J Dent Res. 2020;99:22034520915714.
10. Büttner M, Schneider L, Krasowski A, Krois J, Feldberg B, Schwendicke F. Impact of Noisy labels on dental deep learning-calculus detection on bitewing radiographs. J Clin Med Res. 2023;12(9):3058. https://doi.org/10.3390/jcm12093058.
11. Wilkinson MD, Dumontier M, Aalbersberg IJJ, et al. The FAIR guiding principles for scientific data management and stewardship. Sci Data. 2016;3:160018.
12. Celi LA, Cellini J, Charpignon M-L, et al. Sources of bias in artificial intelligence that perpetuate healthcare disparities-a global review. PLOS Digit Health. 2022;1:e0000022.
13. Krois J, Garcia Cantu A, Chaurasia A, Patil R, Chaudhari PK, Gaudin R, Gehrung S, Schwendicke F. Generalizability of deep learning models for dental image analysis. Sci Rep. 2021;11:6102.
14. Arias-Garzón D, Tabares-Soto R, Bernal-Salcedo J, Ruz GA. Biases associated with database structure for COVID-19 detection in X-ray images. Sci Rep. 2023;13:3477.
15. Rouzrokh P, Khosravi B, Faghani S, Moassefi M, Vera Garcia DV, Singh Y, Zhang K, Conte GM, Erickson BJ. Mitigating bias in radiology machine learning: 1. Data handling. Radiol Artif Intell. 2022;4:e210290.
16. Schneider L, Rischke R, Krois J, et al. Federated vs. local vs. central deep learning of tooth segmentation on panoramic radiographs. J Dent. 2023;135:104556.
17. Gichoya JW, Banerjee I, Bhimireddy AR, et al. AI recognition of patient race in medical imaging: a modelling study. Lancet Digit Health. 2022;4:e406–14.
18. Harrell FE Jr. Regression Modeling strategies: with applications to linear models, logistic and ordinal regression, and survival analysis. Springer International Publishing; 2015.
19. Gebru T, Morgenstern J, Vecchione B, Vaughan JW, Wallach H, Daumé H III, Crawford K. Datasheets for datasets. arXiv [cs.DB]. 2018.
20. Uribe SE, Chaurasia A, Schwendicke F, et al. Availability and specifications of dental images datasets for oral health artificial intelligence applications—study protocol. 2022. https://doi.org/10.17605/OSF.IO/MF897.

Artificial Intelligence: Limitations, Safety, and Regulatory Considerations in Dentistry

11

Rata Rokhshad, Maxime Ducret, Sara Seifi, Melika Mansouri, and Falk Schwendicke

11.1 Introduction

New technologies, especially artificial intelligence (AI), hold significant ethical implications. AI encompasses a wide range of capabilities to replicate human intelligence using algorithmic techniques, allowing vast datasets to be processed and cognitive functions to be performed. Machine learning (ML) and deep learning, which employ multilayer architectures to extract intricate features and patterns from complicated data [1], are at the core of most AI.

R. Rokhshad (✉)
Pediatric Dentistry Resident, Department of Pediatric Dentistry, Loma Linda School of Dentistry, Loma Linda, CA, USA

M. Ducret
Topic Group Dental Diagnostics and Digital Dentistry, ITU/WHO Focus Group AI on Health, Berlin, Germany

Faculty of Odontology, University Claude Bernard Lyon 1l, University of Lyon, Lyon, France

S. Seifi
Student Research Committee, Faculty of Dentistry, Mazandaran University of Medical Sciences, Sari, Iran

M. Mansouri
School of Dentistry, Shahid Beheshti University of Medical Sciences, Tehran, Iran

F. Schwendicke
Conservative Dentistry and Periodontology, LMU Klinikum, LMU Munich, Munich, Germany
e-mail: falk.schwendicke@med.uni-muenchen.de

Integrating AI into healthcare has become increasingly important, an especially prominent example of this dentistry, where AI integration is rising [2, 3]. There is a wide range of applications for AI in dentistry [4]. Dental radiographs and images are subject to AI analysis, yielding valuable and clinically pertinent insights. For instance, in orthodontics, AI aids in identifying landmarks, categorizing malocclusions, and forecasting growth trajectories. Within cariology, AI extends to diagnosing and classifying carious lesions [5]. AI has made notable strides in oral and maxillofacial surgery by enhancing surgical planning and identifying anomalies like jaw osteonecrosis, facial defects, or lesions [2]. Ethics holds a crucial position in all these different applications [6].

Despite recent publications indicating a promising future for AI in dentistry, this revolutionary technical field raises various ethical issues [7]. Ethics is the area of philosophy that examines human behavior to determine its morality, correctness, and potential harm [8]. A simple definition of ethics is the pursuit of what is considered right and good. Normative ethics, meta-ethics, and applied ethics are three categories of ethics [9]. Normative ethics has three aspects: (1) how to act appropriately (good rules, emphasizing adherence to ethical principles, regardless of the outcomes), (2) virtue ethics (good individuals, centering on cultivating moral excellence in individuals and emphasizing the development of vir-

F. Schwendicke et al. (eds.), *Artificial Intelligence for Oral Health Care*,
https://doi.org/10.1007/978-3-031-84047-0_11

tuous qualities to guide ethical behavior), and (3) consequentialism (good results, assessing the morality of actions based on the consequences they produce, prioritizing choices that lead to favorable outcomes or minimize harm) [8, 9]. Meta-ethics examines the nature of right and wrong. Applied ethics defines the use of ethical principles and theories in real-life situations.

AI-based healthcare poses several ethical issues, such as patient privacy, the role of physicians versus machines in patient care, and the future of education required to address the inevitable changes in medicine [10]. To solve the ethical concerns of AI in healthcare, including dentistry, health AI ethics should encompass applied ethics approaches, normative ethics, and meta-ethics [8]. Ethical AI is needed to prevent public trust loss and unwanted outcomes [11].

11.2 Sources of Ethical Challenges

In healthcare, a range of ethical principles towards AI have been defined: transparency, protection of privacy (for both data and patients), nonmaleficence, beneficence, responsibility, diversity and equity, wellness, prudence, solidarity, sustainable development, respect for patient autonomy, and justice [12].

In healthcare, a range of ethical principles towards AI have been defined: transparency, protection of privacy (for both data and patients), nonmaleficence, beneficence, responsibility, diversity and equity, wellness, prudence, solidarity, sustainable development, respect for patient autonomy, and justice [12]. AI technologies should promote individual wellness and improve health (beneficence) and explore the relationship between AI and sustainable dentistry practices (sustainability). Unity and mutual support must be combined with equity and fairness for all (solidarity), and prudence is needed to manage the adaptability of dynamic AI solutions. These key ethical focus areas can and should be developed and applied in dentistry [7].

11.2.1 Data

The performance of AI algorithms is highly associated with data. AI needs significant amounts of high-quality data to be trained with, which contrasts with small and biased data faced by some current medical AI models [13]. In the field of dentistry, data is not as available and accessible as in other fields. Information related to the health of individuals is often locked within isolated, individualized, and limitedly interoperable frameworks [1]. Sampling used in the healthcare realm most of the time involves selection bias, either overly representing the sick (e.g., data gathered from hospitals), the healthy (e.g., data gathered from devices of individuals), or the wealthy (e.g., data people with the ability to afford the costs of dental care). AI trained and built on the mentioned data will be naturally biased [14].

Data processing, measurement, and validation of the outcomes are often insulant replicable in dental AI investigations [15]. In addition, it is often not obvious how datasets were chosen, curated, and preprocessed. Data are used most of the time to train and test the algorithms simultaneously, which leads to "data snooping bias" [16]. The impact of data is particularly relevant for the generalizability of dental AI [17]. Factors like ethnicity, age, or gender may impact tooth anatomy, the structural variation of facial bones, the relationship between dental and oral diseases, and multiple genetic and environmental risk factors such as smoking and diet, which will lead to differences in the clinical manifestations and, hence, the applicability of an AI to different populations [18–20]. Bias emerges not only from how data are gathered but also from the gender, geographical location, age, ethnicity, religion, and socioeconomic background of individuals sampled [21]. In addition, missing data due to nonresponse, data recording problems, or imbalanced dropout introduces bias [22] and performance depreciation [23, 24].

11.2.2 Models

Most AI, particularly when employing deep learning, is hard to explain and understand for humans, limiting the transparency and options for human oversight [25]. Explainability alludes to procedures that help to explain the AI model and foster interpretability, i.e., users (not mainly the developers) understanding the inherent logic of the AI [26]. Different approaches for explainable AI (XAI) include LIME (local interpretable model-agnostic explanations, a method that involves creating an interpretable model specific to each prediction), anchor (a technique that elucidates singular predictions through the identification of a decision rule that anchors the prediction), decision boundary (the distinction that separates different classes or outcomes), a prototype model (a simplified representation of data points from a specific class or category), and a composite method (combining the mentioned approaches for comprehensive interpretability) [27]. The quality, e.g., fairness and generalizability, of AI depends on training data, as outlined. The resulting model will hence reflect the diversity, heterogeneity, and distribution of that data.

11.2.3 Data Loss and Breaches

Similar to all drugs and dental devices, AI needs to be proven to be safe and effective before it can be used in humans [28]. Since AI is essentially a data-driven technology, the risks of data loss and breaches should be considered to protect informational privacy and prevent unauthorized access [29]. Patients should be informed of what personal information is used, for which purpose, and how long the data will be stored. It is also essential that practitioners should only collect data that is strictly necessary and delete or change them at the request of the patient [30].

Another major concern in AI is data leakage, i.e., the unofficial transmission of data [29]. This problem may result from inadequate data security and sanitization, outdated systems, or insufficient employee training.

11.2.4 Potential Loss of Accountability and Oversight

Oversight and audit functions are vital for ensuring AI is safe and used ethically. Through audits, stakeholders can identify and mitigate risks, uphold patient trust, and ensure the responsible deployment of AI technologies in healthcare. Post-deployment surveillance of AI systems is crucial to promptly identify and rectify any issues that arise during real-world use. This includes updating systems in line with new scientific evidence or changes in clinical practices. Auditing machine learning algorithms is crucial because moral (and legal) responsibility ultimately resides with humans. This raises issues when computers are tasked with decision-making that has ethical implications. In this respect, dentists will still have the final decision-making authority, while AI applications mainly serve as an aid to them [31, 32]. However, concerns arise regarding accountability in AI-driven decisions, particularly when they directly affect individuals. Determining who is responsible in such scenarios remains an open question, highlighting the need for clearer regulations in AI governance.

11.3 Overcoming Ethical Challenges in Dentistry

Ethical AI demands to adhere to the FAIR (findable, accessible, interoperable, reusable) principles where possible [33]. The healthcare workforce may need to be trained to command sufficient expertise when dealing with AI and associated data [34].

Various strategies have been employed to address ethical challenges associated with models. Explainable AI enables transparency and accountability and greatly impacts the ethical model. By providing human-understandable insights into its decision-making processes, explainable AI allows users and stakeholders to comprehend how and why certain conclusions or actions are taken by an AI. This level of understanding is essential for building trust in AI applications, especially in critical sectors where the AI's decisions can have significant impacts. Furthermore, explainability supports accountability by making it possible to audit and evaluate AI systems, ensuring they align with ethical standards, legal requirements, and social norms.

Furthermore, some of the concerns for ethical AI in dentistry are fairness, equity, and diversity. By ensuring equitable access to AI, oral health disparities can be reduced regardless of one's demographics. AI developed to avoid discrimination may increase equity and fairness. To achieve diversity, different populations (different nationalities, ages, and genders) must be adequately represented in a training (and test) dataset; diversity is closely related to generalizability which we discussed above. Combining these factors promotes bias mitigation, trust, and compliance with regulatory requirements [35]. Moreover, overfitting is a problem in machine learning which prohibits generalization of AI by learning the structure of data by heart [36]. To reduce the consequences of overfitting and increase generalizability and, hence, fairness, several approaches can be taken, like (1) early-stopping, in which training is stopped before the performance is overly optimized on the training data; (2) network reduction, reducing the complexity and size of a neural network while maintaining its performance by removing unnecessary components; and (3) dataset expansion which focuses on expanding the training dataset, among others [37].

Regarding using AI in daily dental clinics, assessing the potential impact of AI applications on solidarity is important, and ensuring that decision-makers are well-informed is a key step. Moreover, the debate on whether AI can lead to more sustainable dentistry is ongoing. AI could streamline care and reduce travel, yet it also demands significant resources for its development and deployment [35].

In dentistry, patient and clinician autonomy are core principles. The purpose, benefits, limitations, and risks of AI use must be clearly explained to patients to obtain informed consent. Before consenting to AI's involvement in their care, patients must understand the role of AI and have an opportunity to discuss concerns. As they possess contextual knowledge, empathy, and the capacity to make ethical judgments, clinicians must also maintain autonomy. AI should support clinicians rather than replace them [6].

11.4 Regulatory Considerations and Governance

Regulation of AI in healthcare builds on both broad and topic-specific frameworks. Broad regulation encompasses a wide-ranging collection of rules, guidelines, and policies that oversee AI creation, implementation, and operation across multiple sectors and fields. These general regulations are crafted to tackle universal ethical, legal, and safety issues without focusing on a particular use case or sector. Countries have varying regulatory strategies for stakeholder engagement and collaboration on AI use in healthcare. Businesses and research involved in AI development or deployment must adhere to relevant laws covering data protection, privacy, and intellectual property rights.

One of the guidelines for AI regulation in healthcare has been provided by the World Health Organization (WHO). It recommends considering governance management elements such as liability, data access, risk management, data protection, privacy, adoption of education for clinical practice, good practices, standards related to care, governance, interoperability, etc. It also emphasizes the importance of defining the scope of practice for AI model use, creating technical checklists, thorough documentation, and ensuring transparency [38].

The Europe Union adopted a risk-based approach for handling AI, mirroring a similar framework employed for medical products [39–41]. The US Food and Drug Agency (FDA) has played a significant role in guiding global regulatory conversations, setting a precedent with its regulations on new technologies, ranging from 3D-printed drugs to AI-powered medical devices. An article published in 2019 proposed a framework for evaluating AI software as medical devices, emphasizing transparency, safety, and efficacy as important criteria. In 2023, AI functions, training/test data, and tuning were added [42, 43]. In Asia, nations such as China and Japan are formulating regulations for AI in healthcare, focusing on data privacy and algorithm fairness. Likewise, in Africa, countries including South Africa and Kenya are advancing regulatory frameworks, focusing on informed consent and patient safety [44].

Although some countries have taken steps to regulate healthcare AI at the national level, global regulation remains patchy [39, 40, 45]. Current regulations do not consider one of AI's potential key attributes, learning during its use (dynamic AI) [46]. Establishing comprehensive oversight through auditing and monitoring poses a huge challenge worldwide [46]. In healthcare, AI regulation should involve technical aspects, patient outcomes, data security, transparency of decision-making, and ethical issues such as equity of access, bias, privacy, and patient-doctor relationships [47].

11.5 Conclusion

The use of AI in clinical practice requires adherence to certain ethical principles. There is a need for a robust framework that enforces transparency, privacy, harm prevention, diversity, patient benefits, responsibility, fairness, autonomy, and justice. To ensure that AI is ethically developed and integrated into healthcare, governance must be based on these core principles.

References

1. Schwendicke F, Samek W, Krois J. Artificial intelligence in dentistry: chances and challenges. J Dent Res. 2020;99:769–74. https://doi.org/10.1177/0022034520915714.
2. Rokhshad R, Keyhan SO, Yousefi P. Artificial intelligence applications and ethical challenges in oral and maxillo-facial cosmetic surgery: a narrative review. Maxillofac Plast Reconstr Surg. 2023;45:14. https://doi.org/10.1186/s40902-023-00382-w.
3. Mörch CM, Atsu S, Cai W, Li X, Madathil SA, Liu X, Mai V, Tamimi F, Dilhac MA, Ducret M. Artificial intelligence and ethics in dentistry: a scoping review. J Dent Res. 2021;100:1452–60. https://doi.org/10.1177/00220345211013808.
4. Mohammad-Rahimi H, Motamedian SR, Pirayesh Z, Haiat A, Zahedrozegar S, Mahmoudinia E, Rohban MH, Krois J, Lee J, Schwendicke F. Deep learning in periodontology and oral implantology: a scoping review. J Periodontal Res. 2022;57:942–51. https://doi.org/10.1111/jre.13037.
5. Mohammad-Rahimi H, Motamedian SR, Rohban MH, Krois J, Uribe SE, Mahmoudinia E, Rokhshad R, Nadimi M, Schwendicke F. Deep learning for caries detection: a systematic review. J Dent. 2022;122:104115. https://doi.org/10.1016/j.jdent.2022.104115.
6. Ducret M, Mörch C-M. Focus on artificial intelligence ethics in dentistry. J Dent Sci. 2023;18(3):1409–10. https://doi.org/10.1016/j.jds.2022.12.003.
7. Rokhshad R, Ducret M, Chaurasia A, Karteva T, Radenkovic M, Roganovic J, Hamdan M, Mohammad-Rahimi H, Krois J, Lahoud P, Schwendicke F. Ethical considerations on artificial intelligence in dentistry: a framework and checklist. J Dent. 2023;135:104593. https://doi.org/10.1016/j.jdent.2023.104593.
8. Katznelson G, Gerke S. The need for health AI ethics in medical school education. Adv Health Sci Educ. 2021;26:1447–58. https://doi.org/10.1007/s10459-021-10040-3.
9. Chambers DW. A primer on dental ethics: part I. Knowing about ethics. J Am Coll Dent. 2006;73:38–46.
10. Rigby MJ. Ethical dimensions of using artificial intelligence in health care. AMA J Ethics. 2019;21:E121–4. https://doi.org/10.1001/amajethics.2019.121.
11. Morley J, Floridi L, Kinsey L, Elhalal A. From what to how: an initial review of publicly available AI ethics tools, methods and research to translate principles into practices. Sci Eng Ethics. 2020;26:2141–68. https://doi.org/10.1007/s11948-019-00165-5.
12. Jobin A, Ienca M, Vayena E. The global landscape of AI ethics guidelines. Nat Mach Intell. 2019;1:389–99. https://doi.org/10.1038/s42256-019-0088-2.
13. Xiong Z, Cheng Z, Lin X, Xu C, Liu X, Wang D, Luo X, Zhang Y, Jiang H, Qiao N, Zheng M. Facing small and biased data dilemma in drug discovery with enhanced federated learning approaches. Sci China Life Sci. 2022;65:529–39. https://doi.org/10.1007/s11427-021-1946-0.
14. Gianfrancesco MA, Tamang S, Yazdany J, Schmajuk G. Potential biases in machine learning algorithms using electronic health record data. JAMA Intern Med. 2018;178:1544–7. https://doi.org/10.1001/jamainternmed.2018.3763.
15. Schwendicke F, Golla T, Dreher M, Krois J. Convolutional neural networks for dental image diagnostics: a scoping review. J Dent. 2019;91:103226. https://doi.org/10.1016/j.jdent.2019.103226.
16. England JR, Cheng PM. Artificial intelligence for medical image analysis: a guide for authors and reviewers. Am J Roentgenol. 2019;212:513–9. https://doi.org/10.2214/AJR.18.20490.

17. Grewal DS, Khangura RK, Sircar K, Tyagi KK, Kaur G, David S. Morphometric analysis of odontometric parameters for gender determination. J Clin Diagn Res. 2017;11(8):ZC09–13. https://doi.org/10.7860/JCDR/2017/26680.10341.
18. Lee JJ, Ramirez SG, Will MJ. Gender and racial variations in cephalometric analysis. Otolaryngol Head Neck Surg. 1997;117:326–9. https://doi.org/10.1016/S0194-5998(97)70121-9.
19. Parikh RB, Teeple S, Navathe AS. Addressing bias in artificial intelligence in health care. JAMA. 2019;322:2377. https://doi.org/10.1001/jama.2019.18058.
20. Toledo Avelar LE, Cardoso MA, Santos Bordoni L, de Miranda Avelar L, de Miranda Avelar JV. Aging and sexual differences of the human skull. Plast Reconstr Surg Glob Open. 2017;5:e1297. https://doi.org/10.1097/GOX.0000000000001297.
21. Pang C, Humphris G. The relationship between fears of cancer recurrence and patient gender: a systematic review and meta-analysis. Front Psychol. 2021;12:640866. https://doi.org/10.3389/fpsyg.2021.640866.
22. Emmanuel T, Maupong T, Mpoeleng D, Semong T, Mphago B, Tabona O. A survey on missing data in machine learning. J Big Data. 2021;8:140. https://doi.org/10.1186/s40537-021-00516-9.
23. Ayilara OF, Zhang L, Sajobi TT, Sawatzky R, Bohm E, Lix LM. Impact of missing data on bias and precision when estimating change in patient-reported outcomes from a clinical registry. Health Qual Life Outcomes. 2019;17:106. https://doi.org/10.1186/s12955-019-1181-2.
24. Pawlicki M, Choraś M, Kozik R, Hołubowicz W. Missing and incomplete data handling in cybersecurity applications. In: Intelligent information and database systems. Cham: Springer; 2021. p. 413–26. https://doi.org/10.1007/978-3-030-73280-6_33.
25. Papadimitroulas P, Brocki L, Christopher Chung N, Marchadour W, Vermet F, Gaubert L, Eleftheriadis V, Plachouris D, Visvikis D, Kagadis GC, Hatt M. Artificial intelligence: deep learning in oncological radiomics and challenges of interpretability and data harmonization. Phys Med. 2021;83:108–21. https://doi.org/10.1016/j.ejmp.2021.03.009.
26. Fuhrman JD, Gorre N, Hu Q, Li H, El Naqa I, Giger ML. A review of explainable and interpretable AI with applications in COVID-19 imaging. Med Phys. 2022;49:1–14. https://doi.org/10.1002/mp.15359.
27. Das A, Rad P. Opportunities and challenges in explainable artificial intelligence (XAI): a survey. 2020.
28. Benrimoh D, Israel S, Fratila R, Armstrong C, Perlman K, Rosenfeld A, Kapelner A. Editorial: ML and AI safety, effectiveness and explainability in healthcare. Front Big Data. 2021;4:727856. https://doi.org/10.3389/fdata.2021.727856.
29. Murdoch B. Privacy and artificial intelligence: challenges for protecting health information in a new era. BMC Med Ethics. 2021;22:122. https://doi.org/10.1186/s12910-021-00687-3.
30. Safdar NM, Banja JD, Meltzer CC. Ethical considerations in artificial intelligence. Eur J Radiol. 2020;122:108768. https://doi.org/10.1016/j.ejrad.2019.108768.
31. Sounderajah V, McCradden MD, Liu X, Rose S, Ashrafian H, Collins GS, Anderson J, Bossuyt PM, Moher D, Darzi A. Ethics methods are required as part of reporting guidelines for artificial intelligence in healthcare. Nat Mach Intell. 2022;4:316–7. https://doi.org/10.1038/s42256-022-00479-3.
32. Braun M, Hummel P, Beck S, Dabrock P. Primer on an ethics of AI-based decision support systems in the clinic. J Med Ethics. 2021;47:e3. https://doi.org/10.1136/medethics-2019-105860.
33. Marda V. Artificial intelligence policy in India: a framework for engaging the limits of data-driven decision-making. Philos Trans R Soc A Math Phys Eng Sci. 2018;376:20180087. https://doi.org/10.1098/rsta.2018.0087.
34. Choudhury A, Asan O. Role of artificial intelligence in patient safety outcomes: systematic literature review. JMIR Med Inform. 2020;8:e18599. https://doi.org/10.2196/18599.
35. Ducret M, Mörch C-M, Karteva T, Fisher J, Schwendicke F. Artificial intelligence for sustainable oral healthcare. J Dent. 2022;127:104344. https://doi.org/10.1016/j.jdent.2022.104344.
36. Ying X. An overview of overfitting and its solutions. J Phys Conf Ser. 2019;1168:022022. https://doi.org/10.1088/1742-6596/1168/2/022022.
37. DeCamp M, Lindvall C. Latent bias and the implementation of artificial intelligence in medicine. J Am Med Inform Assoc. 2020;27:2020–3. https://doi.org/10.1093/jamia/ocaa094.
38. World Health Organization. Regulatory considerations on artificial intelligence for health. Geneva: World Health Organization; 2023. https://iris.who.int/handle/10665/373421.
39. McKee M, Wouters OJ. The Challenges of Regulating Artificial Intelligence in Healthcare Comment on "Clinical decision support and new regulatory frameworks for medical devices: are we ready for it? A viewpoint paper". Int J Health Policy Manag. 2023;12:7261. https://doi.org/10.34172/ijhpm.2022.7261.
40. Kudina O. Regulating AI in health care: the challenges of informed user engagement. Hastings Cent Rep. 2021;51:6–7. https://doi.org/10.1002/hast.1263.
41. Kieslich K, Keller B, Starke C. Artificial intelligence ethics by design. Evaluating public perception on the importance of ethical design principles of artificial intelligence. Big Data Soc. 2022;9:205395172210929. https://doi.org/10.1177/20539517221092956.
42. Muehlematter UJ, Daniore P, Vokinger KN. Approval of artificial intelligence and machine learning-based medical devices in the USA and Europe (2015–20): a comparative analysis, lancet digit. Health. 2021;3:e195–203. https://doi.org/10.1016/S2589-7500(20)30292-2.

43. Jaremko JL, Azar M, Bromwich R, Lum A, Alicia Cheong LH, Gibert M, Laviolette F, Gray B, Reinhold C, Cicero M, Chong J, Shaw J, Rybicki FJ, Hurrell C, Lee E, Tang A. Canadian Association of Radiologists White Paper on ethical and legal issues related to artificial intelligence in radiology. Can Assoc Radiol J. 2019;70:107–18. https://doi.org/10.1016/j.carj.2019.03.001.
44. Reddy S. Navigating the AI revolution: the case for precise regulation in health care. J Med Internet Res. 2023;25:e49989. https://doi.org/10.2196/49989.
45. Meszaros J, Minari J, Huys I. The future regulation of artificial intelligence systems in healthcare services and medical research in the European Union. Front Genet. 2022;13:927721. https://doi.org/10.3389/fgene.2022.927721.
46. Ayad N, Schwendicke F, Krois J, van den Bosch S, Bergé S, Bohner L, Hanisch M, Vinayahalingam S. Patients' perspectives on the use of artificial intelligence in dentistry: a regional survey. Head Face Med. 2023;19:23. https://doi.org/10.1186/s13005-023-00368-z.
47. Roganović J, Radenković M, Miličić B. Responsible use of artificial intelligence in dentistry: survey on dentists' and final-year undergraduates' perspectives. Healthcare. 2023;11:1480. https://doi.org/10.3390/healthcare11101480.

Artificial Intelligence in Dental Education: Opportunities, Challenges, and Implementation

12

Sergio E. Uribe, Falk Schwendicke, and Carlos González-Cabezas

12.1 Introduction

12.1.1 Overview of Artificial Intelligence (AI) in Education

Artificial Intelligence (AI) is increasingly integrated into education and has the potential to change how students learn and educators teach. AI includes a range of technologies, from machine learning to generative AI models, such as ChatGPT, Gemini, Mistral, or Anthropic, that can analyze data, recognize patterns, and generate content. In education, these tools offer opportunities for personalized learning, where AI can tailor content to individual student's needs and provide targeted feedback based on their progress. This ability to adjust can enhance the learning experience, making it more interactive and personalized. Additionally, AI can support educators by automating routine administrative tasks, facilitating the creation of teaching materials, and offering new ways to engage students through virtual tutors and simulations. However, the use of AI in education must address challenges such as data privacy, algorithmic bias, and the risk of reduced human interaction, all of which require careful oversight. As the role of AI in education continues to grow, it has the potential to support more effective and inclusive learning, but it also requires a balanced approach to implementation.

12.1.2 Relevance of AI to Dental Education

AI has significant potential for transforming dental education by focusing on theoretical learning and hands-on training. Generative AI models like ChatGPT allow students to practice diagnostic scenarios, helping to refine their clinical decision-making in a safe, virtual environment. Additionally, AI assists in research by summarizing relevant literature and identifying emerging trends in the field of dentistry. Despite these benefits, challenges such as maintaining academic integrity and ensuring the ethical use of AI remain critical. Proper implementation of IA in education requires educators and students to be digitally literate to understand how AI works, its benefits, and its limitations. Table 12.1 details

S. E. Uribe (✉)
Department of Conservative Dentistry and Oral Health, Riga Stradins University, Latvia/Conservative Dentistry and Periodontology, LMU Klinikum, LMU Munich, Munich, Germany
e-mail: sergio.uribe@rsu.lv

F. Schwendicke
Conservative Dentistry and Periodontology, LMU Klinikum, LMU Munich, Munich, Germany
e-mail: falk.schwendicke@med.uni-muenchen.de

C. González-Cabezas
Department of Cariology, Restorative Sciences and Endodontics, School of Dentistry, University of Michigan, Ann Arbor, MI, USA
e-mail: carlosgc@umich.edu

F. Schwendicke et al. (eds.), *Artificial Intelligence for Oral Health Care*,
https://doi.org/10.1007/978-3-031-84047-0_12

Table 12.1 Potential applications and key considerations of artificial intelligence in dental education

Aspect	Description	Examples
Enhanced diagnostic training	AI aids in teaching diagnostic skills by analyzing radiographic images, recognizing patterns, and identifying oral pathologies	AI tools that assist in interpreting radiographs, detecting caries, and assessing bone levels
Simulation of clinical scenarios	Generative AI models can simulate patient interactions, enabling students to practice diagnosis and treatment planning in a safe environment	AI-powered virtual patients and chatbots like ChatGPT for role-playing clinical scenarios
Personalized learning	AI provides tailored educational content based on individual progress and understanding, helping students grasp complex subjects	Adaptive learning platforms that adjust quizzes and reading materials according to the student's pace
Support for research	AI aids in summarizing research articles and analyzing data, enabling students to engage with current evidence and trends in dentistry	AI-based literature review tools that extract key insights from large datasets of dental research
Enhanced assessment methods	AI offers new ways to assess student progress, providing data-driven feedback and ensuring consistency in grading	AI tools that evaluate case studies provide personalized feedback on written assignments or analyze practical skills
Administrative support for educators	AI supports administrative tasks such as grading, managing student notes, and filling out forms, freeing up time for direct interaction with students	AI-powered grading software, automated note-taking systems, and digital forms processing tools
Ethical considerations	Integrating AI requires attention to data privacy, academic integrity, and potential biases in AI models	Guidelines for the ethical use of AI in student assessments and ensuring transparency in AI-generated content

how AI can support various educational activities, including analyzing complex clinical data, simulating patient interactions, and customizing learning paths for individual students.

12.2 Understanding AI and Generative AI in Education

Artificial Intelligence (AI) refers to machines simulating human intelligence tasks. **Traditional AI** models are designed to perform specific tasks, such as detecting tooth decay in dental radiographs. To build such a model, developers must collect a large dataset of radiographs, which human annotators then label with the presence or absence of caries (*labeled data*). The algorithm is trained using this data through *supervised learning*, where the model is tested and refined with new radiographs until it achieves the desired performance. This approach is narrow in scope, focusing on a single task, such as caries detection.

Generative AI, on the other hand, does not rely on labeled data for a single, specific task. Instead, it is trained on vast amounts of *unlabeled data*, such as entire pathology textbooks, using complex neural networks. The model learns patterns from the data and can then apply this knowledge to different tasks. Through a process known as *reinforcement learning with human feedback* (RLHF), developers test the model, rewarding correct responses and fine-tuning it when it makes mistakes. Unlike traditional AI, generative AI models like ChatGPT are not limited to one task or pathology—they can generate responses on a wide range of topics. Moreover, because these models are pre-trained (the "P" in ChatGPT), they can produce output tailored to specific audiences, whether a detailed explanation for a dentist, simplified for a patient, or even a creative response like a poem when prompted. The differences are detailed in Table 12.2.

Table 12.2 Traditional AI with generative AI comparison

Aspect	Traditional AI	Generative AI
Task focus	Designed for a single, specific task (e.g., detecting caries)	Capable of performing multiple tasks across various domains
Training data	Requires large amounts of labeled data (e.g., radiographs)	Trained on vast amounts of unlabeled data (e.g., textbooks)
Learning process	Supervised learning: Human-labeled data guides the learning	Unsupervised learning, mostly reinforcement learning with human feedback (RLHF)
Scope	Narrow: Focused on solving a specific problem	Broad; can adapt to various tasks and domains
Data requirements	Requires human annotation (labeled data)	Can work with unlabeled data
Performance tuning	Adjusted for a single task based on testing and tuning	Tuned through feedback across multiple domains
Output flexibility	Limited to one function or outcome (e.g., detecting disease)	Can generate diverse outputs in different formats and styles (e.g., technical or creative)
Personalization	Outputs, such as caries yes/no or tooth number, are standardized	Outputs can be tailored to different audiences (e.g., dentist, patient, etc.)
Examples	Caries detection in radiographs, tooth classification, implant detection, bone segmentation	ChatGPT, generating educational content diagnosing various pathologies

12.3 Current Applications of AI in Dental Education

The dental literature increasingly reports applications of AI in dental education. Some examples of integrating AI into dental education include providing personalized feedback and generating automated case scenarios, creating more engaging learning environments. While AI enhances education through customized content and knowledge acquisition chatbots, challenges such as bias, inaccuracy, and privacy concerns remain. Some institutions have deployed internal versions of generative AI models to prevent misuse and share sensitive data, ensuring a safe AI environment while allowing students and academics to comply with regulations. Table 12.3 provides some examples of AI applications in dental education, with advantages and issues.

Table 12.3 AI integration in dental education: current practices

Example AI in dental education and source	Advantages	Issues
Personalized feedback, generating case scenarios, and creating educational content [1]	Improves the quality of education through personalized and engaging learning experiences	Bias, inaccuracies, privacy concerns, overreliance
AI chatbots for knowledge acquisition, research, and clinical decision-making [2]	Enhances knowledge acquisition, supports research, and aids clinical decision-making	Reduces human interaction, lack of clear guidelines
AI-assisted radiograph mounting [3]	Faster radiograph mounting	Decreased accuracy in mounting by students
Use of AI in orthodontic education [4]	Improves learning experiences with interactive tools	Concerns about potential misinformation
AI-based large language models (LLMs) in periodontal education [5]	High accuracy in answering exam questions supports clinical learning	Risk of misinformation, difficulty with image-based questions
AI in oral hygiene education through synchronous and asynchronous monitoring [6]	Personalized feedback for oral hygiene, potential for non-invasive monitoring	Lack of high-quality studies, privacy concerns
AI in endodontic education [7]	Supports personalized feedback, advanced simulation training	Potential challenges with real-time guidance and data processing
AI chatbots for reflective assignments in dental education [8]	Enables differentiation between AI-generated and student-generated content	Risk of academic misconduct, overreliance on AI
AI for radiograph interpretation in dental education [9]	Supports teaching of diagnostic skills and case assessment	Challenges in integrating with existing teaching methods
AI for essay grading in dental education [10]	Provides detailed feedback, supports formative assessment	Challenges in matching human grading accuracy

12.4 How to Use Generative AI in Dental Education

Where traditional AI is limited to the tasks for which the model was developed, generative AI offers a board of alternative uses and customized content. To use generative AI effectively, educators need to understand the concept of prompting. Prompting refers to how users communicate with AI models by providing specific instructions or queries that guide the AI to produce the desired output. For example, educators can prompt AI systems like ChatGPT to create case studies, simulate patient scenarios, or provide explanations tailored to different learning levels. Educators can tailor AI responses to their teaching goals by creating clear and detailed prompts, whether generating explanations for complex dental procedures or creating engaging, scenario-based learning activities for students. Educators can refine AI output through iterative prompting to ensure accuracy and alignment with educational goals. This approach increases the efficiency and personalization of the dental education learning experience.

12.4.1 Enhancing AI Interaction: The Role of Prompting Techniques in Generative AI

Prompting refers to instructing a generative AI model, like ChatGPT, to perform a task by providing a clear, detailed input or question. The quality and specificity of a prompt can significantly impact the AI's response. In dental education, prompting can be tailored to simulate clinical scenarios, develop quiz questions, or generate personalized feedback. Effective prompting involves asking specific, step-by-step questions and guiding the AI to focus on relevant educational content, enhancing student learning experiences, and supporting instructors in curriculum design.

For a dental educator, instead of simply asking, "Explain the amelogenesis process," an effective prompt should provide context, define the role the AI should assume, specify the task, and outline the desired output. This approach ensures that the AI generates more targeted and useful responses. The previous prompt can be improved by expanding it like this:

1. **Context**: This refers to the background or scenario that frames the interaction. Providing clear context helps the AI understand the topic or situation, leading to more relevant and accurate responses. In this case, the context could involve preparing educational content for dental students.

   Example Context Prompt: "You are helping a dental professor to prepare a 35-min lecture on the process of amelogenesis for first-year dental students."
2. **Role**: This element defines the role the AI should take. Assigning a role helps the AI tailor its response to the required perspective—whether it is a dental expert, a patient, or an educator. For this scenario, the role could be that of a knowledgeable dental educator.

   Example Role Prompt: "You are an assistant professor with expertise in dental biology, explaining the stages of amelogenesis in a way that is easy for first-year dental students to understand."
3. **Task**: The task specifies what the user wants the AI to accomplish. In this case, it could involve explaining the stages of amelogenesis in a structured manner suitable for a classroom setting. A well-defined task ensures that the AI delivers focused content.

   Example Task Prompt: "Your task is to create an outline for a 35-min class, explaining the stages of amelogenesis, including key processes like enamel matrix formation and mineralization."
4. **Output**: The output defines the format of the response. In this case, the output should be an educational outline that matches the class's needs and is suitable for a 35-min lecture.

   Example Output Prompt: "Generate a detailed teaching outline, including major topics, subtopics, and key points, for a 35-min lecture on amelogenesis. Start by providing the first section, and I will give feedback before proceeding."

These strategies can be combined with more advanced prompting techniques for even more specific tasks, enhancing the effectiveness of AI in dental education. Table 12.4 provides more prompting techniques.

Table 12.4 Prompting strategies for dental educators

Prompting technique	Bad prompting	Good prompting
Context	"Tell me about periodontal diseases"	"You must explain the steps for diagnosing periodontal disease to a first-year dental student"
Role	"Help me understand periodontal diseases"	"You are a dental educator explaining the correct procedure for diagnosing and treating periodontal disease"
Task	"Explain periodontal disease"	"Explain the process of detecting and diagnosing periodontal disease, including its stages and treatment options"
Output	"Create a class about periodontal diseases"	"Provide a clear step-by-step explanation of how to assess and treat periodontal disease for dental students." or "provide three questions with four alternatives based on..."
Specificity	"Tell me how AI works in dentistry"	"Explain how AI can assist in diagnosing periodontal issues by analyzing patient gum and bone health for third-year dental students"
Clarity	"What are dental diseases?"	"Describe the key differences between gingivitis and periodontitis for third-year dental students..."
Audience targeting	"Explain periodontal disease"	"As a dental expert, explain periodontal disease in a way that a first-year dental student can easily understand"

(continued)

Table 12.4 (continued)

Prompting technique	Bad prompting	Good prompting
Format of output	"What is periodontics?"	"Write a list of common periodontal diseases and treatment methods for dental students with a brief explanation"
Depth of response	"Give me a summary of periodontal treatment"	"Provide a detailed comparison of the pros and cons of different periodontal treatments for students"
Follow-up clarity	"What about AI in dentistry?"	"How can AI enhance diagnostic accuracy in periodontal procedures, and its limitations?"

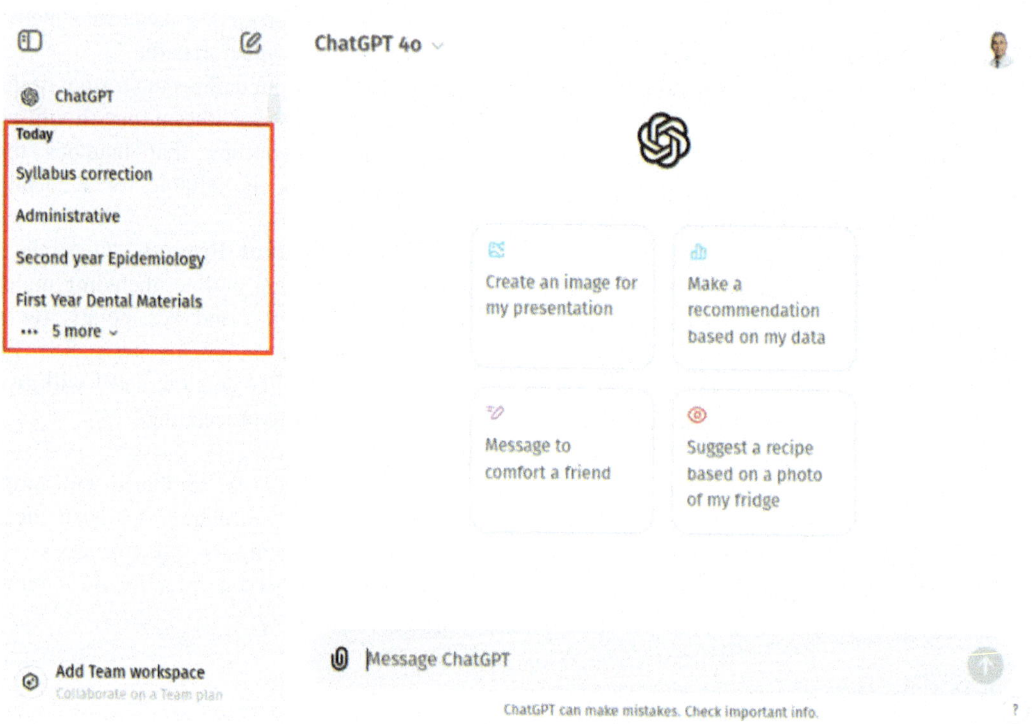

Fig. 12.1 Example of different chats properly named. Screenshot taken from ChatGPT, powered by OpenAI. This screenshot is included for informational purposes and is intended to help illustrate the features and functionality of the ChatGPT interface

12.4.2 Practical Tips for Dental Educators Using Generative AI

In addition to refining dental educators' prompting skills, here are five practical tips for using generative AI effectively in dental education:

1. **Organize and Clean Your Conversations**

   When using AI to generate content or assist with course planning, renaming and organizing your chats can streamline your workflow. Each conversation serves as a fresh context window, so starting a new chat for different tasks—developing lectures or generating case studies—helps maintain relevance and focus. As projects evolve, keeping distinct conversations for different tasks ensures clarity. Archiving or deleting chats you no longer need reduces clutter, makes finding and revisiting relevant threads easier, and keeps AI interactions efficient and organized for ongoing educational activities, as seen in Fig. 12.1.

2. **Set Custom Instructions for Tailored Responses**

   Utilize custom instructions to refine the AI's responses. By specifying your role as a dental educator and outlining what topics or teaching methods you prioritize, the AI can adapt its outputs to your needs, whether you are preparing lectures or designing assignments. This personalized approach helps generate more targeted content. In Fig. 12.2, a customized ChatGPT to answer the administrative questions about the syllabus is shown.

3. **Choose the Right AI Model for the Task**

   Different tasks in dental education may require varying levels of AI sophistication. If using a version of AI with multiple models, choose one that aligns with your goals. For example, advanced models can be used for in-depth diagnostic simulations or research-based assignments, while simpler models work well for routine administrative tasks or quiz generation. Some examples of different models available in popular GenAI chatbots are shown in Fig. 12.3.

4. **Explore Custom GPTs for Specialized Tasks**

   The GPT store offers pre-built models that can be highly useful for dental educators. These models can help automate specific tasks, such as designing visual materials or managing research data, saving time, and enhancing efficiency. Custom GPTs can also

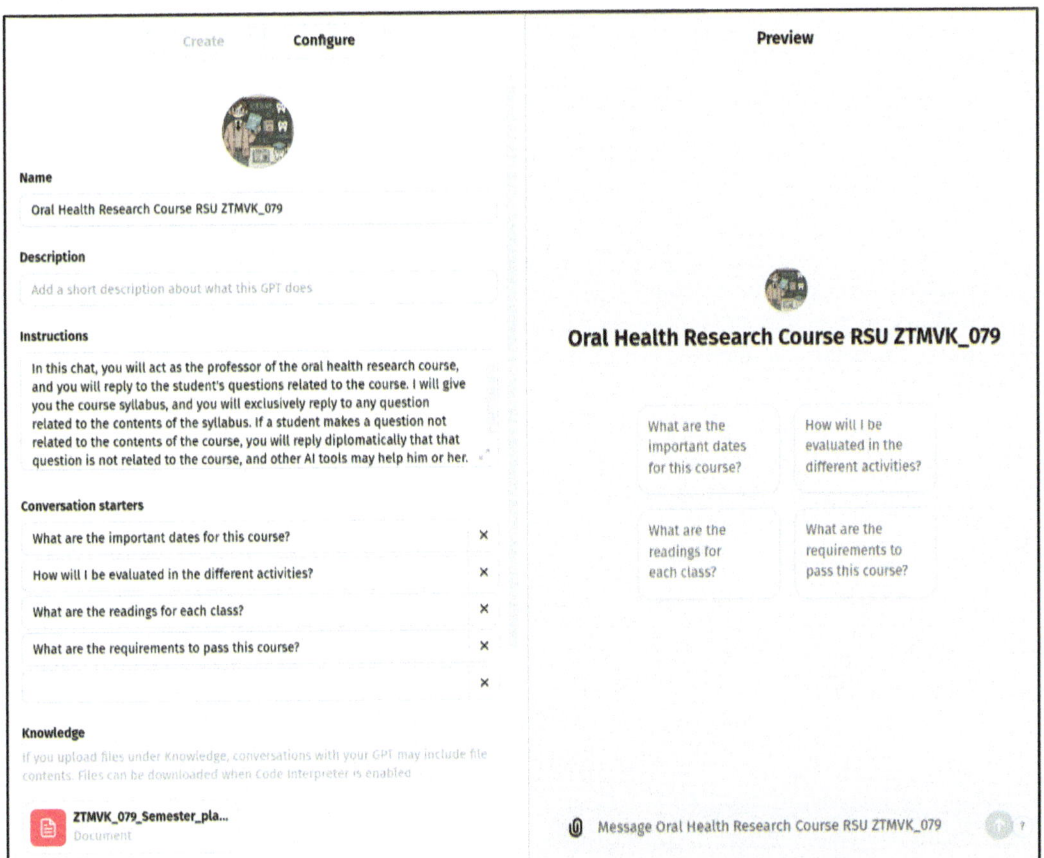

Fig. 12.2 A customized ChatGPT to answer administrative questions about a specific course. Here, the model was fed with the course syllabus, and the prompt limited the answers to the document's content. Screenshot taken from ChatGPT, powered by OpenAI. This screenshot is included for informational purposes and is intended to help illustrate the features and functionality of the ChatGPT interface

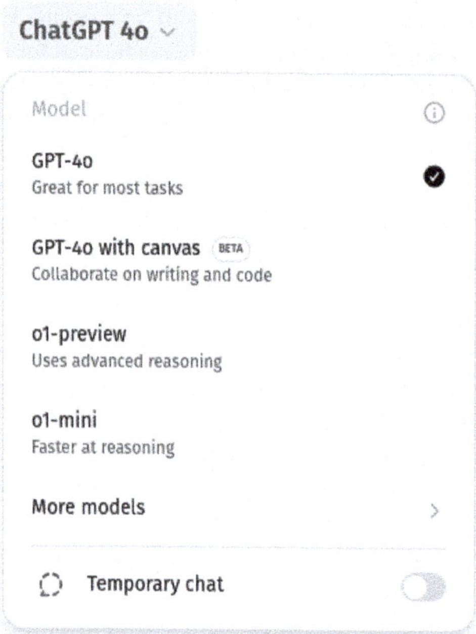

Fig. 12.3 Examples of different models available in ChatGPT. Screenshot taken from ChatGPT, powered by OpenAI. This screenshot is included for informational purposes and is intended to help illustrate the features and functionality of the ChatGPT interface

be created to fit specific teaching needs or workflows. Figure 12.4 shows an example of customized chats available in OpenAI ChatGPT.

12.4.3 Enhancing the Accuracy of Generative AI Outputs with Retrieval-Augmented Generation (RAG) in Dental Education

Retrieval-Augmented Generation (RAG) is a method that integrates the retrieval of specific information from documents with the generative capabilities of AI models to provide more accurate and contextually relevant answers. Rather than relying solely on the AI model's general training data, RAG pulls relevant content from a specific source, such as a research paper or syllabus, to guide its responses. This ensures that the model's output is grounded in the content provided, reducing the risk of misinformation. Figure 12.2 shows an example of a customized chat where the answers are limited to the document's content, in this case the syllabus of a dental course.

In dental education, RAG can significantly improve the accuracy of AI-generated responses by feeding the model-specific documents, such as research papers or course syllabi, and restricting its responses to that content. For example, if a course syllabus is provided, students can interact with it directly, asking administrative questions or clarifications about the course. This targeted use of AI ensures relevance and accuracy, minimizing misinformation. In addition, students can

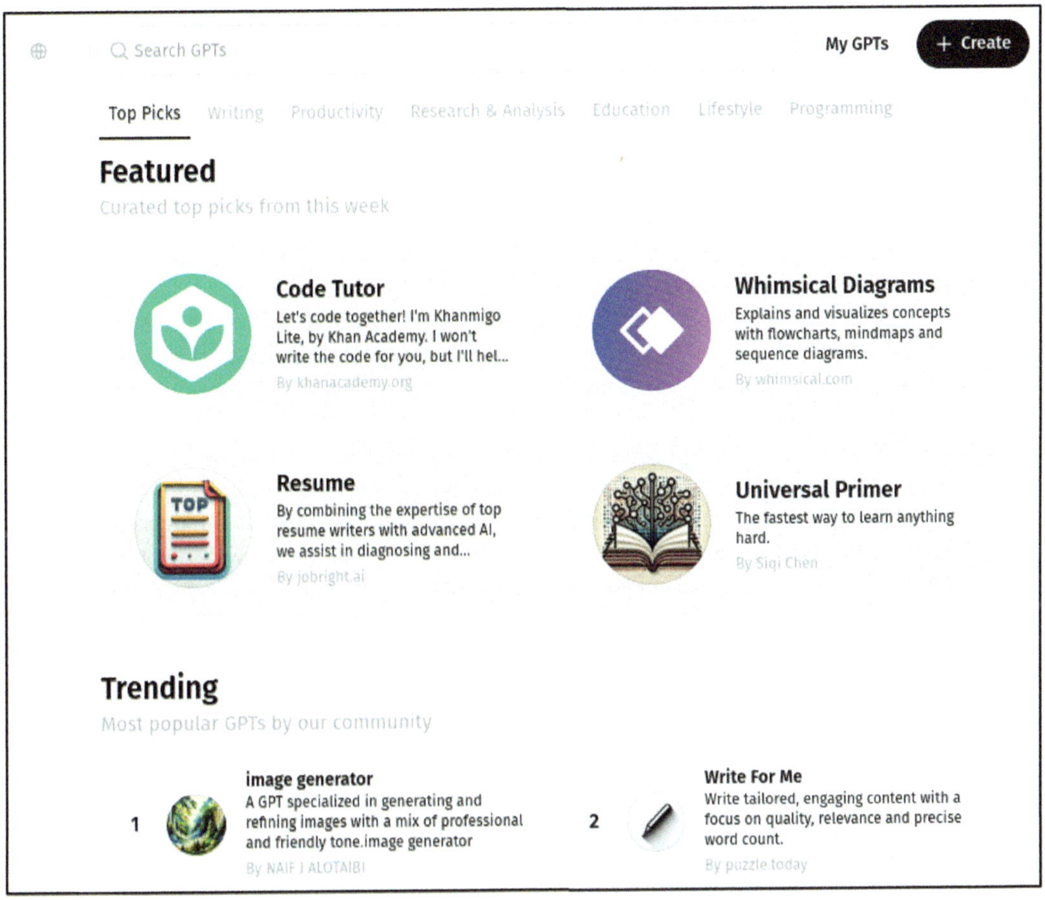

Fig. 12.4 Examples of customized chats available in OpenAI ChatGPT. Screenshot taken from ChatGPT, powered by OpenAI. This screenshot is included for informational purposes and is intended to help illustrate the features and functionality of the ChatGPT interface

use RAG to break down complex material by requesting summaries or explanations of technical concepts from detailed documents, helping to tailor learning to their needs while maintaining information accuracy.

12.5 Challenges and Risks in AI Integration

A global survey of dental educators revealed several challenges and concerns related to integrating Artificial Intelligence (AI) tools, such as chatbots and large language models, in dental education. Although 64% of respondents recognized the potential of AI to enhance knowledge acquisition, research, and clinical decision-making, they also highlighted significant issues. Among these were concerns about AI reducing human interaction, the absence of clear guidelines, and the need for proper training before widespread implementation [2].

12.5.1 Ethical Considerations: Data Privacy, Academic Integrity, and Bias

Integrating AI tools into dental education presents several challenges and risks, particularly concerning data privacy, academic integrity, and bias. One of the key issues is the potential for **bias**, which can manifest when AI systems produce results that unfairly favor certain groups over others or reinforce existing stereotypes. This is especially relevant in education, where biased AI outputs could affect the fairness of assessments or the content generated for students. For instance, if an AI model is trained predominantly on data from a specific demographic or region, it may not represent the diversity found in global dental education.

Data privacy is another critical concern, as AI systems often require vast access to personal information. This raises questions about how student data is stored, shared, and protected. Furthermore, the reliance on AI-generated content for academic purposes, if not properly monitored, can blur the lines of academic integrity, leading to potential misuse, such as presenting AI-generated work as original student output. Also, there is an additional risk that students may inadvertently or deliberately share patient information with commercial companies when prompting AI for diagnosis or treatment planning.

Educators and institutions must address these ethical challenges by fostering critical thinking in students, ensuring transparency in the use of AI, and promoting equitable practices that protect the integrity of education and the rights of students with clear policies on the use of AI that explicitly state what is allowed and what is not.

12.5.2 The Risk of Overreliance on AI and Reduction in Human Interaction

As AI tools like chatbots and large-scale language models become more integrated into dental education, dental educators must be cautious about the potential for overreliance on these technologies. While AI can facilitate grading, content generation, and even answering student questions, it is important to balance technological assistance and human interaction.

Excessive reliance on AI could diminish students' critical thinking skills and reduce the opportunity for meaningful faculty-student engagement. Dental educators should emphasize the role of AI as a supplemental tool, not a replacement for direct interaction and mentorship, to ensure that students continue to develop essential clinical reasoning, communication skills, and ethical judgment. Encouraging students to evaluate AI-generated information critically can also promote a more thoughtful and balanced use of technology in education.

12.5.3 AI's Limitations in Assessing Clinical Skills and Hands-on Training

While AI provides valuable support in theoretical learning, it still faces limitations in assessing clinical skills and hands-on training in dental education. Clinical practice involves complex, real-time decision-making, manual dexterity, and patient interaction, where AI cannot fully replicate human evaluation. However, the future holds promising developments—AI systems integrated into devices such as smart glasses could provide real-time visual aids for dental students, similar to the heads-up displays used by pilots. These AI-enhanced systems could assist in guiding clinical procedures, offering real-time feedback on techniques and diagnostics. Still, human oversight would remain critical to ensure proper judgment and contextual understanding in clinical settings.

12.5.4 Concerns Around AI-Generated Content: Accuracy and Trustworthiness

One of the main concerns when using AI in dental education is the accuracy and trustworthiness of AI-generated content. While AI models like ChatGPT can generate vast amounts of information quickly, there is a significant risk that this content may contain inaccuracies or be outdated, especially in fields like dentistry, where precision is critical. *As a general rule, consider that AI models always present their answers with confidence and are sometimes accurate.* This challenge makes it essential for educators to thoroughly review and fact-check

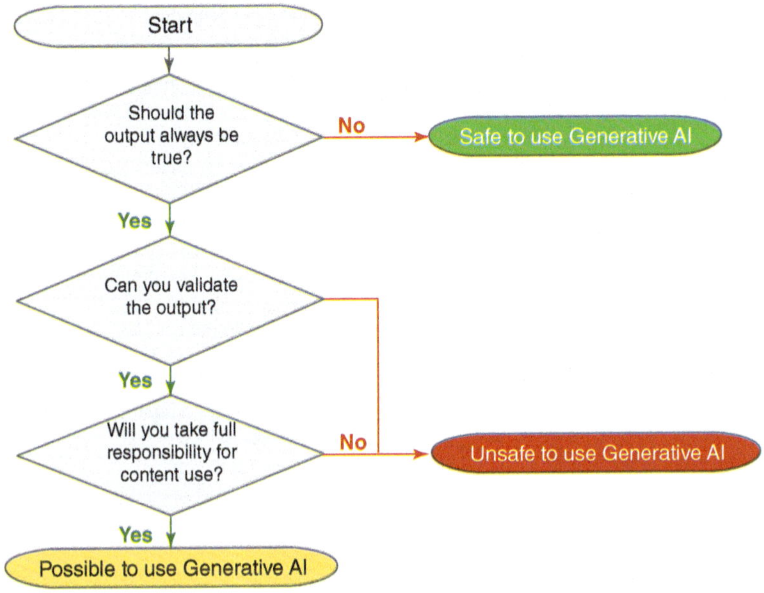

Fig. 12.5 Decision flowchart for the safe use of generative AI in dental education. (Modified image from A. Tiulkanov, licensed under CC BY 4.0)

AI-generated material before using it for educational purposes or sharing it with students. Furthermore, trustworthiness becomes a greater issue when students rely on AI for learning without proper guidance, as AI may inadvertently provide incorrect, biased, or misleading information.

A specific example of this issue is what is known as "hallucinations" in AI. These hallucinations occur when AI generates entirely fabricated or inaccurate content despite appearing plausible and coherent. In dental education, hallucinations can be especially problematic, as they might provide false information on clinical procedures, diagnoses, or treatment plans, potentially leading to confusion or misinformation.

AI-generated content should be used as a supplemental tool, with human oversight and regular verification, to ensure that students receive reliable, accurate information. A key theoretical skill for dental students is the ability to evaluate health information critically, distinguish an opinion, unverified or misleading sources from a fact or validated evidence-based information, ensuring they make informed decisions in their education and clinical practice. This skill is essential in an era where AI will become increasingly embedded in the fabric of society.

12.6 Deciding When to Use Generative AI in Dental Education

When integrating generative AI, such as ChatGPT, into dental education, it is essential to determine whether the generated content is suitable and safe for educational purposes. Figure 12.5 presents a flowchart to help educators assess whether AI-generated outputs can be safely used, emphasizing the need for expert verification and responsibility in content management. Depending on the context and available expertise, generative AI may support learning or pose risks if not properly validated.

Table 12.5 Elements of AI education curriculum for dental students

Element	Description
Basic definitions and terms	Introduce the fundamental terminology of AI, machine learning, and deep learning. Explain the basic concepts such as algorithms, explainability, training models, and external testing
Principles of AI and machine learning	Explain the underlying principles behind AI systems, including how data is used to train AI models and the role of algorithms in learning from data
AI applications in dentistry	Provide real-world examples of AI in clinical settings, such as radiograph interpretation, treatment planning, and diagnostic support systems
Evaluation of AI systems	Teach students to assess AI systems' accuracy, reliability, and applicability in dental care and real-world impact. How to read articles about AI in dental journals: See Dental AI for critical appraisal of AI dental literature [19] and DentalCOMS for technical metrics [20]
Ethics and governance	Discuss the ethical issues surrounding AI use, such as data privacy, informed consent, and the potential biases in AI systems. Address the importance of transparency and accountability in AI tools
Impact on clinical decision-making	Discuss the impact of AI deployment in healthcare, economic analysis, and impact on patients and society
AI and patient care	Highlight the integration of AI in patient care, diagnostic accuracy, and supporting personalized treatment plans
Hands-on AI training	Provide students with opportunities to engage with AI tools through practical exercises, allowing them to experience AI in diagnostics and clinical workflows
Ethical and legal implications	Encourage students to think critically about the ethical and legal frameworks governing AI in healthcare, including patient data management and algorithmic accountability
Future directions and emerging AI technologies	Discuss emerging AI technologies and the future potential of AI in transforming dental education and practice

Modified from Schwendicke et al. [21]

12.7 Guidelines and Recommendations for Implementing AI in Dental Curricula

12.7.1 AI Literacy and Its Importance in Healthcare

Artificial Intelligence (AI) is increasingly integrated into many facets of our daily lives. Whether it is letting our car find a parking space or letting an airline app choose our seats, we use AI without fully understanding how it works. Even in entertainment, algorithms select the next song in our playlists or determine which post appears next in our social media feeds. In all these cases, AI's decisions directly affect us as individuals. In healthcare, however, the implications are far more significant. As healthcare professionals, our AI-driven decisions affect patients' lives—individuals who trust our judgment.

In healthcare, clinicians must often explain diagnostic or treatment decisions to patients. When these decisions are AI-based, understanding and explaining how the AI works becomes critical. Patients may ask why a particular treatment plan or prognosis has been recommended. In scenarios where two clinicians might have different opinions, AI-assisted diagnoses present the challenge of explaining how the model arrived at its decision—which is not always easy due to the complexity of the AI systems used.

A paradox arises: the more complex and powerful the AI model, the more useful it can be because it considers numerous variables. However, this complexity often reduces the model's explanatory power. Clinicians can fall victim to **automation bias**—the tendency to over-rely on AI simply because it seems authoritative. This overreliance on automation led to incorrect diagnoses and potentially harmful treatments. Incorrect automated electrocardiogram diagnoses reduced accuracy by 43.2% for cardiologists and 58.95% for non-cardiologists [11]. In radiography, inexperienced radiologists were more prone to errors when relying on AI-based systems [12]. In mammography, AI improved accuracy for less skilled readers but reduced it for more skilled ones, creating disparities [13]. Treatment decisions were also affected: faulty clinical support systems in e-prescribing increased false prescriptions by 56.9% [14].

Additionally, real-world failures after AI deployment highlight the importance of understanding its limitations. Google's AI system for detecting diabetic retinopathy performed poorly in field trials due to suboptimal conditions, such as poor lighting and low-resolution images [15]. Similarly, IBM Watson for Healthcare failed to accurately diagnose rare cancers because it was trained on a biased and limited dataset [16]. These examples highlight the dangers of blindly relying on AI in critical medical contexts.

Automation bias is not the only risk. If AI systems are trained on biased datasets, they can perpetuate those biases, leading to distorted treatment recommendations. For example, a healthcare prediction algorithm used in the USA was found to be biased against black patients, more often recommending white patients for high-risk treatment programs [17]. Such biases in AI systems can exacerbate health inequalities if clinicians are unaware of how these biases influence decisions.

To use AI responsibly in dentistry, professionals must be educated about how these systems work, their limitations, and their risks. This knowledge will enable clinicians to question AI-generated outputs, cross-check results, and provide transparent and accurate explanations to patients. Interestingly, individuals with low levels of AI knowledge may be more algorithm-averse initially but then fall into automation bias as their knowledge increases to a moderate level. However, as AI knowledge reaches higher levels, users become more cautious and less prone to automation bias [18]. This indicates that advanced AI literacy can help users avoid the pitfalls of overreliance on AI. Such knowledge helps ensure that AI remains a tool for improving care rather than compromising it.

12.7.2 Core AI Curriculum for Dental Students: Key Concepts and Skills

Integrating AI in dental education and practice requires a basic understanding of how these systems operate so students and practitioners can appreciate their advantages, limitations, and risks. Just as using X-rays in dentistry requires a basic grasp of physics without demanding expertise in particle physics, understanding AI does not require mastery of computer science but an essential knowledge of its core principles. Each institution should evaluate its capabilities and needs to determine which areas of AI warrant new content and whether this should be delivered as a standalone course or integrated into existing curricula.

The curriculum must adapt as more AI-driven technologies are adopted—some even replacing clinical tasks. We have witnessed this evolution before when many duties once handled by dentists transitioned to dental laboratories or when digital scanners replaced traditional impression materials. A similar shift has occurred in other fields, like aviation, where even though algorithms manage much of a plane's operations, pilots today need more extensive training than ever before. As AI continues to transform dental education and practice, institutions must anticipate and prepare for these changes, ensuring students are equipped with the skills needed for the future.

These concepts align with the recommendations outlined in the Sect. 12.7.2, which identifies key areas for integration (Table 12.5).

12.8 AI in Dental Education: Key Considerations for Institutional Implementation

As seen during the COVID pandemic, technology implementation issues can arise without careful planning [22], making proactive rather than reactive integration of AI into dental curricula essential. This will require the involvement of all stakeholders: faculty, students, staff, and administration. Institutions must create environments that maximize AI's benefits while addressing the challenges and risks associated with its use [23].

Table 12.6 presents a proposed set of institutional guidelines based on current guidelines from higher education institutions, drawing from industry best practices and recent research. These guidelines focus on promoting the responsible use of AI to enhance learning experiences while ensuring data privacy for students and patients. By following this framework, institutions can implement AI in a way that supports educational goals and maintains ethical standards.

Also, the institutions will face a change in the evaluation process. With the rise of generative AI, the traditional dental education assessment modes may shift significantly [2]. Since AI can easily generate written content, such as essays and reports, we may see a decline in using these formats for evaluation. Instead, oral examinations and interactive assessments,

Table 12.6 Key institutional recommendations for AI implementation in dental schools

Item	Actionable point	Detail
Clear AI policies	Develop and implement clear policies and guidelines for using generative AI in education	These policies should ensure ethical and responsible usage while being flexible enough to encourage creativity. Policies can be customized at the course level, allowing faculty to define AI usage according to specific learning objectives
		These policies should be easily accessible, preferably in PDF and scrollable HTML, with all relevant information on one page
AI literacy	Offer AI literacy courses	Preferable at university level. This would benefit a wider range of students and ensure that foundational AI knowledge is taught consistently across disciplines
	Incorporate AI modules within dental courses	For more specialized applications, dental-specific AI modules can be integrated into the dental curriculum, focusing on the practical applications of AI in dentistry, such as diagnostic support, clinical decision-making, and ethics in dental AI usage
	Continue staff education on AI	Ongoing professional development for faculty and staff should include AI literacy to ensure they can critically evaluate AI technologies, stay informed about new AI developments, and integrate AI effectively into their teaching practices
AI infrastructure investment	Invest in infrastructure and resources to support integrating AI technologies in dental education	This investment will ensure that students and staff can access the tools and platforms to utilize AI effectively and safely in their educational practices
AI multidisciplinary committee	Create a multidisciplinary advisory group to guide AI integration	The group should serve as an advisory body, offering guidance on AI integration to support educational goals, encourage innovation, and address ethical concerns without restricting creativity instead of overseeing and "policing" AI usage
Regular AI policy review	Regularly review and update AI policies to keep pace with technological advancements and regulatory changes	This review will ensure the institution's AI policies remain relevant and effective

From Uribe et al. [24]

where students must demonstrate their critical thinking and problem-solving abilities in real time, may become more prominent. For PhD students, the focus of evaluation could also evolve. Rather than emphasizing the importance of the final thesis, emphasis may shift toward the research process. This includes effective research data management, teamwork skills, adherence to open science principles, reproducibility of experiments, and the generation of valuable datasets or code. These shifts would encourage a more comprehensive view of student competencies, valuing transparency and rigor over final outputs alone.

12.9 The Ultimate Aim: Enhancing Patient Care Through AI Integration in Dental Education

As with any technology in healthcare, the primary objective of integrating AI into dental education is to improve patient outcomes. While AI offers numerous benefits for educators and students—personalized learning and efficient resource management—its true value lies in its potential to enhance clinical decision-making and patient care, reduce the prevalence and severity of oral diseases, and increase dental care coverage. Educators ensure that these technologies deliver higher-quality, evidence-based care by equipping future dental professionals with the knowledge and skills to use AI responsibly and effectively.

As students become proficient in using AI tools, from diagnostic support to patient simulations, they will be better prepared to translate these skills into their practice, improving the accuracy of diagnoses, enhancing treatment planning, and ensuring a higher standard of patient care. This focus on patient outcomes should guide AI's thoughtful and ethical integration into dental curricula, ensuring that technology enhances patients' health and well-being.

Appendix: Common Questions About Generative AI in Dental Education

1. **How does generative AI work?** Generative AI uses a form of generative AI based on language models. It generates text based on patterns learned from vast amounts of data. While useful, it is important to remind students that the model may not always provide accurate information, and its output should be critically evaluated.
2. **Can generative AI help with lesson planning and assessment?** Yes, generative AI can assist dental educators in creating lesson plans, quizzes, and even providing feedback. However, human oversight is necessary to ensure accuracy and educational appropriateness. Educators can prompt generative AI to generate tailored lesson content or evaluate student understanding.
3. **Is generative AI reliable for academic honesty?** While generative AI is a powerful tool for learning, educators should be cautious when students use it for assignments. Current generative AI detection tools are unreliable, as they can fail like any detection device. Digital watermarks for AI-generated content may help in the future, but these could be bypassed. Relying on AI-generated work without proper critical engagement still poses a significant risk to academic integrity.
4. **How can AI support critical thinking?** AI tools like generative AI can encourage critical thinking by generating scenarios, explanations, or counterarguments. Educators can instruct students to analyze AI-generated content to identify biases, inconsistencies, or gaps in reasoning, thereby reinforcing critical thinking skills.
5. **What are the biases and limitations of generative AI?** Generative AI can sometimes reflect biases in its training data, and it might generate inaccurate or incomplete information. Dental educators should guide students

on recognizing these biases and cross-checking information with reliable sources. This is particularly important in dental education, where accuracy is critical for clinical practice.

6. **What is the most efficient way of prompting generative AI models?** The most effective way to prompt generative AI models is to provide clear **context**, ask the model to personify a specific **role**, specify the exact **task**, and indicate the desired **outcome** or give an **example** of a correct output. **Tuning** the prompt based on the initial response can further refine the result. Also, to increase the accuracy of the answer and reduce the risk of hallucinations, the model can be fed with a specific document (e.g., course syllabus or research paper) and instructed to **limit** its answers to the document's content. This ensures the AI's output remains grounded in reliable, accurate information.

References

1. Claman D, Sezgin E. Artificial intelligence in dental education: opportunities and challenges of large language models and multimodal foundation models. JMIR Med Educ. 2024;10:e52346.
2. Uribe SE, Maldupa I, Kavadella A, El Tantawi M, Chaurasia A, Fontana M, Marino R, Innes N, Schwendicke F. Artificial intelligence chatbots and large language models in dental education: worldwide survey of educators. Eur J Dent Educ. 2024;28(4):865–76. https://doi.org/10.1111/eje.13009.
3. Chang J, Bliss L, Angelov N, Glick A. Artificial intelligence-assisted full-mouth radiograph mounting in dental education. J Dent Educ. 2024;88(7):933–9. https://doi.org/10.1002/jdd.13524.
4. Delgado-Ruiz R, Kim AS, Zhang H, Sullivan D, Awan KH, Stathopoulou PG. Generative artificial intelligence (gen AI) in dental education: opportunities, cautions, and recommendations. J Dent Educ. 2024; https://doi.org/10.1002/jdd.13688.
5. Danesh A, Pazouki H, Danesh F, Danesh A, Vardar-Sengul S. Artificial intelligence in dental education: ChatGPT's performance on the periodontic in-service examination. J Periodontol. 2024;95:682–7.
6. Tay JRH, Ng E, Chow DY, Sim CPC. The use of artificial intelligence to aid in oral hygiene education: a scoping review. J Dent. 2023;135:104564.
7. Aminoshariae A, Nosrat A, Nagendrababu V, Dianat O, Mohammad-Rahimi H, O'Keefe AW, Setzer FC. Artificial intelligence in endodontic education. J Endod. 2024;50:562–78.
8. Brondani M, Alves C, Ribeiro C, Braga MM, Garcia RCM, Ardenghi T, Pattanaporn K. Artificial intelligence, ChatGPT, and dental education: implications for reflective assignments and qualitative research. J Dent Educ. 2024;88(12):1671–80. https://doi.org/10.1002/jdd.13663.
9. Schropp L, Sørensen APS, Devlin H, Matzen LH. Use of artificial intelligence software in dental education: a study on assisted proximal caries assessment in bitewing radiographs. Eur J Dent Educ. 2024;28(2):490–6. https://doi.org/10.1111/eje.12973.
10. Shamim MS, Zaidi SJA, Rehman A. The revival of essay-type questions in medical education: harnessing artificial intelligence and machine learning. J Coll Physicians Surg Pak. 2024;34:595–9.
11. Bond RR, Novotny T, Andrsova I, Koc L, Sisakova M, Finlay D, Guldenring D, McLaughlin J, Peace A, McGilligan V, Leslie SJ, Wang H, Malik M. Automation bias in medicine: the influence of automated diagnoses on interpreter accuracy and uncertainty when reading electrocardiograms. J Electrocardiol. 2018;51:S6–S11.
12. Dratsch T, Chen X, Rezazade Mehrizi M, Kloeckner R, Mähringer-Kunz A, Püsken M, Baeßler B, Sauer S, Maintz D, Pinto Dos Santos D. Automation bias in mammography: the impact of artificial intelligence BI-RADS suggestions on reader performance. Radiology. 2023;307:e222176.
13. Povyakalo AA, Alberdi E, Strigini L, Ayton P. How to discriminate between computer-aided and computer-hindered decisions: a case study in mammography. Med Decis Mak. 2013;33:98–107.
14. Lyell D, Magrabi F, Raban MZ, Pont LG, Baysari MT, Day RO, Coiera E. Automation bias in electronic prescribing. BMC Med Inform Decis Mak. 2017;17:28.
15. Beede E, Baylor E, Hersch F, Iurchenko A, Wilcox L, Ruamviboonsuk P, Vardoulakis LM. A human-centered evaluation of a deep learning system deployed in clinics for the detection of diabetic retinopathy. In: Proceedings of the 2020 CHI conference on human factors in computing systems. New York: ACM; 2020. https://doi.org/10.1145/3313831.3376718.
16. Strickland E. How IBM Watson overpromised and underdelivered on AI health care [WWW document]. IEEE Spectrum. 2019. https://spectrum.ieee.org/how-ibm-watson-overpromised-and-underdelivered-on-ai-health-care. Accessed 23 Oct 2024.
17. Obermeyer Z, Powers B, Vogeli C, Mullainathan S. Dissecting racial bias in an algorithm used to manage the health of populations. Science. 2019;366:447–53.
18. Horowitz MC, Kahn L. Bending the automation bias curve: a study of human and AI-based decision making in national security contexts. arXiv [cs.CY]. 2023; https://doi.org/10.48550/arXiv.2306.16507.

19. Schwendicke F, Singh T, Lee J-H, Gaudin R, Chaurasia A, Wiegand T, Uribe S, Krois J, IADR e-oral health network and the ITU WHO focus group AI for Health. Artificial intelligence in dental research: checklist for authors, reviewers, readers. J Dent. 2021;107:103610.
20. Büttner M, Rokhshad R, Brinz J, Issa J, Chaurasia A, Uribe SE, Karteva T, Chala S, Tichy A, Schwendicke F. Core outcomes measures in dental computer vision studies (DentalCOMS). J Dent. 2024;150:105318.
21. Schwendicke F, Chaurasia A, Wiegand T, Uribe SE, Fontana M, Akota I, Tryfonos O, Krois J, IADR e-Oral Health Network and the ITU/WHO Focus Group AI for Health. Artificial intelligence for oral and dental healthcare: core education curriculum. J Dent. 2023;128:104363.
22. Turnbull D, Chugh R, Luck J. Transitioning to E-learning during the COVID-19 pandemic: how have higher education institutions responded to the challenge? Educ Inf Technol. 2021;26:6401–19.
23. Miao, Fengchun, UNESCO, Holmes, Wayne. Guidance for generative AI in education and research [WWW Document]. 2024. https://www.unesco.org/en/articles/guidance-generative-ai-education-and-research. Accessed 11 Oct 2024.
24. Uribe SE, Maldupa I, Schwendicke F. Integrating generative AI into dental education: a scoping review of current practices and recommendations. Eur J Dent Educ. 2025; https://doi.org/10.1111/eje.13074.

Glossary of Key Terms

1.1 Glossary of Key AI Terms in Dentistry

AI term or concept	Definition for health professionals	Comparable statistical concept	Examples in dentistry
Adversarial attacks	Techniques to mislead an AI model by manipulating input data, producing incorrect outputs, and highlighting vulnerabilities	Manipulation of data	CCD's bad pixels can affect AI system accuracy in radiograph disease recognition
AI explainability	The degree to which humans can understand and interpret a machine learning model's behavior	Interpretation of statistical results	Employing explainable AI tools to interpret dental radiograph classifications, highlighting key features behind the detection of periodontal disease
Algorithm fairness	Ensuring AI models make unbiased decisions across different patient groups	Statistical bias/ confounding	Equal accuracy in caries detection for patients of various ethnic backgrounds
Alignment	Ensuring AI values align with human values		Aligning dental AI systems with ethical standards
Anomaly detection	Process of identifying rare or abnormal instances in a dataset, useful for unusual patterns in medical data indicating diseases	Outlier detection	Detecting unusual patterns in dental radiographs indicating diseases like oral cancer
Artificial general intelligence (AGI)	AI system with human-like flexibility and reasoning		An AGI in dentistry capable of diagnosing various conditions with different kinds of data (images, text, speech, lab test, etc.), generate new insights and answers questions in natural language
Artificial intelligence (AI)	A branch of computer science concerned with building smart machines that can perform tasks which typically require human intelligence	Statistical inference	AI systems used for automated detection and classification of oral pathologies
Bayesian classifier	Applies Bayes' rule to calculate probabilities for classification	Bayesian inference	Classifying oral lesions in radiographs

(continued)

F. Schwendicke et al. (eds.), *Artificial Intelligence for Oral Health Care*,
https://doi.org/10.1007/978-3-031-84047-0

AI term or concept	Definition for health professionals	Comparable statistical concept	Examples in dentistry
Bias	Unfairness or discrimination in AI outputs		AI trained on data from group A may miss detecting disease B in a different group, stressing the need for diverse training datasets
Classification	A ML technique categorizing a set of data (structured or unstructured) into classes based on certain attributes	Discriminant analysis	Sort dental radiographies based on criteria or classify panoramic radiographs as "no findings" or "requires human inspection"
Clinical decision support systems	AI systems assisting in making clinical decisions by providing evidence-based recommendations or predictions based on patient data	Decision support tools	A system offering treatment suggestions based on a patient's electronic dental records
Compute	Computational resources for training AI models		As graphic cards become more advanced, disease detection becomes increasingly accurate and faster
Contextual embeddings	Dynamic representations of words that change with context, providing richer semantic understanding	Context-dependent variable analysis	Using contextual embeddings in AI to enhance understanding of clinical notes in different dental cases
Data augmentation	Techniques diversifying training data by applying transformations like rotation, scaling, or cropping, improving model robustness and generalization	Data transformation	Augmenting patient records with additional clinical data to improve the precision of AI-based treatment recommendations
Data leakage	An error where information from the test (or external) data inadvertently influences the model during training, leading to overly optimistic performance estimates. This can occur due to preprocessing steps or other errors in the data handling process	Overfitting due to external data contamination	When developing an AI model to predict tdental caries on bitewing radiographs, if the model is tested on images it has already seen during training, it may mistakenly show higher accuracy, believing it is performing better than it actually would on new, unseen images
Data shift	Data distribution shift occurs when the model's training data differ from real-world data, potentially affecting its performance	Similar to non-stationarity in statistics, where properties of a variable change over time	For instance, an AI model trained on adult dental imaging data might not perform well when applied to children's dental images due to the significant difference (or "shift") in dental structure and development
Decision tree	Generates a tree-like model of decisions for classification	Decision analysis	Diagnosing oral diseases based on symptoms
Deep learning (DL)	DL is a subfield of ML in which algorithms learn from input data through examples (without supervision)	Neural networks	DL used for the detection of oral cancer lesions in CBCT imaging
Diffusion models	Models that learn by destroying and recovering data		Applying diffusion models to enhance dental image analysis
Emergence	Unanticipated behaviors and transparent workings		Exploring emergent features in dental AI for the detection of squamous cell carcinoma mandibular invasion patterns to elucidate survival discrepancies
Example	An instance paired with a label. An example includes the specific case (with its features) and the correct outcome		A set of radiographs for a patient (instance) and the correct diagnosis (label)

(continued)

AI term or concept	Definition for health professionals	Comparable statistical concept	Examples in dentistry
Extracted features	Features that are derived or transformed from the original data	Latent or transformed variables	A feature like the mean intensity of a lesion, derived from an oral CBCT, to detect oral cancer
F1 score	A statistical measure for binary classification accuracy, combining precision and recall using their weighted average	Harmonic mean of precision and recall	Measuring the accuracy of an AI model in oral pathology classification tasks. The higher the F!, the better the performance in a similar dataset
FAIR principles	guidelines for managing and storing data to make it Findable, Accessible, Interoperable, and Reusable, with the goal of facilitating data sharing and collaboration among researchers and organizations	Open science, data management	Implementing the FAIR principles in a dental research project by assigning persistent identifiers to datasets (findable), providing controlled access through authentication (accessible), using standardized data formats and metadata (interoperable), and releasing the data under a clear license for reuse by other researchers (reusable)
Feature	An attribute or characteristic of an instance that can help make predictions	Independent/ explanatory variable	For radiographs, features might include the shape and size of the lesion, bone loss around the lesion, etc.
Feature column	A specific category or group of related features		A feature column might include all features relating to bone loss in oral radiographs
Feature selection	The process of selecting those features which contribute most to the prediction variable	Variable selection	Selecting radionomic features, such as shape, size, and intensity of lesions, from a radiograph for oral cancer detection
Federated learning	A decentralized AI training approach where models train locally on devices, sharing only aggregated updates with a central server	Distributed data analysis	An AI algorithm can learn using data from different healthcare centers without patient data leaving each hospital's server, ensuring patients' privacy and security
Foundation Models	AIs with a wide range of skills across domains		A fine-tuned foundation model to provide accurate answers to questions posed by dental patients using natural language
Gaussian mixtures model	Learns multiple models to classify images into classes	Multivariate distributions	Classifying stages of oral cancer
Generative AI	AI capable of creating new data resembling its training input	Data simulation	Creating synthetic dental images or simulating oral health outcomes
Generative adversarial network (GAN)	A class of artificial intelligence algorithms that uses two neural networks, a generator and a discriminator, working in competition to create new, realistic data instances that resemble a given dataset	Data simulation	Using a GAN to create synthetic dental radiographs that closely resemble real ones, enabling the augmentation of limited datasets for improved AI model training in dental diagnosis
Hallucination	AI confidently providing false information		A LLM-Chatbot generates plausible responses using invented facts
Instance	The specific case for which a prediction is desired		A set of radiographs for a patient, from which we want to predict the presence of oral cancer

(continued)

AI term or concept	Definition for health professionals	Comparable statistical concept	Examples in dentistry
K-nearest neighbor	Classifies input based on similarity with training images	Instance-based learning	Image-based oral cancer detection
Label	The correct answer or outcome for a given instance in the context of a prediction task	Dependent variable	Based on histological examination results, the label could be "cancer" or "no cancer" for a given set of radiographs
Large language models (LLMs)	Advanced AI systems generating human-like language		LLMs powering dental AI chatbots or virtual assistants
Language model prompting	Designing inputs that guide the model to generate specific outputs improves performance on tasks like answering questions without additional training	Input shaping	Using prompts to generate specific dental advice or responses in virtual dental consultations
Linear discriminant analysis	Combines features of training images for prediction	Linear discriminant	Detection of specific oral diseases
Machine learning (ML)	Machines can "learn" information and patterns directly from data without being programmed explicitly	Statistical modeling	ML algorithms applied in predicting oral disease progression based on historical patient data
Metric	A quantifiable measure used to assess the performance of the model		A metric for a model predicting oral cancer could be its accuracy, i.e., how often the model correctly predicts cancer
Model	A computational tool trained on data to make predictions or decisions without being explicitly programmed to perform the task		A model in dentistry might be trained to predict the risk of periodontal disease based on patient's oral hygiene habits, smoking status, and genetic predisposition
Model autophagy disorder (MAD)	This issue arises from repeatedly training AI models on their own generated data, leading to a negative feedback loop that degrades the model's quality and diversity. The model may lose information about the true data distribution, producing less realistic outputs	Overfitting	MAD could potentially occur in AI models used for dental imaging analysis. Here, the model is repeatedly trained on its own generated images, causing a loss of information about the true distribution of dental anatomy and pathology. This may lead to incorrect or missed diagnoses
Model optimization	The process of adjusting a model to improve its ability to predict the label	Model fitting	Tuning a machine learning model to predict the onset better of periodontal disease based on patient data
Multimodal AI	AI systems that integrate and process multiple types of data (e.g., images, text, biosignals) to improve decision-making accuracy and robustness		An AI system that evaluates dental health by analyzing radiographs, patient genetic data, clinical data and also dentist-patient interaction to integrate all the information for a potential diagnosis
Neural network	Learns image representation via gradient descent-based learning	Nonlinear regression	Automated detection and diagnosis in dentistry
Neural network (NN)	A highly structured set of algorithms that models the brain's neural network system (deep learning) designed to recognize patterns from input data	Regression or classification models	Artificial neural networks used in oral cancer prognosis prediction

(continued)

AI term or concept	Definition for health professionals	Comparable statistical concept	Examples in dentistry
Overfitting	A modeling error where an AI system learns the training data too closely, including its noise and outliers, resulting in poor performance on new, unseen data. The model becomes excessively complex and cannot generalize to new data	Overreliance on training data, leading to low bias but high variance	Suppose an AI system is trained to detect caries lesions from dental radiographs and is overly adapted to the peculiarities of a particular set of images (like specific lighting conditions, patient or specific equipment). In that case, it might perform exceptionally on that set but fail to detect cavities effectively in radiographs taken under different conditions or with different equipment
Patch extraction	Deconstruction of an image into smaller pixelated patches known as "sub-images"		Processing whole slides images in oral pathology for further AI analysis
Pipeline	The entire process of a machine learning task from start to end, including data collection, model training, and model deployment		The pipeline in a dental setting might involve collecting patient data, training a model to predict oral cancer, and then deploying that model in a dental clinic to assist in early detection
Pre-training	Training a model on a large dataset in a self-supervised manner before fine-tuning it on a specific task	Initial model training	Training an AI system on general dental images before fine-tuning for oral cancer detection
Precision	The proportion of correct positive predictions	Positive predictive value	In an oral cancer prediction model, precision is the proportion of positive predictions that are truly cancerous
Random forest	Uses a set of decision trees for classification	Ensemble methods	Disease detection in oral radiology
Recall	The ability of a model to identify positive instances correctly	Sensitivity	In an oral cancer prediction model, recall would be the proportion of true positive predictions among all actual positive cases
Reinforcement learning	ML is where an agent learns by interacting with an environment and receiving rewards or penalties based on its actions	Learning with reinforcement	An AI system learning to select the best dental treatment based on reward feedback
Reinforcement learning with human feedback (RLHF)	The model learns from human feedback after making decisions in an environment, similar to teaching a dog a new trick and rewarding correct behavior	Like iterative learning in statistical models, this method continuously improves the AI in dentistry based on received feedback	The AI assists with treatment planning, providing suggestions that improve over time based on dentist feedback on plan quality
Self-supervised learning	A machine learning technique where the model generates its own labels from the data, learning to predict parts of the data from other parts	Feature extraction without explicit labels	Training an AI to recognize patterns in unlabeled dental radiographic images
Semantic segmentation	The process of dividing an image into regions of interest and clustering data into distinct groups based on similarities	Cluster analysis	Segmentation of dental radiographs to identify regions of interest, like restorations, endo, caries, or bone loss

(continued)

AI term or concept	Definition for health professionals	Comparable statistical concept	Examples in dentistry
Semi-supervised learning	Model training on a mix of labeled and unlabeled data, leveraging both to improve performance	Partially supervised learning	Training a dental diagnosis AI on a mix of labeled (diagnosed cases) and unlabeled (undocumented) dental images
Synthetic data	Artificial data generated programmatically, often using machine learning or other artificial intelligence techniques	Simulated data	Generating synthetic dental radiographs using a Generative Adversarial Network (GAN) to augment a limited dataset of real dental radiographs for training an AI model in dental diagnosis. This allows the model to learn from a more diverse set of examples without compromising patient privacy or relying solely on available real-world data
Sugeno fuzzy	An inference system handles uncertainty in data by applying fuzzy (if-then) rules	Uncertainty analysis	Risk assessment in oral health
Supervised fine-tuning (SFT)	This is a process in which a pre-trained machine learning model is refined or "fine-tuned" using a labeled dataset, supervised by a human. It helps the model to perform better on specific tasks	Fine-tune a statistical model	An example might be fine-tuning an AI model previously trained on general oral images to detect specific oral diseases more accurately
Supervised learning	Training of ML algorithms from labelled (e.g., annotations) input and output data	Regression Analysis	Training ML models to classify dental radiographs based on labeled examples
Support vector model (SVM)	A ML algorithm that efficiently separates classes in training images for classification	Plane partitioning	Binary classification in dentistry
Synthetic data generation	Creating artificial data that resembles real data, used to enhance AI model training when real data is sensitive or limited	Simulated data	Generating synthetic dental images for AI training when real patient data is scarce
Target	The specific goal or target that the machine learning model seeks to optimize		In a model predicting oral cancer, the target could be to maximize the sensitivity of cancer detection, even at the risk of producing more false positives
Tensor	A mathematical structure that can represent complex multidimensional data	Higher-Order Matrix or Vector	Tensors could represent 3D dental scans in a deep-learning model for oral cancer detection
Training or learning	The process by which a model learns the relationship between features and the label in a dataset	Model Estimation	Training a model on historical patient data to predict oral cancer
Transfer learning	Leveraging knowledge from one task/domain to improve learning and performance on a different but related task/domain	Learning across domains	Using learnings from general image recognition AI to improve the performance of dental imaging AI
Transformer models	Advanced neural networks that use self-attention mechanisms to handle data sequences, providing flexibility in handling inputs of various lengths		Transformer models analyze dental-patient interactions over time to predict treatment outcomes. Also, ChatGPT and similar are based on transformer neural networks

(continued)

AI term or concept	Definition for health professionals	Comparable statistical concept	Examples in dentistry
Unimodal AI	AI models that process only one type of data (e.g., images, text, or audio) without combining it with other data types		Using only dental radiographs (image data) for detecting caries, without integrating textual patient records or audio
			View multimodal AI
Unsupervised learning	Training of ML algorithms by mining and extracting hidden patterns from input data that has not been labeled	Cluster Analysis	Identifying patterns in patient data to discover unknown correlations or disease groups
Weights	The factors the model learns that determine a feature's influence the prediction	Parameters	In a model predicting gum disease, weights could dictate how much smoking status influences the outcome compared to other factors like age

The manufacturer's authorised representative in the EU is Springer Nature Customer Service Centre GmbH, Europaplatz 3, 69115 Heidelberg, Germany. If you have any concerns regarding our products, please contact ProductSafety@springernature.com

Printed and bound by CPI Group (UK) Ltd, Croydon, CR0 4YY
30/09/2026
02225469-0009